Transhumanism, Ethics and the Therapeutic Revolution

This book explores the impact of developments in pharmaceutical medicine in the twentieth century on a Christian ethical evaluation of transhumanism and future "hi-tech" medical enhancement technologies. It suggests that the Christian ethical assessment of proposed future radical transhumanist biomedical technologies should be conducted in the light of responses to past medical advances. Two specific case studies are featured, focusing on the oral contraceptive pill and on Prozac and selective serotonin reuptake inhibitor (SSRI) antidepressants. Whilst future biomedical technologies may have therapeutic benefits for the relief of disease and contribute to improving human health and welfare, the book considers the implications for society and their acceptability as therapies from a Christian perspective. Stressing the inadequacy of natural law alone, the author proposes an ethical framework for assessing novel biomedical technologies according to the effects on personal autonomy, embodiment and bodily life, and on the *imago Dei*.

Stephen Goundrey-Smith is an applied theologian and ordained minister in the Church of England who has also worked as a pharmacist. He received a PhD in Theology from the University of Exeter, UK.

Routledge New Critical Thinking in Religion, Theology and Biblical Studies

The *Routledge New Critical Thinking in Religion, Theology and Biblical Studies* series brings high quality research monograph publishing back into focus for authors, international libraries, and student, academic and research readers. This open-ended monograph series presents cutting-edge research from both established and new authors in the field. With specialist focus yet clear contextual presentation of contemporary research, books in the series take research into important new directions and open the field to new critical debate within the discipline, in areas of related study, and in key areas for contemporary society.

The Fathers on the Bible
Edited by Nicu Dumitrașcu

The Theological Imperative to Authenticity
Christy M. Capper

The Political Theology of Pope Francis
Understanding the Latin American Pope
Ole Jakob Løland

Transhumanism, Ethics and the Therapeutic Revolution
Agents of Change
Stephen Goundrey-Smith

Fittingness and Environmental Ethics
Philosophical, Theological and Applied Perspectives
Edited by Michael S. Northcott and Steven C. van den Heuvel

Misusing Scripture
What are Evangelicals Doing with the Bible?
Mark Elliott, Kenneth Atkinson, and Robert Rezetko

For more information about this series, please visit: https://www.routledge.com/religion/series/RCRITREL

Transhumanism, Ethics and the Therapeutic Revolution

Agents of Change

Stephen Goundrey-Smith

Routledge
Taylor & Francis Group
LONDON AND NEW YORK

First published 2023
by Routledge
4 Park Square, Milton Park, Abingdon, Oxon OX14 4RN

and by Routledge
605 Third Avenue, New York, NY 10158

Routledge is an imprint of the Taylor & Francis Group, an informa business

British Library Cataloguing-in-Publication Data
A catalogue record for this book is available from the British Library

ISBN: 978-1-032-24400-6 (hbk)
ISBN: 978-1-032-26901-6 (pbk)
ISBN: 978-1-003-29042-1 (ebk)

DOI: 10.4324/9781003290421

Typeset in Sabon
by MPS Limited, Dehradun

Contents

About the Author

Stephen Goundrey-Smith is a scientific theologian and ethicist, and a priest in the Church of England. After training as a pharmacist, and working in hospital pharmacy and in the medical departments of various international pharmaceutical companies, he trained for Church of England ministry at Wycliffe Hall, Oxford. There he gained a Batchelor of Theology degree and developed academic interests in Christian ethics, theological anthropology and the science-religion dialogue. He was subsequently awarded a PhD in theology from the University of Exeter for his work on an ethical re-evaluation of proposed transhumanist biomedical technologies in the light of the impact of widely adopted advances in pharmaceutical medicine in the twentieth century. Stephen Goundrey-Smith is an associate tutor in Christian Ethics at Cuddesdon Gloucester and Hereford, and a course facilitator with the Gateway Theology School. He lives in Chipping Norton, Oxfordshire, United Kingdom.

Acknowledgements

First and foremost, I would like to thank my supervisors, Professor Christopher Southgate and Dr Jonathan Hill for all their advice and support during my doctoral studies, which have been the basis for this project. I would also like to thank Dr Cherryl Hunt for her encouragement and her feedback on the methodology for ethical assessment of medical technology, and Dr Rosalind Marsden for her helpful comments and general scholarly wisdom. I would also like to thank my editor, Katherine Ong, for her help in the book production process. Finally, I would like to thank my parishioners in Chedworth and, above all, my family – my wife, Sally, and children, Archie, Edward, Emily and Sam – for their encouragement over the years and their patience with long hours spent in the office, as I have written this book amidst a busy professional life.

Introduction
Therapy Plus: An Ultimate Cure

I.1 Transhumanism: From Therapy to Enhancement

Transhumanism is concerned with developing human life beyond its current form and limitations using biomedical technologies. Previously, during the modern era, while there has been increasing technology use in society, human social progress has been largely concerned with better education and cultural changes. Transhumanism, however, proposes to transform human life and experience primarily through biomedical technology. This has far-reaching implications for individual citizens and for societies, and raises various theological and ethical issues, which have been extensively discussed elsewhere.[1]

The purpose of this book is to make an ethical assessment of proposed transhumanist enhancement technologies, in the light of advances in pharmaceutical medicine that have already taken place in the modern research-based pharmaceutical industry, during the so-called "therapeutic revolution" years of the twentieth century (1950–1990). The key question that will be addressed here is: what can be learned from theological and ethical engagement with past medical developments, and how does this learning inform an evaluation of proposed future transhumanist biomedical technologies within Christian theological ethics? I will show that some advances by the pharmaceutical industry in the twentieth century – for example, the contraceptive pill and selective serotonin reuptake inhibitor (SSRI) antidepressants such as Prozac – have been distributed on a large scale and have had profound effects on society, and therefore have had, in their time, some of the characteristics of proposed future transhumanist biomedical technologies. An ethical evaluation of future technologies in the light of these past developments would therefore be a useful addition to the literature in this area and would provide an example of a specific dialogue between science and religion.

In recent years, the concept of transhumanism has gained popularity, and a transhumanist "movement" has emerged. Chapter 2 will present a detailed analysis of transhumanism, and the religious and philosophical critiques of it, but, in brief, transhumanism may be described as the use of

DOI: 10.4324/9781003290421-1

biomedical technologies to enhance human life and experience beyond current expected human functions and limitations. Forms of enhancement are already available – for example, the use of caffeinated drinks to improve mental alertness. However, the radical nature of proposed future transhumanist biomedical technologies means they have the potential to provide significant enhancements to human function, longevity and cognitive abilities that were not previously available, and these may have profound effects on the shape of human life. I shall explore definitions of transhumanism in more detail in the next chapter, but note for now that Nick Bostrom, a prominent transhumanist, has defined transhumanism as "an interdisciplinary approach to understanding and evaluating the opportunities for enhancing the human condition that are emerging through advancing technology" (Bostrom, 2005, p. 3).

I.2 Transhumanist Technologies: What They Are

A diverse range of emerging and potential future technologies have been considered transhumanist by advocates of the transhumanism movement. Many of these proposed technologies are radical in their effects on the human body, or highly invasive in nature. While some affirm carbon-based life and embodied humanity – for example, genetic enhancement – others denigrate the body and seek the partial or complete replacement of the body with metal and silicon – for example, cybernetics and mind-uploading. Some of the technologies are not scientifically possible at the time of writing but have been envisaged by some science fiction writers and are of interest because of the ethical implications of their proposed effects.

The proposed technologies that could be considered transhumanist include the following:

1 Nanotechnology – the use of microscopic particles, tools and robots to interact with the body for medical applications. Freitas has discussed nanotechnology in detail, from a transhumanist perspective (Freitas, 2013).
2 Genetic enhancements – including germ-line modifications. The potential applications of genetic enhancements have been discussed by Bailey (2013).
3 Cybernetics – the use of prostheses and robotics to develop and enhance bodily function. There has been much philosophical and ethical debate about the cyborg and what it says about human nature and the human person (Hayles, 1999, pp. 2–5; Haraway, 1991, pp. 149–152).
4 Cryonics – placing the human body in suspended animation using cryogenic techniques, so that a person can be revived in the distant future when radical new medical technologies are available.

5 Mind-Uploading – where all the information in the human brain is uploaded onto a computer, in order that a person can live on "in silico" without the biological substrate of the frail human body (Merkle, 2013).

These technologies are listed above in likely order of adoption, beginning with those that are available now in the early twenty-first century, or that will be available soon, and ending with those that are more distant prospects. This list is not exhaustive, but these are the future technologies which will be considered throughout this book.

Because of their radical nature and far-reaching implications, proposed future biomedical technologies have been subject to scrutiny by theologians and ethicists, to an extent that has not been the case with many previous medical technologies. In some cases, these new biomedical technologies may give rise to hitherto unexpected consequences and new ethical issues; in other cases, these technologies may be treated with suspicion just because they are an unknown quantity culturally, even though they do not clearly raise any new ethical issues. I will explore these themes in more detail in Chapter 5.

I.3 Study Methodology

The methodology I use is a case study analysis of two past cases of pharmaceutical development – the contraceptive pill and SSRI antidepressants – using a series of objective criteria. These comprise general criteria for what constitutes a transhumanist technology and specific ethical criteria to determine whether the technology is ethically acceptable from a standpoint of Christian ethics.

The findings of the case study analysis will be used to answer the following questions:

1 What are the various issues of theological ethics presented by transhumanist developments?
2 To what extent were past medical developments transhumanist technologies in their time, in the same way as proposed future technologies?
3 What were the ethical concerns with past medical developments? Have these ethical concerns been warranted in the light of subsequent experience?
4 How do issues identified with previous medical developments inform the evaluation of future biomedical technologies?

These findings will, in turn, be used to further refine the criteria for the ethical acceptability for a transhumanist technology. The overall implications of these findings for Christian medical ethics and the adoption of biomedical technology in society will then be discussed.

The rest of this section will provide a brief discussion on three aspects of the methodology, namely: 1) the value of case studies in ethical evaluation, 2) the rationale for choosing the two particular cases of previous medical technology, and 3) the importance of objective criteria.

I.3.1 Case Studies

This project uses a case study methodology to assess proposed transhumanist biomedical technologies of the future in relation to therapeutic developments to date, and ethical responses to those developments. Case studies were first adopted in the nineteenth century in the teaching of medicine and the law because teachers found that students learnt general, abstract principles better from the review of specific, actual examples (Schipani, 2011). Case study methodology for teaching and research is now widespread in the social sciences, and has become the most widely used method in practical theology for evaluating formation, faith experience or church or ministerial practice (Schipani, 2011, p. 91). The case study has been particularly beneficial in the clinical pastoral education tradition (Schipani, 2011, p. 93), so it is a natural development for a case study methodology to be used here to evaluate Christian ethical responses to biomedical technologies.

A case study has been described as a unit of human activity embedded in the real world, which can only be studied and understood in context, and where often the boundary between the case and the context is hard to determine (Gillham, 2000). The development of a new drug or medical technology fits well into this definition of a case because it is a specific activity but, in the developed health economies of the United Kingdom and the United States, it takes place in a wider context. Furthermore, in terms of medical technology development, this context has four aspects – the alleviation of human suffering and fulfilment of healthcare needs, the scientific endeavour of the pharmaceutical and bioscience industries, the practice of medicine and finally government financial investment in life sciences research.

Case studies have the following attributes which make them valuable for the ethical analysis of biomedical technologies:

- Case studies are good for answering "how" or "why" questions, rather than questions with quantitative answers (Yin, 2013, pp. 2–5).
- Case studies can be used to assess multiple sources of evidence (Gillham, 2000, p. 1). Thus, the case studies here encompass different domains of evidence from different types of literature – the scientific history of drug discovery, the impact of the drug on society and Christian ethical responses to the drug – in the same case study.
- Case studies are helpful for naturalistic research – the exploration of human phenomena embedded in the real world, which accounts for "real world" complexity (Gillham, 2000, pp. 5–8). The cases used here

are naturalistic, in that they use evidence from the real-world complexity of drug development to develop ethical principles. However, the study methodology used here is not entirely naturalistic, in that it imposes a structure on the case studies, and it assesses the cases according to particular objective criteria, in a way that might be analogous to the experimental conditions of the natural sciences.
- Case studies are reflective, in that they enable theological reflection about a specific, practical situation (Schipani, 2011, p. 92). This, in my view, is an important element of any applied ethical study, and this reflexivity will be developed later in the discussion in Chapter 5, and in the formulation of conclusions in Chapter 6.

However, case study methodology has its drawbacks (Yin, 2013, pp. 10–15). Case studies may lack rigour; they can be constructed in a non-systematic way so that equivocal evidence or biased views could affect the conclusions of the study. Furthermore, they can be hard to define closely and are therefore in danger of being aimless in their scope, resulting in large, unwieldy documentation. In this project, I deal with these potential shortcomings by using specific cases, presented in a carefully structured way, which are queried by specific objective criteria. Each of the two cases is structured in four sections: a) the scientific context, b) the impact of the drug on society, c) the motivations of the developers and d) the theological and ethical critique of the drug according to the criteria for the ethical evaluation of transhumanist developments.

Another criticism of case studies is that they provide little basis for generalisation; the case study is not a statistical "sample", as scientific methodology might use, and it is generalisable only to a theoretical proposition, rather than to a population. This might, at first sight, appear to be a legitimate criticism of this project. Can these two past case studies be representative of all past medical developments? However, as discussed above, these case studies are more naturalistic than empiricist, and their conclusions concerning the ethics of future technological projects are inductive rather than deductive. In any case, as I will argue next, the two case studies in this project have been carefully chosen because they have the potential to be most relevant to transhumanist medical developments.

I.3.2 Choice of Case Studies

What is the rationale for choosing these two particular cases – the oral contraceptive pill and SSRI antidepressants – as the basis of an ethical dialogue with transhumanism? Many of the drug discoveries during the therapeutic revolution years have had significant benefits for human health and well-being – for example, antibiotics to reduce serious systemic bacterial infection, or beta-blocking agents to improve cardiac function and reduce the incidence of heart attacks and strokes. However, the benefits of these medicines have been primarily at an individual and a medical level, and they have only had an indirect effect on human society in totality. The two case studies used in this study, however, have been chosen because, not only have they brought about health benefits for the individual, but they have had an impact on society beyond the practice of medicine, and not merely on the health and well-being of society, but also on societal values and popular culture. Because of this impact, the ethical implications of these medicines are broader than just the medical ethical principles associated with their use in a medical context. In his reflection on the impact of psychopharmacology on the individual and on society, psychiatrist David Healy has pointed out how both psychopharmacological agents (antipsychotics and antidepressants) and contraception have the potential to change human society (Healy, 2000). He claims that contraception has profoundly changed the sexual order, by changing the dynamics of sexual relationships and the role of women in society, and that psychopharmacology has changed the social order, by getting people out of mental institutions and into mainstream society, and eliminating the "hidden" population of mentally ill people. Because these medical interventions have had effects on society, not just the health of the individual, they have come to the attention of the churches and of Christian commentators and have been subject to ethical critique.

The contraceptive pill was the first drug to be widely distributed to a population that was otherwise healthy (Jutte, 2008, p. 288). Consequently, although the pill may have specific benefits as a treatment for a proportion of women with menstrual disorders (Bahamondes et al, 2015), it is largely an "enhancement" for healthy women. For this reason, Elaine May has described the pill as "a flashpoint for social transformation" (May, 2010, p. 168), and the use of the contraceptive pill rapidly came to the attention of Christian ethicists, and the moral theologians of the Catholic Church, in particular. The opposition to hormonal contraception, largely on natural law grounds, by the Roman Catholic church, is well known (Thatcher, 2011, pp. 211–233); it is reviewed in Chapter 3 and its implications for future transhumanist biomedical technologies will be discussed in Chapter 5.

In a similar way, although Prozac and other SSRIs were developed as specific treatments for clinical depression, they have been adopted for use in cases where the person has few or no symptoms of depression, to enhance personality and to help people feel "better than well". This has led to the "Prozac phenomenon", epitomised by the work of psychiatrist, Peter Kramer, which will be discussed in detail in Chapter 4 (Kramer, 1993, pp. 1–21). SSRI antidepressants have had an impact on society as a whole, due to their widespread use and their fine-tuned effects on personality and relationships. For this reason, psychiatrists, such as Kramer and Healy, have highlighted the possible ethical issues with these drugs, and again they have come to the attention of various Christian commentators (Stapert, 1994). The Roman Catholic scholar, John-Mark Miravalle, has developed an ethical evaluation of SSRI use, based on Aquinas and natural law, analogous to the approach taken by the Roman Catholic church with the contraceptive pill (Miravalle, 2010, p. 59). I will evaluate Miravalle's work at length in Chapter 4.

Overall, therefore, the societal effects of these two medical developments and their ethical implications, which are already recognised, make them the optimum cases of previous drug development to use to open an ethical dialogue with future transhumanist proposals.

I.3.3 Objective Criteria

In this project, particular objective criteria are used – general criteria, to evaluate the extent to which a biomedical technology can be considered a transhumanist development, and specific ethical criteria to facilitate their ethical evaluation. These criteria are applied equally to proposed transhumanist technologies in Chapter 2, the oral contraceptive pill in Chapter 3 and SSRI antidepressants in Chapter 4. The objective criteria chosen are an important tool for determining the extent to which the different therapeutic developments may be considered equivalent, and therefore the extent to which ethical issues raised with previous medical developments are applicable to future transhumanist proposals, and might therefore add to, or modify, current Christian ethical views of transhumanism.

Criteria (from the Greek *krisis* – points of judgement) are important because they provide an objective view from which to evaluate specific cases or instances, and they also set limits on, and provide structure to, the resulting discussion. Criteria are a means of making information coherent and intelligible; Thomas Guarino asserts that objective criteria help to provide a framework of rationality and coherence in a world where not all theories are true, and where truth claims differ in their nature (Guarino, 1993). Another important role of criteria is to make existential questions universally intelligible. Jacobsen argues that, for universal and public understanding of existential questions, criteria accessible to all must be used to present their truth (Jacobsen, 2012). I would argue that objective criteria therefore have an important role in the methodology of this study given that, in popular culture, scientific knowledge is often treated as a specialist, esoteric domain and the objective of this project is to formulate a universal and publicly intelligible ethical approach to future technologies based on experience with previous technologies. Moreover, the transhumanist movement might seem like an esoteric sect but, from a preliminary view, the technologies it proposes would appear to have far-reaching implications for how human life might be lived in the future. It is right, therefore, that the issues and ethical questions surrounding these are made publicly accessible and intelligible, and the use of criteria here facilitates this process of clarification.

In this study, two sets of criteria are used to assess the biomedical technologies – one set of general criteria, to assess whether the technology can be considered a transhumanist technology, and a set of specific theological criteria, to facilitate ethical evaluation of the technology and to assess its acceptability from a perspective of Christian ethics.

The general criteria for a transhumanist biomedical technology used in this study are derived from the work of transhumanist scholars, and are as follows:

1 That it is a technology (More, 2013, p. 13) – in other words, it is a material means of effecting a task or process.
2 That the technology is applied to a human person in some way (World Transhumanist Association, 2013). At the core of transhumanism is the transformation of the human condition, and the improvement of human society.
3 That the technology is applied to the human person to improve human function, increase longevity or promote human flourishing (World Transhumanist Association, 2013).
4 That the human person has autonomy in the use of the technology – in other words, the technology is not being applied in a coercive way (More, 2013, p. 13).

These criteria are as broad in scope as the transhumanist movement itself. Furthermore, as I will demonstrate in detail in Chapter 2, these criteria are derived from the literature on transhumanism and so their application to transhumanist technologies is, in a sense, a circular argument. However, it is instructive to apply these general criteria to the two case studies, which concern pharmaceutical products that were developed mainly before the development of transhumanism as a movement – to evaluate the extent to which these pharmaceutical developments were, in their time, transhumanist in character.

In addition, the following theological criteria are used to assess the ethical aspects of the biomedical technologies in this project. These criteria are as follows:

1 Is the project good news for the poor? (Messer, 2007, pp. 229–235).
2 Is the project an attempt to be "like God" (in respect of Genesis 3v5) or does it conform to the image of God? (Genesis 1v26) (Messer, 2007, pp. 229–235).
3 What attitude does the project embody towards the material world (including our own bodies)? (Messer, 2007, pp. 229–235). And how does the technology affect the corporate "body" of society? (Graham, 2006).
4 What attitude does the project embody towards past failures? (Messer, 2007, pp. 229–235).
5 Does the technology enable unbridled autonomy in a negative manner? (Graham, 2006).
6 Does the technology focus too much on the users' subjective experiences? (Graham, 2006).

These criteria have been adapted from the work of theological ethicist, Neil Messer, who has developed "diagnostic questions" about whether a biotechnological project is aligned with God's saving work in the world (2007, pp. 229–235), and the theological critiques levelled at transhumanism – concerning embodiment, autonomy and subjectivity – by theologian, Elaine Graham (2006).

The purpose of these criteria is to define and describe what aspects of biomedical technology are problematic in respect of Christian ethics, and to determine the extent to which each of these technologies is desirable or permissible from a Christian ethical perspective. The utility of these specific ethical criteria, and why they were chosen, will be explored in greater detail in Chapter 2, following a detailed analysis of the transhumanism movement. The final section of this introduction will provide an overview of the content of this book.

I.4 Summary of the Book

The book is structured into six chapters, which will describe the scientific and historical background to both transhumanism and the twentieth-century "therapeutic revolution", discuss the transhumanism movement and theological issues arising from it, present two case studies from twentieth-century pharmaceutical medicine, and then apply the ethical findings from these case studies to the consideration of proposed future transhumanist technologies.

Chapter 1 will present the scientific and ethical context of the project. It will describe the development of modern pharmacology during the years of the so-called "therapeutic revolution" years (1950–1990) and will discuss the impact of the therapeutic revolution on human life and society, in terms of medical and healthcare benefits. The chapter will also describe the historical context of the ethical questions being discussed, by reviewing the history of medical ethics. The wider implications of the research for medical ethics and pastoral care will be briefly discussed.

Chapter 2 will explore in detail the objectives, history and claims of the transhumanist movement. It will examine and critique the various philosophical influences on transhumanism and the approaches taken by different protagonists of transhumanism. This will enable a taxonomy of the transhumanist movement to be developed, so that its diversity can be understood, and common features explored. The chapter will describe three basic classifications of transhumanist scholarship: a) *philosophical transhumanists,* comprising scholars who see transhumanism as a life philosophy; b) *technological transhumanists*, commentators who see transhumanism from the perspective of the effects of technology (computing, artificial intelligence or cybernetics) on human life, and the benefits that it can bring; and c) *ideological transhumanists*, scholars who explore the effects of biomedical technology on human society, but in a way that is neutral to technology *per se*, and which primarily sees these technologies as tools for exploring cultural and ideological issues.

The chapter will then discuss theological critiques of transhumanism from the world faith traditions in general, and from a perspective of Christian theology in particular. The chapter will focus on four specific areas of ethical critique of transhumanism: 1) Autonomy, 2) Nature/Natural Law, 3) Embodiment and 4) the *imago Dei*. Although I discuss these areas from a perspective of Christian theology, I will show that some of the concerns of other faith traditions are also reflected in these four areas of discussion.

The chapter will then present the two sets of criteria listed above – the general criteria, to be used to classify a technology as transhumanist and the specific theological criteria for the ethical evaluation of a transhumanist technology (Messer, 2007, pp. 229–235; Graham, 2006) and will describe the rationale for their use. There will then be a preliminary discussion about how proposed technologies which can be classified as transhumanist should be evaluated against the general and specific criteria.

These two sets of criteria will then be used to assess the two case studies of previous therapeutic developments which took place during the therapeutic revolution years – the contraceptive pill and SSRI antidepressants. Chapter 3 will present the first of these two case studies, the development of the oral contraceptive pill, which was introduced in 1960. The first section of the chapter will describe the history of the contraceptive pill, discussing the events that led to its introduction, and the actions of the protagonists involved. The second section will discuss the effects of the pill on the lives of women and men, on marriage, and on society and will discuss the Roman Catholic Church's theological and ethical concerns with the pill. Finally, the contraceptive pill will be evaluated against the general and specific criteria for transhumanist technologies to determine the extent to which, in its time, it could have been regarded as a transhumanist development, and to evaluate it from the perspective of ethical concerns about transhumanist technologies.

Chapter 4 will present the second of these two case studies – the development of SSRI antidepressants (e.g., Prozac), which took place in the late 1980s. As with the previous chapter, the first section will describe the history of SSRI development, and how SSRIs arose from previous developments in rational psychopharmacology, discussing the events that led to their introduction. The second section will describe and evaluate the effects of SSRIs on society – their therapeutic effect on patients with clinical depression and their use as mood-altering drugs in individuals who are not depressed (the so-called "Prozac phenomenon") – and discuss a theological response to SSRIs, examining in detail the work of Roman Catholic scholar, John-Mark Miravalle (Miravalle, 2010, p. 59). Miravalle's work examines how depression fits into an understanding of human attributes based on the psychology of Thomas Aquinas and of the ethical goods of treating depression, and provides a natural law-based ethical critique of excessive use and over-reliance on antidepressant drugs. The third section of the chapter will then assess SSRI antidepressants against the two sets of criteria for transhumanist technologies developed in Chapter 2, to determine the extent to which, in their time, they could have been regarded as a transhumanist development, and to evaluate them from the perspective of theological concerns about transhumanist technologies.

Chapter 5 will reconsider some current transhumanist proposals and technologies in the light of previous experience with pharmaceutical medicine , as outlined in the two case studies presented in Chapters 3 and 4. The chapter will begin by summarising the findings of the case studies according to the criteria and determining the issues in theological ethics that have arisen through the development and clinical use of these medicines, which are relevant to a Christian response to transhumanist technologies.

The chapter will then answer the four proposed research questions. In terms of the first question, concerning the various issues of theological ethics presented by transhumanist technologies, the discussion will focus on four specific domains – autonomy, nature/natural law, embodiment and the *imago Dei* – which I will show are points of contact between past medical developments and potential future transhumanist technologies. Second, the extent to which the contraceptive pill and SSRI antidepressants were, in their time, transhumanist technologies will be evaluated, according to the general criteria in Chapter 2. Third, there will be a discussion about the ethical issues of these past therapeutic technologies, and whether the ethical issues identified when they were introduced have proved to be of concern with long-term experience. Fourth, the response of Christian theological ethics to future transhumanist biomedical technologies will then be reassessed, in the light of the ethical findings with previous medical technologies, and this reassessment will be used to further refine the criteria for transhumanist technologies used in this project.

Chapter 6 will then draw general conclusions. Transhumanist technologies are often seen either optimistically, as a panacea for all human suffering, or pessimistically, as the gateway to a dystopian future. Based on theological and ethical reflection on past developments in pharmaceutical medicine, using objective criteria, this project will demonstrate that the reality is somewhere in between. With both modern medicine to date and proposed future transhumanist technologies, scientists and practitioners are motivated by the alleviation of suffering, the improvement of human experience and the promotion of human flourishing, and these motivations are consistent with Christian ethics. However, the development of biomedical enhancement technologies, like all science, takes place within a social and cultural context and this affects how the technologies are evaluated by Christians, from a theological and ethical perspective. This project will show that the church should neither accept new biomedical enhancement technologies uncritically nor respond with a knee-jerk rejection of such technologies. Instead, a nuanced Christian ethical critique of such technologies is required, based on the areas identified in this work, namely autonomy, nature, embodiment and the *imago Dei*. In the light of experience with the contraceptive pill and SSRI antidepressants, an ethical evaluation of biomedical technology based largely on natural law, as has happened previously, will no longer be sufficient to ensure an accurate assessment of future, radical biomedical technologies. The concluding chapter will highlight possible further areas for research in the theological ethical evaluation of transhumanism and will end with concluding comments about the impact of biomedical enhancement technologies on society and the church.

Note

1 For example, Ronald Cole-Turner, "Towards a Theology for the Age of Biotechnology", in *Beyond Cloning: Religion and the Remaking of Humanity*, edited by Ronald Cole-Turner (Harrisburg PA: Trinity Press International, 2001); *Religion and Transhumanism: The Unknown Future of Human Enhancement*, edited by Calvin Mercer and Tracy Trothen (Santa Barbara: Praeger, 2015).

References

Adrian Thatcher, *God, Sex and Gender: An Introduction* (Oxford: Wiley-Blackwell, 2011).

Bill Gillham, *Case Study Research Methods* (London: Continuum, 2000).

Daniel Schipani, "Case Study Method", in *The Wiley Blackwell Companion to Practical Theology*, edited by Bonnie Miller-McLemore (Chichester: Wiley Blackwell, 2011), pp. 91–101.

David Healy, "Psychopharmacology and the government of the self", Colloquium at the Centre for Addiction and Mental Health, Nature Medicine, 2000.

Donna Haraway, *Simians, Cyborgs and Women: The Reinvention of Nature* (New York: Routledge, 1991).

Elaine Graham, "In Whose Image? Representations of Technology and the Ends of Humanity", in *Future Perfect? God, Medicine and Human Identity*, edited by Celia Deane-Drummond and Peter Manley Scott (London: T and T Clark International, 2006), pp. 56–69.

Elaine Tyler May, *America and The Pill: A History of Promise, Peril and Liberation* (New York: Basic Books, 2010).

Eneida Jacobsen, "Models of Public Theology", *International Journal of Public Theology*, 6 (2012), pp. 7–22.

John-Mark Miravalle, *The Drug, The Soul and God: A Catholic Moral Perspective on Antidepressants* (Chicago: University of Scranton Press, 2010).

John Stapert, "Curing an Illness or Transforming the Self? The Power of Prozac", *Christian Century*, 111 (1994), pp. 684–687.

Luis Bahamondes, Valeria Bahamondes and Lee P. Shulman, "Non-contraceptive benefits of hormonal and intrauterine reversible contraceptive methods", *Human Reproduction Update*, 21 (2015), pp. 640–651.

Max More, "The Philosophy of Transhumanism", in *The Transhumanist Reader: Classical and Contemporary Essays on the Science, Technology and Philosophy of the Post-Human Future*, edited by Max More and Natasha Vita-More (Chichester: Wiley-Blackwell, 2013), pp. 1–17.

N. Katherine Hayles, *How We Became Posthuman: Virtual Bodies in Cybernetics, Literature and Informatics* (Chicago and London: University of Chicago Press, 1999).

Neil Messer, *Selfish Genes and Christian Ethics: Theological and Ethical Reflections on Evolutionary Biology* (London: SCM, 2007).

Nick Bostrom, "Transhumanist Values", *Journal of Philosophical Research*, 30 (2005), pp. 3–14.

Peter Kramer, *Listening to Prozac* (New York/London: Penguin, 1993).

Ralph Merkle, "Uploading", in *The Transhumanist Reader: Classical and Contemporary Essays on the Science, Technology and Philosophy of the Post-Human Future*, edited by Max More and Natasha Vita-More (Chichester: Wiley-Blackwell, 2013), pp. 157–164.

Robert Freitas, "Future of Medicine", in *The Transhumanist Reader: Classical and Contemporary Essays on the Science, Technology and Philosophy of the Post-Human Future*, edited by Max More and Natasha Vita-More (Chichester: Wiley-Blackwell, 2013), pp. 67–72.

Robert Jutte, *Contraception: A History*, translated by V. Russell (Cambridge: Polity Press, 2008).

Robert Yin, *Case Study Research: Design and Methods*, 3rd Edition (Thousand Oaks: Sage, 2013).

Ronald Bailey, "For Enhancing People", in *The Transhumanist Reader: Classical and Contemporary Essays on the Science, Technology and Philosophy of the Post-Human Future*, edited by Max More and Natasha Vita-More (Chichester: Wiley-Blackwell, 2013), pp. 327–344.

Thomas Guarino, "Between Foundationalism and Nihilism: Is Phronesis the Via Media for Theology?", *Theological Studies*, 54 (1993), pp. 37–54.

World Transhumanist Association, "Transhumanist Declaration", in *The Transhumanist Reader: Classical and Contemporary Essays on the Science, Technology and Philosophy of the Post-Human Future*, edited by Max More and Natasha Vita-More (Chichester: Wiley-Blackwell, 2013), pp. 54–55.

1 Biomedical Science and Medical Ethics

Past and Future

1.1 Introduction: Medicine and Human Flourishing

The practice of medicine has always been of fundamental importance in the relief of human suffering, the promotion of well-being for all people and the provision of humanitarian aid in areas of endemic illness and natural disaster. However, modern science and technology have led to the development of increasingly specific and sophisticated interventions and techniques in medicine, with the potential to have a profound impact on human health outcomes. This has been seen clearly in the field of pharmacology where, since the mid-twentieth century, there has been a so-called "therapeutic revolution", an exponential increase in the number of drug molecules available to health services for the treatment of diseases (Weinshilboum, 1987). The availability of a wider range of drugs, with increasingly specific modes of action has, in turn, enabled more sophisticated medical treatments in different clinical specialties.

This chapter sets the historical context for an ethical evaluation of future transhumanist biomedical enhancement by describing the development of modern pharmacology during the twentieth century and its impact on human life and flourishing, and also the development of medical ethics to date.

1.2 The Twentieth-Century Therapeutic Revolution

This section discusses the development of the modern science-based pharmaceutical industry, describes some of its major therapeutic achievements, and analyses their impact on human mortality and quality of life in the twentieth century. Also, in this section, a definition of the so-called "therapeutic revolution" is given, in terms of the period of history that it describes.

While this book is primarily a work of ethics, I discuss the scientific history of modern pharmacology, and its impact, in some detail in this section. I take a similar approach with the development of the contraceptive pill and selective serotonin reuptake inhibitor (SSRI) antidepressants in Chapters 3 and 4, respectively. This is because, as mentioned in the introduction, this is a multidisciplinary study of theological ethics in science, and readers without a

DOI: 10.4324/9781003290421-2

scientific background would benefit from an understanding of the science behind these developments, in order to appreciate their ethical implications in society at the time of their introduction and since.

The history of the expansion of the manufacturing pharmaceutical industry in Britain during the twentieth century is described in detail by Judy Slinn (2005). Modern pharmaceutical medicine has developed during the twentieth century because of three main factors.

First, during the late nineteenth and early twentieth century, the understanding of, and technological capability in, the molecular sciences increased considerably. The development of drug molecules with specific modes of action became possible because of the discovery of the "receptor" theory of drug action. According to receptor theory, many biological processes are mediated by the action of biochemicals and hormones at specific biochemical receptor sites on the cells in different body tissues.[1] The discovery of receptors paved the way for considerable research on synthetic drug molecules that might exert therapeutic effects by either acting as a stimulant (agonist) or a blocker (antagonist) at the receptor upon which it acted. For example, the anti-asthma drug, salbutamol, exerts its bronchodilator effects by acting as an agonist at beta-2 adrenergic receptors in the lungs (Bryan, 2007). An understanding of receptor theory has enabled a wide range of specific drugs to be developed.

Furthermore, experiments conducted in the nineteenth century demonstrated that particular organs, such as the ovaries and testes, could exert an effect on the whole body, which could only be explained by the existence of chemicals secreted by those organs into the bloodstream. In 1905, Baylis and Starling coined the term "hormone" for these chemical secretions (from the Greek *hormaõ*, meaning "I excite") (Davis et al., 2005). Medical scientists began to see the wider potential of hormonal therapy – for example, to manage menopausal symptoms and improve quality of life, not just to treat disease. In 1910, Arnold Lorand published a book entitled "Old Age Deferred", proposing the use of ovarian extracts to treat menopausal symptoms (Jutte, 2008).

Second, since the beginning of the twentieth century, the pharmaceutical industry has become increasingly socially and academically respectable in both the United Kingdom (UK) and the United States (US) and this has led to its development as a commercial enterprise (Tansey, 1995, p. 6).[2] This enabled the industry to attract highly qualified research staff from academia and ensured further investment in pharmaceutical research (Tansey, 1995, p. 6). Acceptability of drug research to the academic community and indeed to wider society has been an important factor in successful drug development, as will be seen in the case study on oral contraception in Chapter 3.

Third, pharmaceutical medicine has developed to address unmet medical needs, particularly during and after the two world wars in the twentieth century. While German medicinal chemistry was dominant at the beginning of the twentieth century (Slinn, 2005, p. 162), the First World War cut off the supply of German pharmaceuticals to the Allied countries, and this stimulated pharmaceutical research in Britain and the United States (Slinn, 2005, pp. 165–166). Indeed, a key factor in the post-war expansion of new drugs was the effort of wartime therapeutic research during the Second World War bearing fruit. The classic example of this was the development of penicillin in Britain from 1940 to 1944 by Howard Florey and colleagues at Oxford, following the discovery of the Penicillium mould by Sir Alexander Fleming in 1926 (Liebenau, 1990). The work was driven by the need for a specific antibiotic which could be used to treat battle-field infections and therefore aid the war effort. In addition, the pharmaceutical industry, like other industries, benefited economically from the post-war economic boom. There was a significant investment in the biological and scientific industries at this time, and the formation of the National Health Service in Britain in 1948 created a mass market for new drugs, which was a factor in stimulating pharmaceutical development (Quirke, 2005).

The expansion of research and development by the pharmaceutical industry in the decades after the Second World War, a period during which many new drugs were developed, is referred to in the literature as the "therapeutic revolution". This term was coined in retrospect in 1987 by an American clinical pharmacologist, Richard Weinshilboum, in a review of the various drug discovery advances by the pharmaceutical industry during the previous half-century (Weinshilboum, 1987). It should be noted, however, that the term was used more broadly by Rosenberg in 1977 to describe the development of medicine from the beginning of the nineteenth century (Rosenberg, 1977), and by Reekie and Weber in 1979 to describe the development of the pharmaceutical industry since 1935 (Reekie and Weber, 1979). However, Weinshilboum's definition is contextually specific to pharmaceutical medicine and is linked clearly with the post-war economic boom, and for these reasons has been incorporated in the recent work of historians of the pharmaceutical industry, for example, Viviane Quirke (2005) and Judy Slinn (2005). I will therefore define the "therapeutic revolution" as the period between 1950 and 1990, for the purposes of this study.

The so-called "therapeutic revolution" era gave rise to rapid developments in various therapeutic areas, including antibiotics, cardiovascular medicine, respiratory medicine, psychopharmacology, hormonal therapies and various others. The two areas of pharmaceutical medicine studied in this project – the oral contraceptive pill and SSRI antidepressants – both arose from this era of drug discovery.

What is the legacy of the age of expansion of drug discovery known as the "therapeutic revolution"? It certainly led to the growth of the pharmaceutical industry, both commercially and in terms of its marketing activities. There was an exponential increase in pharmaceutical industry business value worldwide, from $600 million before the Second World War, to $4000 million in the mid-1950s (Slinn, 2005, p. 162). Liebenau notes that the world pharmaceutical market continued to expand through the 1960s and 1970s; he states that the worldwide market was worth $10 billion in the mid-60s but increased to $36 billion in the mid-70s and $90 billion by the early 1980s (Liebenau, 1990). This market activity has been dominated by the economies of the developed countries – principally the United States, Britain, Germany, Switzerland and Japan.

While the pharmaceutical industry has certainly been successful commercially because of the "therapeutic revolution", has this revolution had a significant effect on human life, health and flourishing? The demographic and epidemiological evidence available suggests that it certainly has had an impact on mortality and longevity. During the twentieth century, there has been the most rapid decline in mortality in human history. United Nations data show that world average life expectancy (at birth) has increased from 48 years in 1950–1955 to 68 years in 2005–2010 (United Nations, 2011). These averages include data from the developing world; the life expectancies for developed countries alone are higher. For example, life expectancy from birth in the UK in 2012 was reported as 83.3 years for women, and 79.2 years for men (Hicks and Allen, 1999).

As the figures suggest, there is considerable worldwide variation in life expectancy. The United Nations (UN) Population Report indicates that there has been little improvement of life expectancy in Africa, due to political and economic factors, but also due to endemic diseases (HIV, tuberculosis and malaria), because treatments are not being deployed or accessed effectively (United Nations, 2011). It is recognised that improvements in HIV therapy in particular, and wider access to such therapy, are likely to have a major impact on population and life expectancy in Africa over the next 100 years (United Nations, 2011).

As evidenced by the changes in life expectancy reported, mortality rates have been falling during the past century. In the UK, there was a sharp decline in mortality between the late nineteenth century and approximately 1930, and then a more gradual decline throughout the remainder of the twentieth century (Tranter, 1996, p. 64). The Organisation for Economic Cooperation and Development (OECD) attributes this worldwide improvement of life expectancy to better standards of living, better education, better nutrition, sanitation and housing and improved health services – and access to those services (OECD, 2013). The population demographer, Neil Tranter, has discussed the factors contributing to the general reduction of mortality and increased life expectancy during the twentieth century (Tranter, 1996, pp. 71–82). He states that the marked improvements in life expectancy in the first half of the twentieth century have been due to a reduction in communicable diseases, such as influenza, smallpox, measles, cholera and dysentery, but this has been mainly as a result of human factors, such as improved nutrition, cleaner water and improved hygiene.

However, Tranter argues, other factors have come into play to account for the ongoing gradual reduction of mortality during the latter half of the twentieth century (Tranter, 1996, pp. 66–70). The two main factors he cites are a) the development of modern therapeutics from the mid-twentieth century and b) in the UK, increased access to life-saving treatments facilitated by the National Health Service, which was formed in 1948.

Not only have mortality rates fallen over the last century, but the causes of mortality have changed. UK population research indicates that, in 1880, infections and parasitic diseases were the largest single cause of death, accounting for 33% of all deaths (Hicks and Allen, 1999). Furthermore, at that time, around 58% of deaths were classed as "other", and this category included deaths with no symptoms, deaths of "old age" and deaths where the cause was poorly understood. However, by 1997, the leading causes of death were cancer (43%) and cardiovascular disease (26%), and only 17% of people died of infections. These changes in cause of mortality probably reflect the impact of modern sanitation and antimicrobial therapy on the management of infectious diseases, as mentioned earlier. Other factors, however, are a) improved pathological understanding and diagnostic techniques to enable identification and classification of diseases previously classed as "other" (especially non-solid tumour cancers), and b) the replacement of communicable, infectious diseases by "diseases of affluence", such as heart disease and certain types of cancer, as the leading causes of mortality during the twentieth century (Tranter, 1996, pp. 75–76).

As stated earlier, most of the reduction in mortality in developed countries over the last century has been due to factors such as better standards of living, better nutrition, sanitation and housing and improved health services. Nevertheless, modern pharmacology has had a significant impact on mortality and life expectancy in the last 50 years or so. This has been largely due to progress in two areas: a) the use of antibiotics – for example, penicillin and streptomycin – against infectious diseases, and b) the availability of specific cardiovascular drugs – for example, beta-receptor blockers, such as propranolol and atenolol, and anticoagulants, such as warfarin – to prevent heart attacks and stroke.

As well as its impact on health outcomes and the quality of human life, modern pharmacology has also contributed to the development of modern evidence-based medicine (Woolf, 2001). While medicine has always been evidence-based, in the sense that it is empirical (i.e., it responds to observations about the patient), Steven Woolf argues that modern evidence-based medicine seeks to make an explicit link between scientific findings about medicines, and public health policy concerning their use. Woolf asserts that this rational approach has become necessary because of "stirring advances" in pharmacology, which have enabled treatment of a widening range of medical conditions and which, in turn, have meant that health budgets have been unable to keep up with technological advancement. An evidence-based approach to medicine, in my view, also contributes to ethical decision-making about medical treatments, and so I would argue that, as a general principle, future biomedical technologies should also be considered in an evidence-based way, in the same way as past and present medical technologies. I will explore this issue in more detail in Chapter 5.

Following the "stirring advances" in pharmacology in the twentieth century, the scene is set for ever more sophisticated biomedical interventions in the twenty-first century. The use of recombinant DNA technology from the 1980s onwards led to the production of larger biological therapeutic molecules, as opposed to the small molecule medicines of the "therapeutic revolution" years (Culver, 2001). These "biological" therapies affect disease processes at specific points in biochemical and cellular mechanisms. They therefore provide more treatment options, especially for endocrine and autoimmune diseases, and may provide benefits for increasingly specific patient subgroups. Consequently, these biological treatments introduce the possibility of truly personalised medicine – instead of the same medicine being given to everyone with the same illness, medical treatment is customised for the individual patient, according to their specific disease type and personal characteristics – for example, age, sex, weight and metabolic capacity. The next step is "genomic" medicine – the use of agents that are customised to a person's genotype, or that affect the expression of different genes. Because of their specific and potentially far-reaching effects, these new technologies have the potential to radically alter human life and experience in a way that previous forms of medicine have not.

I have shown above that the "stirring advances" of modern pharmacology from the "therapeutic revolution" years have led to a reduction in human mortality, albeit a modest reduction compared to other human welfare factors, such as improved sanitation, housing, nutrition and standards of living. Yet, apart from occasional side effect "scares" and some trenchant media critics of the pharmaceutical industry as a whole, there have been no serious concerns about the overall ethical value of modern pharmaceutical medicine, despite its relatively modest overall mortality benefits, and the risks associated with it. Therefore, it is possible that, because future transhumanist biomedical technologies are potentially more radical in their effects and their scope than past developments, these technologies have the potential to provide proportionally far greater benefits for humanity than past medicines.

Biomedical technologies – both the previous pharmacological advances of the "therapeutic revolution" era, and the proposed transhumanist biomedical enhancements of the future – give rise to medical ethical issues, and the purpose of this project is to provide an ethical re-evaluation of transhumanist technologies, based on ethical findings from past pharmaceutical medicine. It is important, therefore, that the reader is aware of the principles of medical ethics, and how medical ethics has developed, to appreciate how medical ethical insights might be applied to biomedical technologies, past or future. The next section provides a brief history of medical ethics, and an account of how medical ethics has developed in recent times.

1.3 Medical Ethics: Ancient, Modern and Post Modern

Medical ethics as a discipline has its roots in ancient times. Ancient traditions of medical ethics can be determined from the oaths of initiation taken by physicians and healers of that era. Two distinct traditions can be traced – an eastern tradition, based on ancient Indian medicine, and a western tradition, based on the medical practice of ancient Greece (Jackson, 2014, p. 11). This section will focus on the western tradition as this is most relevant to modern western medical practice, and to the ethical principles relating to the modern, and potential postmodern, medical technologies discussed here.

Hippocrates (c. 460–371 BCE) is regarded as "the father of medicine" (Jackson, 2014, p. 2). The Hippocratic Oath, an oath of initiation taken by new medical practitioners, is one of the oldest sources of medical ethics, and the oath still forms part of physician induction in some countries in the modern age. The central ethical tenets of the Hippocratic Oath – which may be summarised as a) do no harm, b) maintain confidentiality and c) do not exploit patients – have not changed since ancient times (Jackson, 2014, p. 198). Nutton notes that an important aspect of the Hippocratic Oath is its emphasis that there is no stigma in doing nothing, if doing nothing is the correct response in that case, and that the primary purpose of the oath is to differentiate good and bad practitioners (Nutton, 1995, p. 29). Nevertheless, although it is well-established, and is a primary source of medical ethics, the Hippocratic Oath has its problems. First, Nutton points out that the oath seems to regard medical ethics solely in terms of the obligations of belonging to a group – that is, of medical practitioners. This is at odds with the multidisciplinary and holistic ethos of healthcare in the modern context. Moreover, Nutton claims that the religious (albeit pagan) language of the oath suggests that it was written for a specific group of physicians and was not used as universally in the ancient world as is popularly thought. Second, Nutton contends that, rather than simply providing guidance to resolve ethical dilemmas, the Oath actually introduced ethical dilemmas. An example of this might be the Oath's prohibition of surgery at all costs. However, I would suggest that this might be a twentieth-century perspective and may not account for the fact that any surgery was highly dangerous prior to the development of modern anaesthesia and disinfection.

Longrigg, though, asserts that the Hippocratic Oath is concerned with ethics in general, not just the ethics of the practice of medicine, and regards the Oath as deontological in nature – that is, it is primarily about the absolute duties of the practitioner (1997, p. 34). Longrigg also suggests, correctly in my view, that the adoption of the Hippocratic Oath by Galen, a Roman physician of the second century, has contributed to its centrality in the Western medical tradition. Nevertheless, despite a clear ethical and cultural tradition of medicine in the ancient world, the operation of the human body at that time was understood solely in pre-modern terms, with the theory of the "humours" – that supposedly chemical substances called "humours" regulated the body, and that illness was caused by an imbalance of humours (Jackson, 2014, pp. 17–18).[3]

Elsewhere in the world of classical philosophy, the thought of Plato had implications for embodied human life. Plato argued that the virtues of this world – for example, the triad of truth, goodness and beauty – could not be fully experienced in this world – and were, in fact, only expressions of perfect "forms" of these virtues in another heavenly world. This led to dualistic thinking, in which the body and materiality were a separate realm from the spirit. This posed one of the greatest challenges to the Christian message of the early church; because of the incarnation of Christ and the coming of the Holy Spirit, there was no body-spirit divide inherent in Christian anthropology, and this supported a monistic, and holistic, view of the human person. I will explore the implications of this for embodied human life in subsequent chapters.

Aristotle was a student of Plato, but he moved away from Plato's theory of forms and, instead, asked the question: what are the goods of human life? In other words, what are the things of life that have moral currency and value, and lead to fulfilment, happiness and flourishing? Aristotle equated "happiness" with function. He argued that, by the application of reason, functions could be achieved, and the goods of life could be realised. Aristotle's *Nicomachean Ethics* was an example of how his theory worked out in practice. The work of Aristotle is particularly significant in medical ethics because his thinking was highly influential for Thomas Aquinas, and the medieval development of natural law theory (Pope, 2012, pp. 67–86).

Bryant, Baggott la Velle and Searle outline the principles of Judaeo-Christian ethics (Bryant et al., 2005, pp. 20–21). They state that the ethics of the Judaeo-Christian tradition are based on the revelation of God, and obedience to God's revealed commands and covenant, obedience which brings with it moral tenets. The particular contribution of Christianity to medical ethics has included the notion of a healing and reconciling God (e.g., Exodus 15v26), and the concept of *shalom*, which is often translated "peace", and is concerned with human wholeness and flourishing, in its broadest sense. The idea of *shalom*, with connotations of health, is seen in Old Testament passages such as Psalm 32, Jeremiah 8v15 and Isaiah 53v5. O'Brien and Harris quote Cornelius Plantinga's helpful definition of *shalom* as

> Universal flourishing, wholeness, and delight—a rich state of affairs in which natural needs are satisfied and natural gifts fruitfully employed, all under the arch of God's love.
>
> (O'Brien and Harris, 2012)

Moreover, passages from the New Testament portray Jesus – the Messiah and the Prince of Peace – as the bringer of *shalom* and healing (Luke 10v5–9;

Hebrews 12v13–14). Jesus performed healing miracles (Mark 2v1–12; John 5v1–15) and by his death on the cross, Jesus provided the ultimate healing, by forgiving sins and reconciling the world to God. Thus, a message of healing appears to be central and integral to a Christian understanding of salvation.

The development of natural law is especially important for the development of medical ethics, as the natural law approach to ethics has underpinned Roman Catholic moral responses to modern medical developments, including both the cases described in this book. Bryant, Baggott la Velle and Searle give an account of natural law, as it relates to medical ethics (Bryant et al., 2005, pp. 21–22). Natural law, they state, originates as far back as the Stoics in the fifth century BCE. The central principle of natural law is, to quote Bryant, that "a good life is a life based in accordance with nature". This was combined with the principle, derived from Aristotle, that nothing in nature is produced without a purpose, and that if a creature can fulfil its nature, then it is directed to morally good ends. Drawing on Aristotle and the Stoics, the medieval theologian Thomas Aquinas (1225–1274) developed natural law theory most fully. He developed Aristotle's idea of the functions of life into a classification of general and specific human functions. According to Aquinas, reflection on human nature shows the ends or purposes to which human beings are naturally inclined, and this indicates moral imperatives in human life. Much Roman Catholic thinking on medicine is still based on natural law – so, for example, because procreation is the natural end of sex, the Roman Catholic Church has objected to contraception on theological grounds. This will be explored in greater detail in Chapter 3.

The Renaissance was a significant time for the development of medicine, as a discipline. The establishment of the "new" universities, and their medical curricula led to an expansion of experimental knowledge of medicine at that time (Jackson, 2014, p. 61).[4] And led to the gradual rejection of the humouralism of the Hippocratic and Galenic medical traditions, in favour of physiological mechanisms, based on the new empirical, experimental, observations.

Consequently, during the seventeenth century, a new type of medical practitioner emerged – one who used material treatments, for example, herbal or natural products, instead of relying on humoural theory. Wear terms such practitioners "iatrochemists" (*iatros* = doctor) and these were the forerunners of both apothecaries (specialists in pharmaceutical medicine) and pharmacists (Wear, 1995, pp. 320–325). Wear has described the development of iatrochemical medicine, which has traditionally been based on the principles of Paracelsus, the sixteenth-century scientist and mystical writer, who strongly opposed traditional ideas of medicine from the ancient world (Wear, 1995, pp. 310–312). In the seventeenth century, the Puritans empathised with iatrochemical medicine because a search for personal knowledge in the natural world aligned well with the Reformed ideal of a personal relationship with God. Furthermore, the Puritans found iatrochemical medicine attractive because it did not have the "pagan" foundations of the Hippocratic tradition (Wear, 1995, p. 323).

The era from the Renaissance to the Enlightenment was a time of seismic change in medical ethical thinking. Bryant, Baggot la Velle and Searle argue that the Copernican revolution undermined religious understandings of the universe, which in turn, undermined traditional Christian moral thinking, based on religious revelation and an immutable natural law (Bryant et al., 2005, p. 22). The general approach to ethics therefore shifted from God revealing ethical principles to humanity, to humanity determining ethical responses with the power of reason. A key ethical development for medicine in the modern era was consequentialism, which came to prominence in the eighteenth and nineteenth centuries. The best-known form of consequentialism was utilitarianism, which was developed by Jeremy Bentham and John Stuart Mill (Bryant et al., 2005, p. 23). The consequentialist approach is that the rightness or wrongness of an action is determined by the consequences of the action, not by the duty or the motivation of the actor. Therefore, in principle, an act is good if it produces the greatest good for the greatest number of people. Consequentialism, in its various forms, is potentially problematic from a Christian perspective for various reasons. First, because of revelation, the Christian ethical tradition has a clear deontological basis, and also stresses the importance of virtue, so is by no means a solely consequence-based ethical system. Second, consequentialism seems to have a limited perception of the scope of human good. Third, there is the problem of whether consequences can be anticipated. The fourth and possibly greatest difficulty is that a consequentialist approach could, for example, justify the murder of one person (prohibited in Christian terms), for a greater good (Messer, 2006, p. 80).

Nevertheless, consequentialism plays a major part in modern bioethics, since many medical economic arguments about cost-utility of medical treatments and distribution of healthcare resources are, in practice, made on consequentialist grounds. Consequentialism has also been significant for the development of the concept of autonomy in the modern era, which I will discuss in Chapter 2.

However, a purely consequentialist approach to ethics of biomedical technology is problematic, because of the issue of "unintended consequences" that may be observed with newly introduced treatments, for which there is limited experience. The issue of unintended consequences is an important one in the ethical evaluation of newly developed medical technologies and therefore highly relevant to proposed transhumanist technologies and will be discussed in more depth later in this book.

Another key influence on modern bioethics has been the Second World War, and its aftermath (Bryant et al., 2005, pp. 23–24). After the Nuremberg War Crimes Trials, there was a subsequent international awareness and condemnation of the Holocaust and Nazi atrocities during the war. Under the Nazi regime, non-consensual medical experiments had been conducted on prisoners – Jews, but also children and other vulnerable groups, and prisoners of war. At an ideological level, this experimentation was justified by the Nazi racial purity ideology, and the fact that these groups were regarded as sub-human (*Untermenschen*), so "did not count" as human beings. As a consequence of the subsequent international outcry, ethical standards for scientific experimentation and international human rights agreements were developed, such as the Nuremberg Code (1947), the World Medical Association's Declaration of Geneva (1948), and the Helsinki Declaration (1964) (Jackson, 2014, p. 171). Duffin contends that the Nuremberg Code had little impact on the development of US life sciences research after the war (Duffin, 1999, p. 323); nevertheless, as well as providing a framework for human rights, these standards also provided the foundations for modern, ethical clinical trial methodology (Duffin, 1999, p. 105).

Other stimuli for the development of modern bioethics as a discipline were: a) the perceived inadequacies of traditional forms of ethical thought; b) the rapid advance of biomedical technology (evidenced by the post-war development of the pharmaceutical industry in the "therapeutic revolution" era, as discussed); c) decreasing paternalism in medicine, and decreasing deference to the authority of the medical profession and d) an increasing concern for the environment and the sustainability of the earth's resources (Bryant et al., 2005, p. 24).

Modern bioethics is therefore concerned not just with the practice of medicine and the behaviours of medical practitioners, but with the appropriate distribution of healthcare services in society, and the political and financial implications of this distribution. New medical technologies (e.g., transplantation, genetic and reproductive technologies) have introduced new ethical issues, such as 1) how much intervention is ethically justified, when radical forms of medicine are technologically possible? 2) at what point does death occur? and 3) how can scarce resources be distributed equitably? (Jackson, 2014, p. 193). The first and third of these issues are especially important in any ethical evaluation of future transhumanism and enhancement technologies. Indeed, I will show in Chapter 5 that, similarly, the ethics of transhumanist medical technologies are far broader than the ethics of individual medical intervention and in addition relate to the equitable distribution of medical technologies in society, and the extent to which the whole of human society is affected by their use.

To conclude this section, I would argue that, in its long and illustrious history, medical ethics has developed through three phases, a Hippocratic phase, a Renaissance/Enlightenment phase and a Late Modern phase. Initially, with the Hippocratic tradition of ancient Greece, medical ethics focused on the duties and behaviours of the medical practitioner. As the scientific knowledge and methods of medicine were undeveloped at that time, the conduct of the practitioner was the key determinant in the moral good and reputation of the practice of medicine. Then, following the Renaissance and Enlightenment, when greater experimental knowledge of the human body gradually brought more sophisticated methods of medical treatment, ethical questions in medicine began to focus on the techniques of medicine and the consequences of these techniques for the patient. Finally, in the late modern and post-modern era, with the developments of modern bioethics, the ethical questions of healthcare and medicine are no longer solely restricted to those concerning the practice of medicine. They now encompass questions about the distribution of healthcare resources in society – budget, staffing, medicines and equipment - the relationship between healthcare and human rights in society and the extent to which medical intervention is appropriate in an age where increasingly radical medical technologies are available.

It is within this context that the ethical implications of proposed future transhumanist biomedical technologies must be evaluated, and I will perform a preliminary ethical analysis of future radical biomedical technologies in Chapter 2. However, in the light of the impact of modern pharmaceutical medicine to date, we should now consider the potential benefits of future radical biomedical technologies.

1.4 Agents of Change: Learning From Past Successes

While the next chapter will provide a detailed history of transhumanism and an account of religious criticisms of the transhumanism project, this section will give an outline of some of the potential benefits of radical transhumanist biomedical technology, as claimed by various commentators on transhumanism.

Commentators highlight the potential benefits of radical biomedical technologies for human health and well-being (Bostrom, 2005). If the ideological aspects of transhumanism are put to one side, the fact is that many proposed future biomedical technologies would indeed lead to a radical improvement in human health, commensurate with the radical nature of the technologies. For example, all the technologies outlined in the Introduction would have profound benefits for human health:

- Medical nanotechnology offers the possibility of detailed mechanistic treatment of systemic diseases which invoke inflammatory processes, for example, cancers and autoimmune disorders.
- Germ cell genetic manipulation could, in a generation, completely eradicate some inherited diseases – for example, cystic fibrosis and haemophilia.
- The routine use of sophisticated cybernetic limbs has the potential to considerably reduce morbidity due to chronic musculoskeletal and joint pain.
- Cryopreservation would preserve the lives of those whose diseases could not be treated in the foreseeable future. Indeed, those whose bodies have been cryogenically frozen because they have incurable

diseases could constitute disease registry populations for clinical trials of new treatments for those diseases. Put simply, people would be reanimated when a treatment for their condition became available.

- Finally, human bodily suffering could be eradicated altogether by eliminating its locus – the human body – using mind uploading. However, this would render the pharmaceutical industry obsolete, rather than advance it, and it raises considerable questions concerning personal identity and the significance of bodily life, which we will explore in later chapters.

Many of these benefits are clearly consistent with the contribution of modern pharmaceutical medicine to the reduction of mortality and the alleviation of chronic suffering, as described previously in this chapter. Furthermore, some technologies that have been described as transhumanist – for example, genetic manipulation and nanomedicine – are feasible developments from medical interventions that have already been prototyped at the time of writing. And yet such technologies, if developed in an equitable way, would have a potentially greater impact on human suffering than those currently available, improving well-being for a possibly greater proportion of citizens.

If this is the case, the question we should perhaps be asking is why we would *not* use some transhumanist technologies to improve human health and well-being? Transhumanism commentators often describe the adoption of transhumanism as a moral imperative (Bostrom, 2005, p. 10); surely using radical biomedical technology for a more extensive eradication of human disease would be an important moral motivation for society, industry and health practitioners? McNamee and Edwards argue that forms of technology are already being used to improve human life – for example, drainage and sewerage systems, drug therapy and computers – and that transhumanist technologies are, in a sense, no more than extensions and advances on some technologies already in use. Moreover, they argue that technological advances give humanity the opportunity to make positive future plans, and to proactively deal with risks to human life (McNamee and Edwards, 2006).

There might, therefore, be a positive ethical argument for the appropriate use of transhumanist technologies in future, based on their radical therapeutic potential. Yet this positive ethical argument for transhumanist technologies as medical treatments is seldom articulated even by transhumanist scholars, and certainly not by Christian theologians. Consequently, it is all the more important that the ethical issues with transhumanism are fully examined, and then re-evaluated in the light of previous medical developments, to gain an insight into the true ethical status of future transhumanist technologies. The potentially far-reaching therapeutic benefits of future transhumanist biomedical technologies on human health and flourishing, compared with the relatively modest impact of past therapeutic developments, is a factor in the ethical evaluation of medical technologies presented in Chapter 5.

One potential complicating factor is whether a biomedical technology is considered a therapy – that is, it corrects a disease-related deficiency in a person – or an enhancement – that is, it confers an additional characteristic to person who is already healthy. I will discuss this issue in much more detail in Chapter 2. However, in brief, I argue that, if a biomedical technology is considered a treatment, then its use in human society is considered within a culture of healthcare, whereas if it is considered an enhancement, it is not seen as a healthcare issue culturally. This is a barrier which prevents people from recognising the "therapeutic" value of a biomedical intervention that is considered an enhancement, as far as current norms of human function are concerned.

The proposal of this book is that, regardless of the debate about whether a biotechnology is an enhancement or a therapy, some radical biomedical interventions may have considerable potential in relieving human suffering and improving human welfare in a way that might exceed the benefits of widespread pharmaceutical medicine to date.

There is therefore a moral argument for deploying some proposed future biomedical technologies in an appropriate way, regardless of cultural concerns. In fact, failure to explore the use of some of these technologies to meet the most pressing human health needs would be inconsistent with the importance of the scientific endeavour in human society over the last four hundred years, and would not do justice to the "stirring advances" of the pharmaceutical industry during the twentieth century.

However, it will be important to determine whether the biomedical developments with the most humanitarian benefits are ethically acceptable. The Christian ethical evaluation of therapeutically beneficial biomedical technologies, in the light of past therapeutic developments, is the key focus of this book.

1.5 Medical Ethics and Christian Pastoral Care

The final section of this context-setting chapter provides a brief discussion of the pastoral significance of medical ethics. Radical future biomedical technologies may have implications for medical ethics – the goods of human life, the values of society and the distribution of healthcare resources – but what are their implications for human well-being and welfare, and the pastoral task of the Christian church?

Ronald Cole-Turner has argued that medical technology is imposing a new metaphysics on human nature (Cole-Turner, 2001). Commenting on Peter Kramer's book "Listening to Prozac", Cole-Turner argues that reductionist biological arguments have caused humanity to conflate natural and spiritual considerations and that human society is now trying to solve spiritual problems with pharmacological solutions. Similarly, Michael Burdett has argued that transhumanism applies biomedical technology directly to the human being in a way that transcends traditional Christian understandings of humanity (Burdett, 2014). Transhumanist biomedical technologies therefore go beyond the purview of medicine and seek potential solutions to metaphysical issues.

A brief overview of pharmaceutical medicine and its effects on the human population suggests that pharmaceutical medicine to date has had a significant impact on human health outcomes and well-being, but that proposed transhumanist biomedical technologies might have a yet more radical effect on human life, and could therefore potentially have a greater positive effect on human health and well-being than current pharmaceutical developments. It is possible that, during the twenty-first century, there will be an "enhancement revolution" that will be more far-reaching than the "therapeutic revolution" of the twentieth century. However, this "enhancement revolution" will have medical implications. Transhumanist biomedical technologies may reduce mortality rates more significantly than pharmaceutical medicine to date and may lead to another shift in causes of death in future.

During this "enhancement revolution", it will be important from an ethical perspective that what is good about the human person – and human society – is upheld and preserved. This would be a goal for people of goodwill of all religious traditions and none – although, in this book, I will examine this primarily from a perspective of Christian theological ethics.

This study has two important ethical implications. First, it will place the ethical evaluation of transhumanist technologies into its proper historical context, namely recent developments both in modern medicine and within the discipline of medical ethics. This will enable a nuanced and comprehensive – and realistic – ethical evaluation of future technologies, which will limit any unhelpful, "brave new world" popular perceptions and cultural assumptions, and put any dystopian fears into perspective. In my survey of medical ethics earlier in this chapter, I indicated that to date there have been three phases of medical ethics, the Hippocratic phase, the Renaissance/Enlightenment phase and the Late Modern phase. It may be that, in historical context, a new, fourth phase of medical ethics is needed to address the issues of transhumanism.

Second, this study will provide an ethical framework which will allow theologians and scientists to consider the merits of future medical technologies that have not yet been discovered, and to consider ethical issues with medical technologies in a proactive and reflective way, when they are at the discovery, design and prototyping stages.

The study also has important pastoral implications. The church's reaction to medical developments is often a dissonant one. At an individual level, Christians seek health technologies to heal and control disease and improve quality of life, as much as any citizen in wider society. However, in preaching and public discourse, churches may give mixed messages about medical technology. On the one hand, medical technology is heralded as a gift to humanity from a God who is the creator and sustainer of all living things. But, on the other, churches are wary of exploring medical advances in any depth - because of a lack of scientific knowledge about them, a cultural fear of their implications, or a theology that understands healing to be the prerogative of God alone. For this reason, there is little shared understanding of medical issues in the church, which leads to two pastoral issues. First, individual Christians may be left to face ethical decisions about medical treatment alone and without the church's support – typically when these decisions are urgent and relate to serious illness or end-of-life care for themselves or their family. Second, the lack of coherent engagement of churches with medical technologies means that, unless they work in medicine and healthcare, individual Christians may not have the confidence to speak about medical issues from a Christian perspective, openly and with an appropriate vocabulary, at a time when such medical technologies are the subject of much popular speculation.

My hope is that this project will make some contribution to all these important issues. These ethical and pastoral implications will be reviewed, based on the findings of this work, in the concluding chapter of this book. The next chapter, however, will develop this evaluation by describing transhumanism in its different forms, and applying the general and specific criteria described earlier to proposed future transhumanist technologies.

Notes

1 For a history of receptor theory, see John Parascandola and Ronald Jasensky, "Origins of the Receptor Theory of Drug Action", *Bulletin of Medical History*, 48 (1974), pp. 199–220.
2 Tansey maintains that the campaign to enable commercial organisations to be licensed for animal experimentation was a key factor in this academic acceptability.
3 It is interesting to compare the idea of "humours" with modern therapeutic science, based on circulating hormones and the balance of chemical action of drug molecules at cell receptors.
4 The new medical curricula of the Renaissance involved the dissection of human bodies.

References

Andrew Wear, "Medicine in Early Modern Europe, 1500–1700", in *The Western Medical Tradition 800BC–1800AD*, edited by Lawrence Conrad, Michael Neve, Vivian Nutton, Roy Porter and Andrew Wear (Cambridge: Cambridge University Press, 1995), pp. 215–362.

Charles Rosenberg, "The Therapeutic Revolution: Medicine, Meaning and Social Change in Nineteenth Century America", *Perspectives in Biology and Medicine* 20 (1977), pp. 485–506.

Graham O'Brien and Timothy Harris, "What on Earth Is God Doing? Relating Theology and Science through Biblical Theology", *Perspectives on Science and Christian Faith*, 64 (2012), pp. 147–156.

John Bryant, Linda Baggott la Velle and John Searle, *Introduction to Bioethics* (Chichester: Wiley, 2005).

Jenny Bryan, "Ventolin Remains a Breath of Fresh Air", *Pharmaceutical Journal*, 279 (2007), pp. 404–405.

Jacalyn Duffin, *History of Medicine: A Scandalously Short Introduction* (Toronto: University of Toronto Press, 1999).

Joe Hicks and Grahame Allen, "A Century of Change: Trends in UK Statistics since 1900", *House of Commons Research Paper*, 99/111 (1999).

Jonathan Liebenau, "The Rise of the British Pharmaceutical Industry", *British Medical Journal*, 301 (1990), pp. 724–728, p. 733.

James Longrigg, "Medicine in the Classical World", in *Western Medicine: An Illustrated History*, edited by Irvine Loudon (Oxford: Oxford University Press, 1997), pp. 25–39.

Judy Slinn, "The Development of the Pharmaceutical Industry", in *Making Medicines: A Brief History of Pharmacy and Pharmaceuticals*, edited by Stuart Anderson (London: Pharmaceutical Press, 2005), pp. 155–174.

Kenneth Culver, "A Christian Physician at the Cross-roads of New Genetic Technologies and the Needs of Patients", in *Beyond Cloning: Religion and the Remaking of Humanity*, edited by Ronald Cole-Turner (Harrisburg PA: Trinity Press International, 2001), pp. 14–34.

M.J. McNamee and S.D. Edwards, "Transhumanism, Medical Technology and Slippery Slopes", *Journal of Medical Ethics*, 32 (2006), pp. 513–518.

Mark Jackson, *The History of Medicine: A Beginner's Guide* (London: Oneworld, 2014).

Michael Burdett, *Technology and the Rise of Transhumanism* (Cambridge: Grove, 2014).

Nick Bostrom, "Transhumanist Values", *Journal of Philosophical Research*, 30 (2005), pp. 3–14.

Neil Tranter, *British Population in the Twentieth Century* (Basingstoke: MacMillan, 1996).

Neil Messer, *SCM Study Guide: Christian Ethics* (London: SCM, 2006).

Organisation for Economic Cooperation and Development (OECD) (2013), "OECD Factbook 2013: Economic, Environmental and Social Statistics", 2013, 10.1787/factbook-2013-95-en (accessed May 2015).

Ronald Cole-Turner, "Towards a Theology for the Age of Biotechnology", in *Beyond Cloning: Religion & the Remaking of Humanity*, edited by Ronald Cole-Turner (Harrisburg PA: Trinity Press International, 2001), pp. 137–150.

Robert Jutte, *Contraception: A History*, translated by V. Russell (Cambridge: Polity Press, 2008).

Richard Weinshilboum, "The Therapeutic Revolution", *Clinical Pharmacology and Therapeutics*, 42 (1987), pp. 481–484.

Steven Woolf, "Evidence-Based Medicine: A Historical and International Overview", *Proceedings of the Royal College of Physicians of Edinburgh*, 31 (2001), pp. 39–41.

S.R. Davis, I. Dinatale, L. Rivera Wall and S. Davison, "Postmenopausal Hormone Therapy: From Monkey Glands to Transdermal Patches", *Journal of Endocrinology*, 185 (2005), pp. 207–222.

Stephen Pope, "Natural Law and Christian Ethics", in *Cambridge Companion to Christian Ethics*, edited by Robin Gill (Cambridge: Cambridge University Press, 2012), pp. 67–86.

Tilli Tansey, "Pills, Profits and Propriety: The Early Pharmaceutical Industry in Britain", *Pharmaceutical History (London)*, 25 (1995), pp. 3–9.

United Nations, "Department of Economic and Social Affairs, Population Division (2011). World Population Prospects: The 2010 Revision", 2011, http://esa.un.org/wpp/ (accessed May 2015).

Vivian Nutton, "Medicine in the Greek World: 800-50BC", in *The Western Medical Tradition 800BC–1800AD*, edited by Lawrence Conrad, Michael Neve, Vivian Nutton, Roy Porter and Andrew Wear (Cambridge: Cambridge University Press, 1995), pp. 11–38.

Viviane Quirke, "From Alkaloids to Gene Therapy: A Brief History of Drug Discovery in the 20th Century", in *Making Medicines: A Brief History of Pharmacy and Pharmaceuticals*, edited by Stuart Anderson (London: Pharmaceutical Press, 2005), pp. 177–201.

W. Duncan Reekie and Michael Weber, *Profit, Politics and Drugs* (London: McMillan, 1979).

2 Transhumanism

Losing Our Humanity?

2.1 What Is Transhumanism?

This chapter describes the history and development of the transhumanist movement, discusses religious responses to transhumanism and describes some social and theological critiques of transhumanism. The chapter then presents general and specific criteria used to assess biomedical technologies; these criteria will then be applied to some of the proposed transhumanist medical technologies mentioned in the Introduction to determine whether they can be classed as transhumanist technologies, and to evaluate their ethical implications. These criteria will be used in the same way subsequently in Chapters 3 and 4 to assess the two previous pharmaceutical developments – the contraceptive pill and selective serotonin reuptake inhibitor (SSRI) antidepressants.

However, this opening section defines transhumanism and describes the origins and intellectual landscape of the transhumanism movement. Because of the diverse nature of the transhumanist movement, a wide range of scholars will be evaluated here. This will enable a taxonomy of the transhumanism movement to be developed, which will assist readers in understanding the key concepts of transhumanist thought, together with religious and ethical engagement with them.

As I have discussed elsewhere, notwithstanding socio-cultural influences, the development of modern medicine has been largely a scientific and technological endeavour. By contrast, transhumanism is essentially a philosophical and intellectual movement, mainly because many of the technologies it envisages are not yet scientifically feasible and have not yet been developed.

Thus, Max More has defined transhumanism as,

> Philosophies of life … that seek the continuation and acceleration of the evolution of intelligent life beyond its current human form and human limitations by means of science, technology, guided by life-promoting principles and values.
>
> (More, 2013, p. 5)

DOI: 10.4324/9781003290421-3

More helpfully states that the name "transhumanism" implies that transhumanism goes beyond what is currently considered to be human. Therefore, it is not just about the use of education or culture to refine human life, but about using biomedical technology to go beyond the current biological limits of human life (More, 2013, p. 5).

In its literature, the World Transhumanist Association is slightly more specific, describing transhumanism as,

> The intellectual and cultural movement that affirms the possibility and desirability of fundamentally improving the human condition through applied reason, especially by developing and making widely available technologies to eliminate ageing and to greatly enhance human intellectual, physical and psychological capacities.
>
> (World Transhumanist Association, 2003)

Another prominent transhumanist, Nick Bostrom, has defined transhumanism, more succinctly, as,

> An interdisciplinary approach to understanding and evaluating the opportunities for enhancing the human condition that are emerging through advancing technology.
>
> (Bostrom, 2005a, p. 3)

The term *transhumanist* tends to be used to describe the process or technologies for human change, while the term *post-human* (as a noun) is used to describe the end point of transhumanism – the transformed human entity. Thus, More states that *transhumanist* technologies are applied so that humans may become *post-human* – that is to say, no longer recognisably human by current standards, but with greatly enhanced characteristics, such as greater physical capability, cognitive capacity, and extended life expectancy.

Confusingly, the terms *transhuman(ist)* and *post-human* are sometimes used interchangeably in the literature; for example, Anthony Miccoli refers to "post-humanist scholars" in a way that suggests that, in fact, he is using the term *post-humanism* to describe the process, instead of *transhumanism* (Miccoli, 2010, pp. 123–133).

These definitions indicate that, while proposed transhumanist technologies may be biomedical in character, they are applied with the intention of transforming human life in more radical and different ways than has happened with medical technologies to date.

2.2 Origins of Transhumanism

This section examines the origins and historical development of the transhumanist movement. Human beings have sought to acquire immortality or new capacities since time immemorial (Bostrom, 2005b, p. 1). The pseudo-science of alchemy was concerned with the notion of human transformation, and More has described the alchemists from the thirteenth century onwards as "proto-transhumanists" (More, 2013, p. 9). At the time of the Renaissance, nature and the human body became seen as legitimate objects of study and, subsequently, the Enlightenment focused on rationalism and empiricism. These intellectual changes enabled transhumanist aspirations to be envisaged, and the rise of modern science has made these aspirations realistic possibilities.

There have been various influences on the development of transhumanist thought. The work of Charles Darwin on evolution and natural selection has understandably been foundational to the development of transhumanism (Bostrom, 2005b, p. 3) as it represented a sea change in the understanding of humanity, introducing the idea that there was no "fixed" human nature, but that human nature was still evolving and emerging. Accordingly, some transhumanists – for example, Ray Kurzweil and Hans Moravec – describe transhumanist technological development as continuous with, or analogous to, the process of human evolution.

Nietzsche and the existentialists were also significant for the development of transhumanist thought (Bostrom, 2005b, p. 4). While Nietzsche was not interested in the role of technology in humanity *per se,* his ideas of individualistic experience and personal growth arising from the incommensurability of human existence align well with the aims of the transhumanist movement. In addition, the works of scientist J.B.S. Haldane (*Daedalus: Science and the Future*), and of science-fiction writer Aldous Huxley (*Brave New World*) have described the use of technology to transform human life radically, and have therefore fed the imagination of transhumanists (More, 2013, p. 8, p. 11). During the 1960s, philosopher and author, F.M. Esfandiary, who subsequently changed his name to F.M. 2030, ran a series of classes entitled *New Concepts of the Human*. He described a transhumanist as a "transitional human who, by virtue of their technology usage, cultural values and lifestyle, constitutes an evolutionary link with the coming era of post-humanity" (Bostrom, 2005b, p. 11). F.M. 2030 said that a transhumanist was characterised by; a) their use of technologies, b) their absence of religious beliefs and c) their rejection of traditional family values. In 1998, the World Transhumanist Association was formed by Nick Bostrom and David Pearce, to provide a respectable academic outlet for transhumanist ideas. The transhumanist movement began in North America, but transhumanism is gaining adherents throughout the western world (McNamee and Edwards, 2006), which is significant for the future of medicine, and for sociocultural attitudes to healthcare in developed countries, an issue I will reflect on in Chapters 5 and 6.

2.3 Approaches to Transhumanism

Different protagonists of the transhumanist movement have taken different approaches to the transhumanist project, depending on their academic interests, and the worldviews underlying those interests. Nick Bostrom is a philosopher, and he rightly takes a holistic approach, viewing the transhumanist movement as part of the wider intellectual, cultural and social development of humanity, rather than simply a biotechnology project.[1] Bostrom argues that transhumanism has its roots in secular humanism; he appears to understand transhumanism as a means of improving the human condition, in the tradition of liberal optimism and progress (Bostrom, 2005a, p. 10).

Bostrom – perhaps naively – appears unconcerned about any potential loss of human values due to technology adoption, or about the possibility of the loss of human identity. He refers to the incompleteness of humanity when he describes the transhumanist desire to make good the "half-baked" project of human nature (Bostrom, 2004). He states that, from a transhumanist perspective, moral status is independent of species membership, but is related to intellectual capacity, rather than human embodiment (McNamee and Edwards, 2006). As well as the theological concerns this raises in respect of embodiment, this view is also troublesome when considering the theological status of human beings who lack intellectual capacity for whatever reason, which has implications for the *imago Dei*, the understanding of how human beings bear the image of God. Both these theological issues will be explored later in this chapter. Bostrom has been described as transhumanism's "most intellectually robust proponent" (McNamee and Edwards, 2006), and the social objective of transhumanism that he cites – the use of technology to improve the well-being of all people – is one that is indeed in keeping with the optimism of liberal humanism.

Max More, too, takes a philosophical view of transhumanism (More, 2013, p. 4). As described earlier, he defines transhumanism as a *life philosophy* which, he argues, is about actively seeking a better future, rather than praying to a deity to provide one. More is therefore dismissive of religion – inappropriately so, in my view, given its cultural significance, irrespective of any specific theological commitments. More's *life philosophy* is devoid of any supernatural beliefs about physical transcendence, and yet his approach to transhumanism is, in fact, quasi-religious, inasmuch as he presents transhumanism as a life philosophy – a good way, or rule, for living life – in a way that seems analogous to religious belief and observance.

More is famous for his slogan, "No more gods, no more faith, no more timid holding back. The world belongs to post-humanity". This suggests technological optimism, confidence about the importance of the transhumanist project, and perhaps humanistic hubris. More asserts that transhumanists do not fear death or loathe their physical bodies, and they are not interested in Utopia. Also, in apparent contrast to Bostrom, More states that transhumanism is not about predicting the future, but is about seeking goals for humanity, rather than writing a schedule for human history.

Unlike scholars with a technological background, such as Kurzweil and Moravec, More claims – again perhaps naively – that transhumanist technologies will not inevitably change humanity (More, 2013, p. 4). That said, More still has a provisional view of humanity, arguing that human nature is not an end in itself; that it is not perfect, nor is it a given (More, 2013, p. 5).

More has also discussed some key terminology of transhumanist thought (More, 2013, pp. 4–6). He states that, as well as greater physical capability, cognitive capacity and extended life expectancy, the post-human may also have *morphological freedom* – freedom of form – meaning that they may not necessarily take on a recognisable humanoid body shape (More, 2013, p. 4). For example, the post-human person may be a cyborg – a human/robot hybrid – or they may be completely disembodied, as would happen with mind-uploading.

More also describes the idea of *singularity* – a point in history that might be reached when, due to environmental conditions or scientific discoveries, humanity can no longer continue in its current form of existence (More, 2013, p. 6). Lastly, More describes the concept of *extropy*, a term that he himself has coined (a term complementary to the physicochemical idea of entropy), which describes the drive to extend humanity beyond its current form and constraints (More, 2013, p. 5).

Julian Savulescu is an ethicist, and his espousal of transhumanist enhancements arises from his consequentialist ethics (Savulescu, 2009). He makes ethical arguments in favour of enhancements, based on what he considers to be the consequential benefits for humanity. For example, he has proposed the concept of *procreative beneficence*, which states that parents have a right to select the "best possible" child available to them, based on the best available evidence (Savulescu, 2001). Savulescu has a permissive attitude to the idea of biological enhancement – so, for example, he claims that the use of the drug modafinil to achieve greater mental alertness is no different ethically to drinking caffeinated drinks, which is a normal part of daily life at present (Maslen, 2014). Savulescu is therefore interested in the ethical issues surrounding the enhancement potential of drugs that are already in use – for example, the possible use of SSRIs, such as citalopram, for moral enhancement – not just the radical and biologically invasive forms of biomedical enhancement which might be available in the future (Kahane and Savulescu, 2015).

Savulescu argues that biomedical enhancement will promote autonomy but, interestingly for someone taking the consequentialist ethical approach, does not seem to acknowledge the valid criticism that transhumanist enhancements may lead to injustice, or even oppression, in human society, an issue that will be discussed later in this chapter (Sparrow, 2014). Furthermore, Savulescu argues against "species-ism" – which he defines as any kind of privileging of human life over animal life for any reason (Savulescu, 2009). He rejects the idea that humanity intrinsically has greater significance than any other species. He argues that species-ism is morally equivalent to racism and sexism and makes the dubious claim that species-ism can reinforce exclusivist attitudes – racism, sexism – within human society (Savulescu, 2009), a claim that seems hard to support.

By contrast, Hans Moravec is a computing and cybernetics specialist, rather than a philosopher. Moravec points to the increasing sophistication of computers, the development of artificial intelligence (AI) and the fact that computing power is increasing exponentially (Moravec, 1988, p. 6). He argues that a "break-even" point of computer usefulness will occur at some point in the future, after which there will be rapid adoption of sophisticated computers and robotics in all areas of life, and a closer symbiosis between computers and humans will develop (Moravec, 1988, p. 2). He asserts that intelligent machines already exist, and that humans must embrace the technological era, rather than shy away from it. Moravec claims that, although robots are limited in their applications now, humans often *want* robots to be limited – because of their egos, humans don't want to be upstaged by robots (Moravec, 1988, p. 108).

Moravec discusses the potential loss of personal identity, a problem that might arise from *morphological freedom*, as described earlier – for example, with someone whose brain was uploaded onto a computer (Moravec, 1988, pp. 109–110). He addresses the identity issue by appealing to a distinction between *body identity*, where the person is defined by the material matter of their human body, and *pattern identity*, where a person is defined by their thought patterns and processes (Moravec, 1988, p. 116). This enables Moravec to address the embodiment problem that mind-uploading presents; however, he equates the mind with brain, and makes the erroneous assumption that thought processes are the sum of human experience, when there are many other bodily, material and cultural aspects of human life. A criticism of the concept of pattern identity, as opposed to body identity, is that it can be described in computing/AI terms as a simulation, rather than real life. However, Moravec has countered this argument by questioning whether a simulation has less moral value than "real life", and the difficulties, in some scenarios, of distinguishing between real life and simulation (More, 2013, p. 8).

Moravec's argument is rich with science-based speculation and technical possibilities, but details of the socio-cultural impact of transhumanism – what it will actually mean for human experience – are notably absent from the discussion. This, in my view, is a significant limitation of his work.

Ray Kurzweil is a computer specialist, and his scientific premise is similar to that of Moravec. Kurzweil argues that computer memories are doubling in size every twelve months and, although computer intelligence currently exceeds human intelligence only in some narrow domains (e.g., playing chess), this will change as computers become more sophisticated and, in future, it will be hard to see the difference between the computer and human abilities (Kurzweil, 1999, pp. 2–3). Kurzweil acknowledges the role of evolution in human development to date, and he argues that eventually computers will be able to evolve in a similar way to humans (Kurzweil, 1999, p. 18).

Like Moravec, Kurzweil deals with the identity issue of the disembodied person by appealing to pattern identity, rather than body identity (Kurzweil, 1999, pp. 51–55). However, unlike Moravec, Kurzweil acknowledges the problem of disembodiment, stating that many of our human activities – for example, eating, sex and sport – don't make sense without a body (Kurzweil, 1999, pp. 133–134). He therefore explores how synthetic bodies, built with nanotechnology and sophisticated virtual interfaces, will enable future post-humans to have sexual, creative and spiritual experiences (Kurzweil, 1999, p. 146). He proposes a timescale of technological change and suggests that, by 2099, the "reverse engineering of humanity will be complete, and carbon-based human life will be obsolete" (Kurzweil, 1999, pp. 188–190). However, while Kurzweil's vision is compelling scientifically and he seriously tries to picture human experiences in a post-human context, he too provides little ethical assessment of the benefits and risks of technology in a post-human future.

N. Katherine Hayles is a literary scholar, rather than a technologist, and her view of transhumanism is based on her study of the cyborg – the human/robot hybrid – in literature, and the semiotics of the human condition that emerge from that study (Hayles, 1999, p. 1). She is highly critical of Moravec's espousal of mind-uploading, and his vision of a disembodied post-human person. Hayles argues that, while embodiment does not secure gender distinction, it shows that the function of the mind is dependent on embodied life (Hayles, 1999, p. xi). Hayles examines the meaning of human embodiment through a study of the cyborg and cybernetics in the texts of the science-fiction novelists Bernard Wolfe and Phillip K. Dick. For Hayles, like other scholars of the transhumanist movement, transhumanism is more than just about science and technology. Concerning Phillip K. Dick's work, she observes that, "Dick is drawn to cybernetics themes because he understands that cybernetics radically destabilises the ontological foundations of what counts as human" (Hayles, 1999, p. 23). Because it introduces the concept of hybridisation of flesh and machine in the human physical form, the cyborg appears to challenge the notion of body-mind dualism that, in one form or another, has often been significant in the understanding of human ontology from ancient times.

She subsequently observes that "Moravec's dream of downloading human consciousness into a computer would likely come in for some hard knocks in literature departments" because they "tend to be sceptical of any kind of transcendence, but especially of transcendence through technology" (Hayles, 1999, p. 284). On the contrary, transcendence is an important issue for theologians, but the idea of transcendence through technology alone is one that theologians would be wary of because of their commitment to the Christian account of eschatology through relationship with Christ.

Hayles concludes that embodiment is an important aspect of humanity, and that the post-human person need not be anti-human or apocalyptic but can simply be a survivor of the human race. She states that, while post-humanity might evoke either the terror of human extinction, or the pleasure of a new way of being human, evolutionary history affects every aspect of humanity, so embodiment cannot be simply cast aside (Hayles, 1999, p. 284).

Hayles' view of the importance of embodiment in human history and culture seems at first sight to be consonant with the Christian message of God who became embodied as Christ in human history. This contrasts with the problem of disembodiment seen with some transhumanist technologies, for example, mind-uploading. However, Hayles' claim that humans can "re-flesh" themselves with technology could suggest that all material human life is just "informational instantiation", as Miccoli has argued (Miccoli, 2010).

Donna Haraway is a biologist, a feminist and a historian of science and, in her work, she discusses the cyborg as a tool for mapping social and bodily reality (Haraway, 1991, p. 149). Like Hayles, Haraway also identifies the potential of the cyborg to challenge dualism. Technological culture, she claims, challenges various dualisms in Western thought – between male and female, nature and culture – because, with the cyborg, it is not clear who makes, and who is made (Haraway, 1991, p. 177).

This review of transhumanist thinkers suggests that, although they might be diverse in their views, the main protagonists of transhumanism might be classified into three main groups. The first group of transhumanist thinkers might be classified as *philosophical transhumanists*. These are scholars who see transhumanism as a life philosophy, which will enrich human experience and provide a good way of life for adherents to follow. This group would include Max More and Nick Bostrom, and might also include ethicist, Julian Savulescu.

The second group of transhumanists might be classified as *technological transhumanists*. These are scholars from a technological background – computing, artificial intelligence and cybernetics specialists – who see transhumanism from the perspective of the effects of technology on human life, and the benefits that it can bring. This second group includes Ray Kurzweil and Hans Moravec. These thinkers discuss the seemingly inexorable advance of technology, and how humanity needs to respond to this development, and harness it in a positive way. They might, however, differ in their ideas about how exactly humanity might adopt technology to enhance human experience.

The third group of transhumanist scholars might be termed *ideological transhumanists*. This group explores the impact of transhumanist technology on human society; however, they do so in way that is neutral to technology *per se* but which, in my view, sees these technologies primarily as a tool for exploring cultural and ideological issues. So, for example, Katherine Hayles uses the cyborg in literature as a means of exploring embodiment as an element of gender identity, and Donna Haraway presents the cyborg as a means of challenging patriarchal and anti-liberationist tendencies in Western scientific thought.

Some transhumanists, such as Kurzweil and Moravec, are primarily interested in how technology will change humanity, but less interested in the social and cultural effects of the application of technology. By contrast, other transhumanists, such as Hayles and Haraway, are interested in technology precisely as a tool for exploration of ideological issues, such as feminism.

However, despite the divergent trajectories and worldviews of specific transhumanist scholars, various common themes emerge across the transhumanist movement. One key theme, seen in the work of Bostrom and More, is that human nature is somehow "unfinished". As stated earlier, More asserts that transhumanists believe that human nature is not an end in itself, and that it is not perfect, nor a given (More, 2013, p. 4). Similarly, Nick Bostrom refers to the incompleteness of humanity, when he describes the transhumanist desire to make good the "half-baked" project of human nature (Bostrom, 2004). The technological transhumanist writers, Ray Kurzweil and Hans Moravec, both cite the evolution of computing and artificial intelligence and suggest that the development of transhumanist technology is analogous to human evolution. Furthermore, the philosopher and author, F.M. Esfandiary acknowledged the unfinished-ness of human nature, when he described a transhumanist as a "transitional human who, by virtue of their technology usage ... constitutes an evolutionary link with the coming era of post-humanity" (Esfandiary and FM-2030, 1989, p. 149). While these views are consistent with the Darwinian notion that there is no fixed human nature (Bostrom, 2005b, p. 3), they are in stark contrast to the concept of natural law in Christian theology, and this will be explored in greater detail later in this chapter.

Another important theme in transhumanism is how biomedical technology will enable humanity to transcend itself. More's concept of *extropy* describes the use of transhumanist technology to help humanity reach beyond its current constraints, and to extend beyond its current form (More, 2013, p. 5). Similarly, in his critique of transhumanism, McNamee and Edwards have observed that a key characteristic of the transhumanist movement is its refusal to accept the traditional limitations of humanity (McNamee and Edwards, 2006). Transhumanism, they state, "deplores the standard paradigms" – cultural expectations, political expedience, religion – "that seek to make the world comfortable at the expense of human enhancement and advancement". Again, the implications of this for Christian eschatology will be explored later in the chapter.

A third theme is that transhumanists will often cite a moral imperative to embracing transhumanist developments. For example, Bostrom has argued that scientists have a moral obligation to develop new medical technologies to eradicate disease and extend life (Bostrom, 2005a, p. 10). Similarly, Freitas has emphasised the moral duty of humanity to explore new medical technologies, arguing that the loss of human life to disease is not only tragic at a personal level, but represents a tragic loss of knowledge and human capital (Freitas, 2013). Here there is some common ground with medical science, where there is equally a moral imperative to use pharmaceutical medicine to alleviate human suffering and improve human welfare and the human experience. This aspect will be explored further in Chapters 5 and 6.

A fourth theme is the progressive spirit of transhumanism. The transhumanist movement has its roots in secular modernity (More, 2013, p. 4), and so it stresses the importance of being proactive, rather than reactive, about human goals, of creating better futures with technology, rather than praying to a deity to bring a better future. However, while modernity has been largely concerned with improving the lot of humanity through education and culture, transhumanism seeks to radically transform humanity specifically with technology (Bostrom, 2005a, p. 4). Although development of technologies, such as transportation, medicine and electronic communications, have indeed been a feature of the era of modernity, transhumanism applies biomedical technology directly to the human being in a way that profoundly changes human function and experience.

Fifthly, transhumanist thought raises issues concerning personal identity. More states that *transhumanist* technologies are applied so that humans may become *post-human* – that is to say, no longer recognisably human by current standards (More, 2013, p. 4). The post-human person may have greater physical capability, cognitive capacity, and extended life expectancy, but they may also have *morphological freedom* – freedom of form – so they may not take on a recognisable humanoid body shape. As noted above, this may be problematic for body identity, but some transhumanists address this by appealing to *pattern identity*, that a person's identity is defined by their thought patterns and processes, rather than their bodily form. This seems to be at odds with the idea of embodiment, and importance of the body, as a material, biological entity, in Christian theological ethics, based on the doctrine of the incarnation and the New Testament accounts of the bodily resurrection of Christ. This issue will be discussed in more depth in a later section of this chapter.

Sixthly, transhumanists emphasise personal autonomy and choice, as might be expected because of transhumanism's alignment to liberal modernity. Thus, the Transhumanist Declaration states that every human being should have the choice about whether to enhance their body and, if so, what enhancements to make (World Transhumanist Association, 2013). However, in contrast with the modern era, the potential influence of personal autonomy is much more far-reaching in a world where there are radically invasive biomedical technologies. In their critique of transhumanist medical technologies, McNamee and Edwards have advised caution if there is no clear medical end to the application of a technology, stating that biomedical enhancements cannot simply be libertarian extensions of free choice and consumption (McNamee and Edwards, 2006).

However, despite these common themes, More has rightly pointed out that the epistemology and metaphysics underlying transhumanist thought is mixed (More, 2013, pp. 6–8). He argues that many transhumanists are materialists, in that they see the functions of the physical human body as the sum of all reality. He also states that many transhumanists are functionalists, who believe that human mental function constitutes the person, and must be instantiated in a physical medium, but not necessarily a biological one, hence the idea of morphological freedom and the espousal of mind-uploading by Kurzweil and Moravec.

Another area of variation among transhumanist scholars is their attitude to the risks associated with biomedical technologies. For example, on the one hand, Moravec provides a bold vision of a technologically enabled future whereas, on the other, Kurzweil provides a more considered analysis of the problems of human experience in such a world. Transhumanists are sometimes perceived as gung-ho technological optimists, as is suggested by Max More's slogan "No more gods, no more faith, no more timid holding back" (McNamee and Edwards, 2006). However, in fairness, some transhumanist sources acknowledge the risks of technology as well as proclaim the benefits. The Transhumanist Declaration, which was developed as a "mission statement" by the World Transhumanist Association in 1998, and was revised in 2002 and 2009, states that,

> We need to carefully deliberate how to reduce risks ..." [of technology], and that "policy making ought to be guided by responsible ... moral vision, taking seriously both opportunities and risks ... .
>
> (World Transhumanist Association, 2013)

Both Bostrom and More state that transhumanists admit that technology can be misused (Bostrom, 2005a; More, 2013). Furthermore, Bostrom asserts that transhumanists condemn the use of technologies for any state-sponsored eugenics programmes, whether motivated by race, gender or any ideological purpose (Bostrom, 2005b). Bostrom's view is that human beings are valuable, and that the development of transhumanism does not mean that humanity must forego its currently established values - which would include abhorrence of genocide (Bostrom, 2005a).

Another interesting area of variation among transhumanists concerns attitudes to religious beliefs. More states that, although acceptance of transhumanist principles does not rule out religious belief, there are very few Christians who are transhumanists (More, 2013, p. 8). Some of the points of conflict between transhumanism and Christianity will already be evident in this discussion and will be explored in greater detail later in this chapter.

2.4 Therapy or Enhancement?

Much discussion of future transhumanist technology is concerned with enhancement – the application of biomedical technologies not primarily to heal the human being of disease or disorder, as has been done during the modern era, but to enhance the human being, to extend their function, cognition and longevity. Consequently, a definition of what constitutes a biomedical enhancement will be helpful in assessing both proposed future transhumanist developments and past medicine case studies. The next section will therefore provide a definition of an enhancement, and a discussion about the moral status of enhancements.

Bailey cites Chan and Harris's definition of an enhancement as:

> A procedure that improves our functioning; any intervention that increases our general capabilities for human flourishing.
>
> (Bailey, 2013)

However, this definition of "enhancement" requires further exploration. The *prima facie* approach is to say that a therapy is an intervention that restores normal function in a person who is ill (dysfunctional), whereas an enhancement is something that gives a healthy, functional person additional function and makes them "better than well". Shapiro, however, argues that there are many things which could be considered enhancements at present – for example, drinking caffeine to improve alertness – but they are not perceived as enhancements, because they are already accepted by society (Shapiro, 2013). Shapiro points out that a "disorder context" needs to be present for a technological intervention to be perceived as an enhancement – in other words, it may not be clear that an intervention is an enhancement, unless the context of the intervention is medicine or healthcare. For example, consumption of caffeinated drinks may be considered a means of enhancing mental function, but as it is an occurrence in everyday life, rather than only in the context of a healthcare service, it is not perceived as an enhancement.

Furthermore, the line between a therapy and an enhancement is sometimes an indistinct one. Brent Waters argues that a therapy given to an eighty-year-old with heart failure that restores their cardiac function to that of a healthy eighty-year-old would be regarded as a treatment, but if the person responded very well to this therapy and cardiac function improved to that expected in a healthy 40-year-old, the therapy would be considered an enhancement (Waters, 2006a). Shapiro also notes that the ethical doctrine of double effect can apply with therapies and enhancements; a steroid can be taken with the intention of treating a bad knee, but have the unintentional "side-effect" of building muscles (Shapiro, 2013). Enhancements are therefore relative; while Bailey suggests that only enhancements that take a person well beyond normal human functioning are interesting (Bailey, 2013), Kahane and Savulescu take the view that even modest enhancements can be of ethical and social significance (Kahane and Savulescu, 2015).

The other consideration is how "natural" the enhancement appears to be. Shapiro observes that it is common to classify a therapy as "natural" and an enhancement as "un-natural" (Shapiro, 2013). However, he argues, this is unhelpful because the link between nature and moral status is flawed, and natural law cannot apply universally. He gives the example that it is not, in fact, natural for humans to wear clothes, but it is certainly traditional for them to do so. However, he concedes that the question of how natural an enhancement is, provides a useful entry-point to the discussion. Hopkins argues that natural law advocates are often the most vociferous opponents of enhancements, but that their objections are not to technology *per se*, but to the anti-essentialist views of humanity often seen in the social sciences (Hopkins, 2013). He asserts that most advocates of enhancement agree that there is a biologically-grounded human nature – otherwise, the concept of enhancement would be meaningless as there would be no "basic" humanity to be enhanced. The significance of nature and natural law in the ethical evaluation of both past biomedical therapies and proposed future biomedical enhancements is a major theme in this book, and will be explored at length.

If operating from the principle of natural law – that is, asking how natural a proposed enhancement is – is an unhelpful way of ascertaining an enhancement's moral status, how can the morality of an enhancement be adequately determined? The fact that enhancements may be relative – what is an enhancement for one person is a treatment for another (see Waters' argument about cardiac function above) - suggests that the moral status of an enhancement is predicated on social factors, rather than simply on individual biological dysfunction.

Where a person has a disease, which prevents them from functioning normally in society, then a just and humane society has a moral obligation to offer a therapy via its health service. Correspondingly, if they are a good citizen, the person who is ill arguably has some moral obligation to avail themselves of the therapy (notwithstanding any extenuating factors concerning the person's circumstances and the nature of the therapy) so as not to be a burden to the health service and to society in general. For an enhancement – a biomedical procedure that increases a person's function to greater than normal – the moral framework is slightly different. Society does not have a moral obligation to provide enhancements to normally functioning individuals, in the same way that it has a moral obligation to provide therapies to dysfunctional individuals. Furthermore, an individual who is functioning normally in society does not necessarily have a moral obligation to seek enhancement.

However, if the baseline for normative human function in society were higher – for example, if a particular enhancement was used universally in society to provide an increased level of function in some way – then there would be an obligation for society to provide the enhancement for all citizens. Consequently, ter Meulen argues that any discourse about enhancement should be considered in terms of societal goals and within the context of human rights (ter Meulen, 2013), an approach which is certainly consistent with the increasing importance of human rights in medical ethics in the late twentieth century. Moreover, Wolbring suggests the possibility of discussing enhancements outside of the framework of health and disease. He suggests that assessments of human abilities should be developed to determine able-ism, rather than diagnose disease and assess disability and that the concepts of able-ism and ability should be used as objective tests for the need for enhancement (Wolbring, 2010).

If, as argued here, the difference between "therapy" and "enhancement" is not always clear when a medical technology is being used in practice, then the fairest ethical position for a society is to deploy a biomedical technology to ensure that all citizens meet the same standard of ability, regardless of whether the technology should be defined as a therapy or an enhancement. In this scenario, the state does have a moral duty to provide biomedical "enhancement" technologies on the principle of citizen equity, to ensure that all citizens can achieve the same standard of function and well-being. Furthermore, in this scenario, citizens may have a moral obligation to avail themselves of biomedical technology, on the principle of participation in a democratic society where equality is valued. I conclude therefore that there is a moral imperative for the use of biomedical technology by a society to benefit human health and well-being, irrespective of whether the technology is considered a therapy or an enhancement.

In theory, in a just society, access to enhancements should be possible either for all citizens equitably, or for no citizens. In practice, however, technologies become available and are marketed by the corporations that invent them, so what is needed is a regulatory system that enables fair access to enhancements by the citizens who need them most, according to transparent, objective and verifiable criteria.

2.5 Evaluating Transhumanist Technologies

Given the range of potential technologies that could be described as transhumanist, and the differing worldviews of the advocates of the transhumanist movement, there is a need to define objective criteria for what constitutes a transhumanist biomedical technology, and how the technology might be evaluated ethically.

The criteria for what would constitute a transhumanist technological intervention, as derived from the transhumanist literature, are very broad and wide-ranging. In summary, the key principles seem to be as follows:

1 That it is a technology – in other words, it is a material means of effecting a task or process (More, 2013, p. 13). This, of course, will include any physical or chemical effect or intervention – including pharmaceutical medicine – but may also include processes, policies and organisational methods. Bostrom notes that technology does not just include gadgets but "all instrumentally useful objects and systems that have been deliberately created" (Bostrom, 2005a).

2 That the technology is applied to a human person in some way. Article 1 of the 1998 Transhumanist Declaration states that humanity will in future be transformed radically by technology (World Transhumanist Association, 2013). In addition, More argues that transhumanism is not just about using education or culture to improve the human condition, but using technology to change it (More, 2013, p. 6). At the core of transhumanism is the transformation of human life and experience, and the improvement of human society.
3 That the technology is applied to the human person to improve human function, increase longevity or promote human flourishing. The Transhumanist Declaration specifies the moral right of an individual to extend his or her capacities (World Transhumanist Association, 2013). Both Bostrom and Bailey point to the significance of technology to extend human capacities and enable humans to flourish (Bostrom, 2005a; Bailey, 2013).
4 That the human person has autonomy in the use of the technology – in other words, the technology is applied in a self-determined way and not in a coercive way (More, 2013, p. 13). Bostrom notes the emphasis that transhumanists place on individual freedom and choice in the use of enhancement technologies (Bostrom, 2005a). McNamee and Edwards also note that transhumanists advocate free choice and that this perhaps reflects the western free market economy (McNamee and Edwards, 2006).

According to these criteria, a wide range of biomedical technologies could be classified as transhumanist in character. Furthermore, given the secular assumptions of the transhumanist movement, as outlined so far in this chapter, it is unsurprising that radical biomedical technologies have attracted criticism from various religious traditions. For this reason, criteria for a theological and ethical evaluation of transhumanist technologies are required, to determine the acceptability of these technologies, and these will be discussed later in this chapter. First, however, I will explore religious responses to the transhumanism movement, and some of the ways in which transhumanism has challenged faith traditions.

2.6 Transhumanism and Religions

Given that transhumanism makes significant claims about human perfectibility, the possibility of immortality, the relief of suffering and the transformation of human experience, it is unsurprising that transhumanism has been scrutinised in some detail by scholars of different world faith traditions. There has been evaluation of the claims of transhumanism by commentators on Islam (Bouzenita, 2018; Hejazi, 2019), Judaism (Tirosh-Samuelson, 2015), Buddhism (Evans, 2014; LaTorra, 2015; Sarbacker, 2020), and Chinese religious traditions (Redmond, 2015), as well as in relation to Christian traditions.

While the focus of this book is primarily on a Christian ethical evaluation of transhumanism, it is important to note that many of the world religions have themes in common – for example, beliefs about creation, human nature, what constitutes moral life for the human person, and about eschatology and post-mortem destiny. This section will therefore draw out these themes in the reactions to transhumanism by the faith traditions of the world. This will identify critiques of transhumanism from these faith traditions which are also relevant to a Christian ethical engagement with transhumanism.

However, before embarking on this survey, it is worth pointing out some important caveats. First, all the religions discussed here have different traditions and subtypes, and there will be diversity in beliefs and views between different adherents of the same religion. This means that the most meaningful engagement of religion with transhumanism is at the level of core beliefs only. Second, while all literature is necessarily interpreted by readers, I am assessing the literature from scholars of various world religions as a Christian theologian and practicing protestant Christian believer, with a limited personal knowledge of other faith traditions. Third, transhumanism, as we have seen previously in this chapter, is largely a product of western modernity. For this reason, there have been varying degrees of cultural inertia in engagement of non-western religions with transhumanism, despite the quasi-religious claims of transhumanism. On the one hand, Ahamad et al claim that transhumanism is attractive to Buddhists, due to the cultural influence of the Indian technological business sector and its entrepreneurial spirit (Ahamad et al., 2019). This claim, however, is contentious in the light of a thoroughgoing analysis of Buddhist beliefs, as will be seen later in this section. On the other hand, Hejazi has commented on the relatively recent engagement of Islamic scholars with transhumanism, and offers three reasons why Islamic engagement with transhumanist thought has been slow (Hejazi, 2019). These are a) the fact that technology is regarded as a western invention and therefore seen as a tool of colonisation by many Muslims, b) the emergence of political Islam since the 1960s (which has emphasised that society may be improved, not by technology, but by application of Sharia law), and c) the association of Islam with anti-western ideology, a narrative that has emerged in global discourse since 9/11. Indeed, there is some historical evidence for all three of these claims.

I will now examine the responses from scholars of faith traditions in some detail. Sarah Hejazi has made a detailed study of the implications of transhumanism for Muslim doctrines of the human person, quoting extensively – and apparently appropriately – from Qu'ranic material (Hejazi, 2019). She notes that the western view of the human person is centred on the self, whereas for Muslims, all human thought has a social and corporate element. This is perhaps a generalisation, and I think that her perception of the western view of the human person may conflate ideas of cultural individualism and the psychological notion of the self as personal subject. Furthermore, she argues that the Islamic view of the human person is that the physical and metaphysical aspects of a human person are inseparable, and that embodied human life is of prime importance in Islam. Embodied life also has significance in Christianity, however, as previous mentioned, and I will discuss this in detail later in this chapter. Hejazi goes on to claim that, given the transhumanist emphasis on the individual, the potentially dualistic nature of some proposed transhumanist technologies and their potential to denigrate the significance of the body, the beliefs she has outlined are all reasons why Muslims might be cautious about transhumanist technologies, as indeed a Jewish or Christian believer might (see Tirosh-Samuelson, 2015 and Waters, 2009, respectively).

Hejazi outlines the Islamic doctrine of humankind as "God's Deputy" (*khalifa*), entrusted by God with the well-being of the earth (Qu'ran 7.20) (Hejazi, 2019). This idea appears to be similar in some respects to the functional understanding of the Christian doctrine of *imago Dei* – that, because humanity is made in God's image (Genesis 1v26), humans have a particular vocation in relation to care of the creation, an idea that I will discuss at length later in this chapter. She argues that, since Islam has a high view of bodily life, and of the importance of living a bodily life pleasing to God, some Muslims might be positive about transhumanism, if they saw it as correcting deficiencies in creation for the common good – that is, for a social end.[2] Therefore, she concludes, Muslims might not object to life extension for social reasons. However, she cautions that Muslims would not approve of complete removal of bodily limitations, as this would constitute self-aggrandisement and self-deification, in opposition to God's sovereign rule. Avoiding hubris is an important factor in the adoption of technology, and this is reflected in the criterion for the ethical assessment of transhumanist projects that is concerned with attitudes to past failures.

Anke Bouzenita also cites the doctrine of humanity as "God's deputy" in her analysis of transhumanism from an Islamic perspective (Bouzenita, 2018). She describes the "God's deputy" concept in terms of human dignity and of service of the world. She concurs with Hejazi that Muslims would not object to life-extending medical technology *per se*, as it could provide people with more opportunities to do good works. She argues that enhancement – extension of creation rather than correction of creation – would not be acceptable to Muslims because of the idea that Allah had created humanity "in the best shape". However, she also acknowledges the potential lack of distinction between enhancement (improvement) and therapy (correction), as discussed earlier in this chapter. Furthermore, Ghergikov has argued that it would be acceptable for Muslims to exercise control over nature, appealing to the "God's deputy" doctrine (Ghergikov, 2020). He concurs that life extension might be acceptable to the Muslim due to the significance of the body, but that absolute immortality would conflict with Islamic beliefs about death, resurrection and the afterlife.

Hava Tirosh-Samuelson has examined transhumanism from a Jewish perspective (Tirosh-Samuelson, 2015). In respect of the doctrine of creation, he cites Elliot Dorff, a leading conservative Rabbi, who argues that human beings are made in the image of God, but are not themselves God, which again seems to align with the Christian doctrine of *imago Dei*. For these reasons, Dorff argues, a) the body is "on loan" from God, and this is the rationale for healing and medicine, and b) humans have an obligation to be partners with God in creation, which would be a motivation for research into use of stem cells and reproductive technologies. In this respect, healing is a *Mitzvah*, a religious obligation.

Nevertheless, Tirosh-Samuelson goes on to argue, even though many Jews would advocate the use of biotechnology for the purpose of healing, they would not be happy with transhumanist projects that denigrate the body. He claims that embodied life is significant to Jews, as it is to Muslims and Christians, because for Jews, embodied human life provides a basis for sociality and a locus for obeying the religious law. Tirosh-Samuelson notes that, while transhumanism is utopianism, it is a very different kind of utopia to that envisaged by Jewish (or indeed Christian) eschatology. Jewish utopia, he claims, is social,[3] whereas the utopia of transhumanism is individualistic, mediated by the personal application of biomedical technology. He then notes – correctly, in my view – how the transhumanist worldview invests technology with a salvific value; technology becomes an alternative form of salvation, and therefore ultimately, an alternative eschatology. The Jewish view of the future, he contends, as understood by the Jewish apocalyptic tradition, is open, unknowable and uncontrolled – but transhumanism attempts to impose an alternative destiny on human life, where the future is controlled by technology. However, he argues, this approach actually denigrates the body and denies the wisdom of mortality. This objection is very much consistent with Christian eschatological critiques of transhumanism from scholars such as Celia Deane-Drummond and Brent Waters (Deane-Drummond, 2006; Waters, 2006b). Moreover, with the application of transhumanist biotechnology, humans undergo a process of self-deification, which is distinct from the Orthodox theological idea of *theosis* (participation in the divine nature). I will explore both these aspects later in this chapter.

Ghergikov, too, notes that, from a Jewish perspective, the human search for transcendence cannot be reduced to the technological (Ghergikov, 2020). Jewish people value efforts to improve health, longevity and cognitive function, not for their own sake, but as a means to a better society. This is a broadly similar argument to that presented by Hejazi, in relation to Islam and transhumanism (Hejazi, 2019).

Geoffrey Redmond has reviewed the implications of transhumanism for three Chinese spiritual traditions – Confucianism, Daoism and Chinese Buddhism (Redmond, 2015). Redmond notes that both Confucianism and Daoism (in its later form) have valued longevity of human life and view old age as an honoured state, and so the possibility of life extension by biomedical technology might be appealing to some adherents of these traditions. However, there are some dissimilarities between these traditions.

For the Confucian, old age is associated with greater wisdom and capacity for moral decision-making; as these characteristics may be the goal of some forms of enhancement – for example, moral enhancement - this might make transhumanism particularly attractive. However, while respect for longevity became a feature of later Daoism, the emphasis in this tradition has largely been on living life the natural way. For this reason, Daoists might be more sceptical about the use of artificial biomedical technology to extend human life, or for the human person to be treated as an artifice, to be moulded at will by technology. Furthermore, Daoists emphasise the importance of spiritual practices – asceticism and monasticism – as a gradual means of achieving a transcendental state, whereas for transhumanists, transformation is achieved in a relatively rapid way, using biomedical technology. As such, transhumanism has the potential to undermine the entire spiritual practice of Daoism.

Redmond states that, while both Confucians and Daoists might endorse transhumanism to some extent, the situation with Chinese and Japanese Buddhism is much more ambiguous and complex. Buddhism, Redmond argues, has always been characterised by the concept of rebirth (reincarnation), with an understanding that death is an inevitable part of life. Accordingly, Buddhism – especially in Japan – is very much a funerary religion, Redmond claims. The prospect of biomedical immortality, mediated by technology, would render this idea of rebirth obsolete. Transhumanism therefore would not only undermine a central Buddhist belief, but would also have significant implications for the cultural requirements concerning death and the funeral industry in countries where Buddhism was prominent. However, absolute biomedical immortality may be problematic for Buddhists for other reasons. Another key emphasis of Buddhism is on the relief of human suffering, and, on this basis, transhumanist technologies may be attractive to Buddhists because of their apparent ethical goal of relieving suffering and improving human experience (Bostrom, 2005a; More, 2013). However, Buddhists deal with suffering through transcendentalism and the practice of meditation, whereas the transhumanist approach is the "quick fix" of biomedical technology. Consequently, universal use of transhumanist technologies has the potential to completely remove the motivation for the Buddhist religious life.

All in all, Redmond's analysis of these Chinese spiritual traditions is helpful in that it identifies some points of engagement between transhumanism and these religions. However, the scope of this study is limited to the use of biomedical technology to extend life (and possibly the associated purpose of relieving suffering). Both these are factors relating to the material world, but it would be interesting to see the implications of transhumanism for these religious traditions in terms of metaphysical beliefs and assumptions. Redmond notes briefly that it is hard for Buddhism, or indeed any religion, to argue against life extension on the grounds of metaphysical beliefs. However, transhumanism is by no means devoid of metaphysical assumptions, as we have seen (More, 2013), and more understanding of the implications of these for different faith traditions would be helpful.

In addition, some scholars have engaged with transhumanism from the perspective of Buddhism in more general terms. The ambiguous relationship between transhumanism and Buddhism, already alluded to by Redmond concerning Chinese Buddhism, is evidenced by the variety of responses by different scholars. Woody Evans states that, while transhumanism and Buddhism may have similarities, Zen Buddhism is particularly about being "fully present" rather than transcendentalism (Evans, 2014). Consequently, for Zen Buddhists, there would be less attraction to the ability of transhumanist technologies to provide a radical transformation of the human experience. While Redmond highlighted how Buddhists might be wary of transhumanism because of their doctrine of rebirth, other commentators – for example, James Hughes and Sarah Ahamad et al. – have argued the opposite: that Buddhists might be more open to transhumanism precisely because of its offer of transcendence through biomedical immortality (Hughes, 2007; Ahamad et al., 2019) In particular, as already stated, Ahamad et al. note that Indian Buddhism may be more culturally open to transhumanism, because of the perceived shared objective of human self-improvement.

Indeed, Michael LaTorra sees no conflict between Buddhism and transhumanism at all (albeit from an American cultural perspective) (LaTorra, 2015). He proposes the idea of Buddhist Transhumanism, which seeks to attain the traditional Buddhist objectives of the relief of suffering and "realising awakening" – presumably a reference to a transcendental state – by using science and technology. LaTorra points out – reasonably – that both Buddhism and transhumanism are essentially practical disciplines, and for this reason, they have some common ground. Interestingly, however, he also argues that, while western people are wary of Buddhist transcendentalism and the idea of Nirvana – the final transcendent state – because it implies annihilation, the spiritual transcendence of Buddhism and the technological transcendence of transhumanism are aligned and compatible. However, I am not sure that annihilation is uppermost in the minds of many western people when they think of Buddhist transcendentalism. To conclude, while LaTorra proposes an appealing synergy between Buddhism and transhumanism, I would suggest that his analysis of the metaphysical aspects of both worldviews is superficial, and complexities become more apparent on closer inspection.

On the other hand, Sarbacker takes a more cautious view of the compatibility of Buddhism and transhumanism (Sarbacker, 2020). He examines the implications of enhancement technologies for Buddhism, with particular reference to the fluidity of the human/divine boundary, and the Buddhist notion of the "Noble Person", which he describes as someone who is enlightened by Buddhist practice to the point where their bodily existence is disrupted, and they have esoteric insights. Sarbacker argues, that, while the "Noble Person" state could be achieved with technology, the person thus technologically enhanced would still be a sentient human being, albeit with what he describes as "altered compositional factors". Such an enhanced person would still therefore be a transient being in the material world (albeit with extended life expectancy) and therefore still be vulnerable to the suffering and evil of the world, even if they had more powers to counteract it. These arguments, to my mind, are persuasive, given the fact that absolute immortality is not scientifically feasible, and of questionable value philosophically (Williams, 1973).

Sarbacker further argues that, while human transformation, either by meditation or technology, might lead to deification of the individual,[4] the power that this confers is not only still temporary, but morally ambiguous. In other words, enhanced capabilities, however they are attained, may be used for virtuous or non-virtuous purposes, a theme which we will explore in detail in Chapter 5. To put it bluntly, the enhanced person may not be as "noble" as the enhancer expects.

Reflecting on these issues arising from the engagement of world faiths with transhumanism, some common themes emerge:

- People of faith are respectful of the created world, and the monotheistic religions in particular, value embodied human life. Some transhumanist technologies, however, denigrate bodily life – so embodiment will be a key constraint on the use of transhumanist technologies for many people of faith. Embodiment is one of the ethical domains explored in this book.
- The idea that humanity has an important role in looking after the world on God's behalf. This is seen in the Islamic belief of "God's Deputy" (*khalifa*), and in a functional understanding of the *imago Dei* in Christianity. This notion of humanity as God's representative carries with it an ethical obligation on the part of humanity for the care of the world, and this will include determining an appropriate use of technology. Again, the significance of biomedical technology for the *imago Dei* will be explored in this book.
- The importance of healing and the relief of suffering – seen in both western and eastern religious traditions – which is unsurprising given that healing and relief of suffering are universal humanitarian concerns. These are motivations for people of faith to explore appropriate use of biomedical technology, and the appropriate use of such technologies within a religious ethical framework is the central consideration of this book.
- For western religious traditions in particular, emphasis is on the social aspects of human life rather than the human being as an individual, and the utopian ideals of these religions are social rather than individualistic. Concerns about individualism will be a key critique of transhumanism

for adherents of various religious traditions, and this issue is explored further in Chapter 5.

- Various religions – from Islam to Buddhism – value longevity of human life, which is why some commentators conjecture that they might be accepting of transhumanism. However, the value of longevity for people of faith is related to the increased opportunities to gain wisdom and superior moral reasoning, whereas this is not always emphasised by advocates of human enhancement for life extension.
- A key issue expressed by some religious commentators is the way that transhumanism provides an alternative secular soteriology and eschatology to religious faith. The "quick fix" of biomedical technology becomes a person's destiny, and the means by which they are "saved", instead of the promises of the religious faith. This is an issue explored by various Christian critics of transhumanism, notably Brent Waters, and will be explored later in this chapter (Waters, 2006b).

In this section, I have reviewed some of the responses of world religions to transhumanism. These responses are varied; as well as reasons why these religions might be cautious about transhumanism, there are also reasons why they might be accepting of transhumanism. However, I have shown that some common themes emerge, and these are consistent with some of the responses of Christianity to transhumanism, which I shall now explore.

2.7 Transhumanism and Christianity

Some transhumanist commentators have proposed positive points of contact between transhumanism and Christian faith. For example, Campbell and Walker argue that both transhumanism and religious faith offer a means of transcendence and perfectibility (Campbell and Walker, 2005). However, for Campbell and Walker, the transhumanist project is re-contextualising humanity in terms of technology. They argue that those who embrace transhumanist technologies have a theological mandate to do so as co-creators with God, referring to Philip Hefner's concept of humankind as a "created co-creator" (Hefner, 1993) – that is, created by God, yet sharing with God in other creative acts within the world. However, Campbell and Walker say, the use of technology to transform humanity should be limited by other theological parameters, such as embodiment and eschatology, and should be consistent with ethical principles, such as justice and respect. Campbell and Walker admit that, with transhumanism, attributes of personhood – embodiment and gender – are sacrificed in favour of biological attributes, such as strength, memory, and longevity.

Garner explores the link between the application of transhumanist technology and the *imago Dei*, the idea that humanity is created in the image of God, and argues that both transhumanism and religious faith create social visions that engender hope for their adherents (Garner, 2005).

On the one hand, he argues that there is a disconnect between transhumanism and the *imago Dei*, because transhumanism, he claims, rejects species-ism, whereas (substantive) approaches to the *imago Dei* have often, in the past, been used to define humanity (Garner, 2005). On the other hand, however, he argues that if human society does not embrace transformative biomedical technology, it will be rejecting the social transformation that is inherent in the concept of *imago Dei* (presumably in a relational, functional or eschatological view of the *imago Dei*, as will be discussed later in this chapter). Nevertheless, Garner correctly identifies that the *imago Dei* is relevant in both a Christian and a transhumanist social vision and this will be explored in greater depth, in a theological critique of transhumanism in respect of the *imago Dei* later in this chapter, and then subsequently in relation to the case studies.

Jeanine Thweatt Bates has engaged with Haraway's work on the cyborg and has explored the possibility of developing a theological "post-anthropology" that would be inclusive of the cyborg (Thweatt Bates, 2012). In her methodology, Thweatt Bates draws a sharp distinction between the cyborg and transhumanist technologies, such as mind-uploading, stating that the cyborg is not a subset of transhumanism (Thweatt Bates, 2012, p. 68). I disagree with her categorisation; the cyborg and mind-uploading both represent radical biomedical technologies, but with differing degrees of altered embodiment. Thweatt Bates' theological post-anthropology has several elements. She notes that the functional approach to the *imago Dei,* seen in Hefner's created co-creator concept, provides a helpful means of dialogue between theology and the concept of the cyborg (Thweatt Bates, 2012, p. 143). She also notes the recent emergence of "body theology", in contrast to previous approaches to human nature which she claims have been dualistic and have deprecated the body. Body theology has been important in recent theological developments on gender and sexuality – and such an approach, she contends, is important in understanding the cyborg because it takes seriously the theological significance of bodily experiences (Thweatt Bates, 2012, p. 149). Turning to the issue of hybridity, she examines the Garden of Eden account and notes that Adam and Eve were, in fact, both hybrids, consisting of material dust and spirit from God. In the light of the first humans' distinctive relationship with God, and the account of the Fall, she argues that, in the same way, cyborgs – who are hybrids – could, in a sense, have both relational capacity and moral agency (Thweatt Bates, 2012, p. 172). Thweatt Bates concludes her cyborg theology with a Christological reflection exploring the potential of redemption for the cyborg (Thweatt Bates, 2012, p. 175). She notes that Jesus, the divine-human hybrid, is a cyborg, and therefore represents the "ultimate" human. If this is the case, she argues, then Christ can still be a saviour in a future world of transhumanist technologies. While her observations are interesting, especially those concerning soteriology in scripture, all she seems to demonstrate is that cyborg nature can be accounted for theologically using "body theology", and that hybridity is common in a material world (something that Elaine Graham has already observed (Graham, 2006)). In my view, Thweatt Bates' cyborg theology may provide some grounds for theological inclusion of cyborgs within humanity, but it does not provide any ethical basis for adopting cybernetic enhancements, in the way I am seeking to do here.

Some commentators advocate a qualified acceptance of transhumanism by Christians, and have sought to reconcile transhumanism with Christian faith. Benedikte Göcke contends that a modified form of transhumanism should be acceptable to Christians, and makes the somewhat sweeping contention that "there is nothing in Christian faith that is in contradiction to [transhumanism]" (Göcke, 2017). He presents the concept of a "Christian cyborg" – which he does not define, but which presumably denotes an enhanced person who is a Christian believer. He argues that the immortality of the "Christian cyborg" is relative, since even a cyborg can be destroyed, or cease to exist, and therefore has no bearing on the immortality provided by the Christian hope. He also appeals to a distinction between quantitative enhancements – those that extend current human capabilities – and qualitative enhancements – those which lead to entirely new human capabilities – as a means of ruling out radical transhumanism. Markus Lipowicz's critiques of Göcke's argument (which I generally endorse) are that 1) transhumanism is by definition radical rather than moderate, and 2) that Göcke's argument does not take into account the Christian metaphysics of the person, namely the concept of the "soul", which Lipowicz regards as fundamental in theological anthropology (Lipowicz, 2020).

Fuller and Lipinska make a case for accommodation of transhumanist philosophy within Christian theology by appealing to the need for *theomimesis* – "playing God" – to promote human well-being and improve human flourishing (Fuller and Lipinska, 2014). They describe the transfiguration of Christ (Mark 9v2–8) as a typology for the transformation of a person using biomedical technology. Their approach is an interesting one but, in my view, it is deficient in two ways; first, they interpret the transfiguration in an unorthodox manner, and second, they do not discuss the idea of humanity as a "created co-creator", which has been significant in theological discussions of technology adoption to date, and which is clearly relevant to their argument (Hefner, 1993).

Although these scholars have sought to find common ground between transhumanism and religion, many of the parallels identified – for example, by Campbell and Walker, and Garner, concerning personal transcendence, perfectibility and a vision for the improvement of society – are, in my view, at a superficial level only; closer inspection of the values of transhumanism shows significant divergences from Christian theological ethics.

Christian critiques of transhumanism and proposed transhumanist technologies have focused on the following areas:

a social ethical and justice issues arising from the economic impact of widespread immortality, or at least significant increases in longevity, due to transhumanist biomedical technologies,
b the effects of transhumanist technologies on personal autonomy, and the risk of oppression in society due to effects of enhancement technologies on individual autonomy,
c the extent to which transhumanist biomedical technologies are contrary to nature and natural law,
d the challenge of transhumanist biomedical technologies to the notion of embodiment, and the importance of embodiment from a Christian perspective,
e the implications of transhumanism for the *imago Dei*, the doctrine that human beings are made in the image of God and in particular, the criticism that transhumanism provides an alternative eschatology.

I will discuss these issues in detail in the forthcoming sections of this chapter.

2.7.1 Immortality and Social Justice

Many commentators have urged caution about the transhumanist project from the perspective of social ethics, and they have been labelled – rather pejoratively – as "bio-conservatives" by advocates of transhumanism.[5]

Francis Fukuyama, a social philosopher, has famously dismissed transhumanism as "the world's most dangerous idea" because, in his view, it eliminates any notion of a "human essence" and thereby undermines any defence of legal and political equality of human beings based on a common understanding of humanity (Fukuyama, 2002, p. 149). This idea of a human essence, or an essential human nature, has been important in Christian theology in the past, in the scholastic natural law tradition, and also in substantive approaches to the doctrine of *imago Dei*, which have sought to understand what specific human attributes the *imago Dei* consists of. Both these will be discussed in later sections of this chapter.

Leon Kass, Chair of the US President's Council for Bioethics from 2001 to 2005, has warned of the possible social and ethical consequences of extended life, saying that "Finitude is a blessing for everyone, whether he knows it or not" (Kass, 2001). Similarly, Stock and Callaghan have stated that "no social good will come from the conquest of death" and, in a pointed critique of the transhumanist principle of free exercise of personal autonomy, they add, "and the worst possible way to resolve the question of life extension is to leave it to individual choice" (Stock and Callahan, 2004).

There are various possible social consequences of increased longevity (Bailey, 2013). These include a glut of able-bodied people, with increasing numbers of older people in society, a consequent loss of innovation in society (because this is often driven by generational change), increased pressure on marriage as a means of emotional support for each partner, and on monogamy as a way of life. All these are valid concerns, which are already being observed to an extent in western society because of increasing longevity due to the availability of increasingly sophisticated medical techniques. These factors relating to longevity are likely to have an impact on personal relationships, the workplace and social care and welfare.

These concerns about immortality are shared by Christian theologians, albeit for slightly different reasons. Celia Deane-Drummond argues that human finitude is a positive good of life,[6] and asserts that, where individual choice and consent are elevated as ethical norms, immortality is inappropriately privatised (Deane-Drummond, 2006). Furthermore, while human perfectibility is seen by some transhumanists as a shared goal between transhumanism and religious belief (see, e.g., Campbell and Walker, as discussed (Campbell and Walker, 2005)), Deane-Drummond argues that, in the western Christian tradition, perfectibility is only possible in union with God in the next world. She concludes that, in this world, a Christian vision of perfection must find a focus in good medical and bioethical decision-making, if it is to avoid anti-materialist Gnosticism (Deane-Drummond, 2006).

Furthermore, theological ethicist Brent Waters has argued that, ultimately, human finitude and medical care are opposed (Waters, 2006a). A human being will die and, as a means of preventing death, medical therapy will always be ultimately thwarted. The proper ethical end of medical care, he argues, is in the alleviation of suffering and the care of the vulnerable person. Waters concludes that Christians should place their hope in the resurrection of the body of Christian theology, not the immortality of the soul that transhumanism offers. The former, he claims, completes and fulfils creation, while the latter ultimately rejects it. The former is true to nature, while the latter negates nature.

A significant objection to the transhumanist project arising from these issues is that transhumanist enhancements will lead to social inequality, injustice and even oppression, due to the socioeconomic differences between the enhanced and the unenhanced in society. Again, these are valid concerns, albeit ones that could in theory be offset by wise public policy and good regulation of technology. In reply to this, Bailey has argued that there are many instances where political and moral equality have not rested on biological equality in the past, citing social systems in history, such as feudalism and slavery (Bailey, 2013). However, in my view, these past social inequalities are not a good reason for perpetuating social injustice in the future through inequitable biological enhancement.

2.7.2 Autonomy

As already indicated, the use of transhumanist biomedical technologies raises significant questions concerning the exercise of personal autonomy. A stated aim of the transhumanist movement, as described earlier, is that individuals who are seeking biomedical enhancement can choose to use the biomedical technology, or not, autonomously, as a matter of free, personal choice. The corresponding theological response to this, raised by Elaine Graham, is that transhumanist biomedical technologies therefore are problematic because they enable unbridled autonomy in a negative manner (Graham, 2006). This section will therefore define autonomy, examine in detail the concept of personal autonomy and describe the possible effects of biomedical technologies on autonomy. It will also explore related issues of authenticity and the possibility of moral enhancement (the use of medical interventions to enhance moral decision-making itself).

The notion of personal autonomy has become the standard of participation in the healthcare system, from the perspective of the recipient of care, and a central concept of modern medical ethics. Autonomy is one of the so-called Four Principles of medical ethics described by Beauchamp and Childress in 1979 (Beauchamp, 2007), along with beneficence, non-maleficence and justice. The exercise of autonomy is essentially about an agent's capacity for self-government and may be defined as "to be one's own person, to be directed by considerations, desires, conditions and characteristics that are not simply imposed externally upon one but are part of what can somehow be considered one's authentic self" (Christman, 2015). I have chosen this definition as it is general in context, worded in non-technical language and yet is sufficiently nuanced to take to account different aspects of personal autonomy.

The concept of autonomy as self-government, or self-rule, appears to be in tension with the Christian belief that God is sovereign over all creation and that humans are invited to live under his kingly rule (e.g., Psalm 95v3–7, Isaiah 43v15). Furthermore, the modern notion of autonomy has come from secular origins, in the thought of Immanuel Kant and J.S. Mill, whom I will discuss later in this section. As a result, Christian ethicists have expressed caution about autonomy. Oliver O'Donovan notes that, while liberal political thought has been a feature of western society for a long time, the use of medical technologies on the otherwise healthy body has highlighted the problem of unhindered personal autonomy in the healthcare context (O'Donovan, 1984, pp. 6–7). Neil Messer, too, has critiqued autonomy as a factor in biomedical decision-making (Messer, 2017). He notes, correctly, that there are limits to the goodness of autonomy. Autonomy might be in tension with beneficence – for example, when a person chooses to refuse a life-saving treatment. Messer is also sceptical about the conditions for true personal autonomy.

It might seem inappropriate, then, that the exercise of autonomy should be a criterion in a Christian ethical evaluation of biomedical technologies. However, I would argue that autonomy, defined in terms of self-determination, is a necessary prerequisite to the exercise of Christian moral responsibility. Personal autonomy is not necessarily in opposition to divine sovereignty, because the scope of human actions is ultimately limited in comparison that of God's actions. The idea that God gives humanity limited autonomy – for example, naming the animals – as a gift is seen in

Genesis 2–3. Furthermore, although autonomy may not appear to be a Christian concept, freedom certainly is. The New Testament emphasises the concept of personal freedom in Christ, through the work of the Holy Spirit (see 2 Corinthians 3v17 and Galatians 5v13–26). This freedom would not be possible – or valuable – if a person were unable to choose it because their ability to exercise self-determined choice was limited by other factors.

Consequently, I contend that personal autonomy – the ability to make a self-determined decision – is compatible with a Christian understanding of divine authority and is a prerequisite for the exercise of moral agency of any type, which would include Christian moral responsibility. The functional approach to the *imago Dei* – the idea that humans display the image of God because of their function, their role and vocation in the world - implies that a person must make ethical decisions about their actions in the world to fulfil their vocation. For this to be possible, the person would need a degree of autonomy. Indeed, Christian moral responsibility and personal autonomy can be seen as part of the process of Christian ethical action in the world. Moral responsibility provides the motivation for ethical action, and personal autonomy provides the ability for ethical action.

As stated earlier, the idea of autonomy as a factor in a Christian ethical study of transhumanist biomedical technologies may be particularly problematic given the associations of transhumanism with modernity. However, the concept of autonomy is important in contemporary medicine, and a discussion of autonomy in relation to future biomedical technologies will ensure that ethical issues about such technologies are intelligible from the perspective of contemporary bioethics as well as from theological ethics.

However, in understanding personal autonomy, there are two complicating factors. First, it is hard to assess the extent to which external factors affecting self-government are truly external to the person. An externalist view of autonomy will acknowledge that a person's motivation to act is in response to a wide range of arguably external factors (Buss, 2018). These may be coercive socio-political pressures which are clearly external, or the constraints of acting in someone else's best interest, which is an external factor, yet with internal causation, because of the emotional commitment to the act. These are factors that, for example, may influence a woman's choice to take the contraceptive pill; there may be social pressures to do so, or she may feel that she is acting in the best interests of her partner or family by doing so.

Second, it is often difficult to distinguish empowering and coercive factors that arise from within the person, and their effects on self-government (Buss, 2018). At the most basic level, an agent who can make a decision has the authority to determine how he or she will act (if at all) in response to the decision, regardless of the external factors that may have contributed to it. The person's motivation to act may be aligned with, or coherent with, the person's character as a moral agent, or it may not. According to a coherentist account of autonomy, an act is autonomous if it is coherent with the values, motives and desires that arise from the character of the person, as a moral agent. However, even if the person's motivation is coherent with their desires or wishes, this does not necessarily mean that the decision is made in a truly autonomous way. For example, according to a coherentist view, a drug addict's decision to take an addictive drug may be classed as autonomous because their action is aligned with their desires (their craving of the drug), but it cannot be regarded as truly autonomous because of the addictive nature of drug use. Drug addiction and brain washing are two scenarios cited in philosophical literature as being problematic to the concept of personal autonomy (Buss, 2018). Both these scenarios are clearly relevant with the use of psychopharmacological agents and will be explored further in Chapter 4, in relation to the case study of SSRI antidepressants.

Recently, philosophical discussions about autonomy have focused on the concept of authenticity, which concerns the capacity of an individual to act in accordance with their true self and real character (Tennison, 2012). The autonomous person should not only be able to control their actions, but should also be able to express their character, and their actions should be consistent with their character. However, Bublitz and Merkel note that, while concerns have been expressed about the ability of neuroenhancements to affect authenticity, the meaning, scope and ultimate value of authenticity is vague and poorly defined (Bublitz and Merkel, 2009). They describe the two main theories of authenticity; first, the essentialist theory, which states that a person has an essential character, and their personhood is therefore threatened by anything that causes them to depart from "who they really are"; and second, the existentialist theory, that a person's character may be self-defined. Bublitz and Merkel argue that ultimately autonomy is more concerned with control than authenticity. I think that this view is realistic, given the difficulties of teasing out genuine internal and external factors and therefore of attributing a person's decisions to the subtleties of their character. Authenticity is therefore not an absolute pre-condition for autonomy. Bublitz and Merkel argue that, if a person has what they consider to be the basic conditions for autonomy – a) ability to discern right from wrong, b) responsiveness to reason, c) awareness of their environment, d) self-control, e) no external manipulation, and f) identification with their true character traits and desires – then they cannot be considered non-autonomous just because they are inauthentic. On this basis, they conclude that new neuroenhancements pose no threat to autonomy. This conclusion, however, is a problematic extrapolation in my view, given that new neuroenhancements might affect one of their other stated conditions for autonomy.

Huang has discussed the issue of authenticity in relation to autonomy (Huang, 2015). She notes that, whereas Carl Elliot argues from a bioconservative position that identity is central to authenticity (Elliot, 2000), De Grazia's view is that identity is secondary to authenticity (DeGrazia, 2000). Huang goes on to argue that it is problematic to base identity on authenticity. For example, she contends, it may not always be appropriate for the true self to be preserved; what if a person's true self is a psychopath? It is also difficult to distinguish between interventions that lead to self-improvement, which might be desired, from those that would be unwanted alterations, even though both these would affect a person's identity. Furthermore, she argues, all chemical interventions are alterations, of one form or another, but no one would consider that a person might become inauthentic by taking paracetamol for a headache. In this respect, this argument about the effects of biomedical intervention on authenticity runs parallel to that concerning biomedical intervention and natural law. Many biomedical interventions could be considered unnatural, but only a few have been subject to ethical critique on natural law grounds, as will be discussed later. Huang concludes that a satisfactory theory of authenticity cannot be based on identity, and she cites Charles Taylor's concern that, if authenticity is equated with identity, it could be diminished at a societal level by utilitarian calculation (Huang, 2015).

Before further consideration of the problems concerning autonomy that biomedical technologies present, it is worth considering the nature of personal autonomy in the context of healthcare provision. In a healthcare context, personal autonomy is endorsed when a person can give informed, explicit and non-coerced consent for a medical intervention.

Saad has provided a concise review of the development of autonomy in modern medicine, from its origins in the Hippocratic tradition, through its development as a modern concept in the Enlightenment thought of Rousseau and Kant, to its primacy in contemporary medical ethics (Saad, 2018). While the survey of the history of medical ethics in Chapter 1 suggests that the Hippocratic tradition was concerned primarily with the actions and motivations of the practitioner rather than the autonomy of the subject, Saad argues persuasively that the dominance of paternalism in ancient medical practice is a caricature and that the concept of autonomy was in fact present in the Hippocratic code, but simply not made explicit. She argues that the idea of autonomy has been made explicit in the Enlightenment era through new ways of expressing morality independently of religious revelation. She describes two Enlightenment views of autonomy; Rousseau's vision of autonomy as a personal, rational attribute, rather than a political one, where morality is worked out by social contract, and Kant's view, where morality can be discerned from within, objectively deduced from a universal moral law (the categorical imperative). She then charts the establishment of the concept of autonomy in modern bioethics, in the work of Paul Ramsey (Ramsey, 1970) and Thomas Beauchamp (Beauchamp, 2007).

As well as Rousseau and Kant, another key figure in the development of the modern idea of autonomy was John Stuart Mill. In his great work, "On Liberty", Mill described the nature of individual liberty – the exercise of personal autonomy - in relation to authority (Mill, 1966 edition). Gillon notes that, for Mill, personal autonomy was important on utilitarian grounds, as the means of assuring the greatest good for the greatest number in human society (Gillon, 1985). However, this depends on a majority of people having the freedom to act in a manner that will lead to a good outcome for the greatest number. A consequentialist might argue that the greatest good for the greatest number in society would, in fact, be better served by no one in society having personal autonomy – that is, a totalitarian state. I contend, though, that autonomy is an innate good of human life, regardless of how it is exercised.

Saad notes three important characteristics of autonomy as described by modern bioethics:

a Choices made by autonomous subjects in modern healthcare scenarios may not be inherently moral choices.
b Autonomy in the modern healthcare context is often individualistic in nature, about the wishes of the individual, and does not reflect society's response. She notes that the duty derived from personal autonomy is, in fact, the duty of others (healthcare practitioners) to respect the subject's person's autonomy.
c The sanctity of choice and the principle of non-interference in that choice.

This introduces the issue of the role of relationships in the autonomy of an individual. As mentioned previously, when understanding autonomy, it is hard to distinguish internal motivational – or demotivational – factors, from external reinforcement or coercion factors. However, commentators have rightly pointed out the deficiency of a notion of autonomy based only on individual informed consent, and have emphasised the significance of a person's relationships and broader social context for their personal autonomy.[7]

This reduction of personal autonomy to the process of informed consent in medicine and healthcare also has wider political implications. Onora O'Neill has argued that public trust in science and medicine has declined, despite efforts to respect persons and to promote autonomy in society (O'Neill, 2002, pp. 1–10). She contends that this is due to self-interest on the part of various stakeholders, such as the medical profession, politicians and the healthcare industries and that, with the increasing emphasis on personal autonomy across society, the autonomy of the powerful increases as well as, if not more than, that of the less powerful and marginalised. She notes that debate, especially on social media, about new medical procedures is shrill, and there appears to be a widespread culture of blame in society concerning medical errors, even though the risks of medicine are no greater than in earlier generations. O'Neill concludes that this decline of public trust in medicine is partly because scientific education of the public is lacking, and partly because doctors and scientists do not always communicate in an accessible way. She also notes that the contemporary team approach to healthcare undermines trust, because the patient is unable to develop a relationship with a single practitioner. I would challenge

O'Neill's observation about the risks of medicine; in my view, the risks of medicine are greater currently because of the availability of more invasive procedures - and will become more so as even more radical biomedical technologies become available. However, I agree fully with her analysis of the reasons for loss of public trust in medicine, and her overall argument that the exercise of autonomy in healthcare decision-making is not the sole determinant in public trust in the healthcare system.

The application of "high-tech" biomedical technologies, such as some of those proposed by transhumanism – for example, mind-uploading, cybernetics or genetic enhancements – has the potential to make radical changes to human function and longevity. These changes may undermine individual moral agency – and therefore personal autonomy. For example, a cybernetic arm with complex computer control software, could include an anti-tamper mechanism which might cause the prosthesis to automatically shut down and stop functioning – against the will of the person to whom it is attached – if a surgeon interfered with it. Also, with a person whose mind has been uploaded on a computer, their personal identity may be preserved, but their ability to act in a certain way as a person in the world – which is the basis of moral agency – will be to some extent compromised by the loss of their body, even if there are some artificial interfaces that might compensate to enable the uploaded person to engage in some ways with material life.

The use of such technologies could therefore over-determine the attributes of human life for those in whom they are deployed. Miccoli argues that transhumanism leads to an abdication of human responsibility, and with an eschatological flavour, he asserts that, in the technology-enabled world, "technology is God, and all will ultimately submit to it" (Miccoli, 2010). Consequently, in a future technologically enhanced world, individual autonomy and responsibility may be subverted by the will of those who develop, distribute and apply radical technologies, and the individual themselves may collude with this loss of moral agency by their acceptance and use of these technologies.

Given the above reflections on autonomy in the use of technology, control of medical technologies by humanity, and their critical assimilation into human society, is a valid Christian response to their availability, and is consistent with current approaches to evidence-based medicine (Woolf, 2001). The polar alternative is the situation that Miccoli describes; where the technology – or, at least, the culture surrounding the technology – controls humanity instead. There are indications that this is already happening with the adoption of digital media and personal devices, which are now highly pervasive in human society, and have considerable potential to manipulate human behaviours (Ley et al., 2014).

However, as well as a definition of personal autonomy and the conditions for autonomy in the healthcare setting, there is the separate question of the morality of the choice made by the autonomous person. The capacity for autonomous choice may be consciously exercised by a person for good ends or for bad ends. The moral agent may choose to do good works in human society, creating a just and fair society and nurturing a positive and generous culture. Alternatively, the agent may choose to act selfishly, for vanity or personal gain, or to exploit the weak and marginalised in society for their own benefit. While the fact of having autonomy might have some innate moral value, the choice made by the autonomous individual will also contribute to the moral significance of the situation. One way of dealing with this issue of the appropriate use of autonomy might be to use biomedical technology for "moral enhancement", to ensure people always make good moral choices (Douglas, 2008). I will now therefore consider the issue of moral enhancement.

The terms "cognitive enhancement" and "moral enhancement" are often used interchangeably, but in this and subsequent discussions, I use these terms to denote the enhancement of non-moral cognitive processes and specific moral reasoning respectively (if indeed it is possible to make an absolute distinction).

Cognitive enhancement – the enhancement of cognitive abilities in general terms, rather than moral reasoning specifically – has been in view for some years. For example, Rizutto and Frost argue that human beings are uniquely cognitive creatures, and that cognitive decision-making – for example, about choice of sexual partner or the assessment of risky situations – guides evolutionary outcomes (Rizutto and Frost, 2012). This seems a simplistic claim, which does not account for the way that humans are affected by circumstances that are external to them. They note that cognitive enhancement is already taking place with, for example, the use of caffeine and other stimulants by students, and argue that cognitive enhancement by pharmacological means is no different to cognitive enhancement by means of education or culture. They advocate a progressive approach to the adoption of cognitive enhancement agents in society, with appropriate societal safeguards, such as cognitive enhancement guidelines for health and educational bodies, and careful legislation to maximise social benefits and minimise risks.

The question of whether moral reasoning specifically can be enhanced is an even more complex one, because of the relationship between moral decision-making and the exercise of moral agency, and cognitive processes. Adam Willows considers the possibility of moral enhancement from the perspective of virtue ethics. He argues that, while there may be a *prima facie* argument for moral enhancement (how can anyone argue that being a better person is not a good thing?), moral enhancement cannot ensure that a person is virtuous, because it cannot create prudence (practical wisdom), which is needed to act virtuously in the context of a specific situation (Willows, 2017). Willows contends (correctly from a classical Aristotelian perspective) that virtues are habits, whereas biomedical interventions that affect moral behaviour do not involve the development of habits. Consequently, with the proposed use of moral enhancement agents, the formation of virtue is decoupled from the practice of virtue. He notes that, while some drugs have been shown to affect dispositions – for example, citalopram increases pro-social behaviour and paroxetine reduces hostility – there is more to being virtuous than having good dispositions, and that the role of prudence is vital in the inculcation of virtue. He concludes that biomedical enhancements may affect virtues by their effects on dispositions, they cannot replace the agential experience and situational understanding that prudence enables. My view is that Willows' analysis is sound, and consistent with the views of other scholars.

Alfred Archer discusses the social implications of moral enhancement – in particular, whether these technologies would have negative consequences for those who either choose not to adopt them, or who cannot access them, and therefore would lead to division and injustice in society (Archer, 2016). He cites Thomas Douglas's claim that moral enhancement technologies would benefit the unenhanced in society (Douglas, 2008), because the unenhanced would be influenced positively by the enhanced people around them. Archer argues, however, that in reality, the situation is less straightforward. He contends that the existence of moral enhancement technology would raise the bar for moral behaviour in society, and would affect standards of blameworthiness in society. In addition, he notes that the existence of two statuses in society would be problematic for those who valued egalitarianism, and that there was no guarantee that the morally enhanced would have any empathy or understanding of the unenhanced. He conjectures, persuasively, that the morally unenhanced might be treated like children, in a way that undermined their dignity and autonomy.

However, in keeping with their advocacy of other aspects of transhumanism on consequentialist grounds, Savulescu and Persson have argued that moral bio-enhancement is needed urgently because, they claim, current moral psychology is unequal to the existential threats facing humanity (Persson and Savulescu, 2017). They argue – somewhat stridently – that human civilisation is threatened if humans don't become more moral. In addition, they argue that moral enhancement of humanity could be at the expense of biological species identity because, in their view, being human is not necessarily a determinant of moral significance. This view is unsurprising given the authors' stance on the "privileging" of humanity in other publications.[8] However, this is at odds with a Christian view of humanity having a specific relationship with God and a specific vocation, as engendered by their possession of the *imago Dei*.

SSRI antidepressants have been commonly reported as potential agents for moral enhancements (Levy, 2014). However, some authors have instead advocated the use of psychedelic agents for moral enhancement, such as psilocybin (magic mushrooms) and ayahuasca (Earp, 2018; Tennison, 2012). While these drugs may hold some promise because of the profound and lasting "reset" effect they can have on dispositions that affect moral behaviour, their legal status and the need for carefully controlled use probably limit their usefulness as moral enhancements for widespread use in human society.

Nevertheless, moral enhancement is problematic for understanding autonomy. If the moral enhancement agent changes the individual's desires and will so that they always want to make the right choice – and therefore they do always make the right choice – then with a coherentist understanding of autonomy (the course of action chosen is aligned with the person's desires), the person's autonomy would not actually be compromised, even though the person is indeed being influenced by an external factor. However, the problem with biomedical interventions for "moral enhancement" is their potential to short-circuit the process of a person reacting to, and reflecting upon, a situation where a moral decision needs to be made – for example, a career change.

The role of reflexivity in genuine personal autonomy in a world where autonomy can be influenced by biomedical enhancements has been discussed by Robert Sparrow (Sparrow, 2014). In response to Persson and Savulescu's proposal that pharmaceutical products can be used for moral enhancement and increasing individual autonomy (Savulescu and Persson, 2012), Sparrow contends that the autonomy provided by pharmaceutical enhancements is illusory and that there is a risk that enhancements simply provide a "fig leaf" for abuse of power and vested interests in a technically advanced society. He argues that possible inequalities between enhanced and unenhanced persons could infringe the autonomy of the unenhanced, and concludes that humans would be less free in a future, technological world than in the world as it is at present.

Sparrow compares "moral enhancement" – development of moral agency – by pharmacological means, with moral agency inculcated by moral and cultural education, and concludes that these two modalities for developing moral agency cannot be ethically equivalent. Moral advancement by education has implicit in it the freedom provided by education, with the potential for debate, dialectic and counterargument. By contrast, drug enhancement is a technical intervention. It is instrumentalist – that is, it is a pragmatic intervention towards a specific end, rather than something of moral value in itself – and it treats the person enhanced as an object to be manipulated, rather than a personal subject who is able to make decisions freely as a moral agent. Sparrow argues persuasively, therefore, that personal autonomy is, in fact, reduced after moral enhancement by pharmacological means. If biomedical technology were regularly applied to human beings in this instrumentalist manner, this would be morally deficient as it would make personal autonomy and the exercise of the will routinely dependent on the effects of a biomedical technology, which could be deployed in society in an oppressive way.

The effects of biomedical technologies on personal autonomy and the ability of these technologies to objectify a person as an artefact to be manipulated at the expense of their subjectivity as an authentic self are both important themes in this book and will be explored in detail in subsequent chapters. However, I will now explore in more detail natural law objections to radical biomedical technologies.

2.7.3 *Nature*

Although the concept of natural law (as distinct from civil law) was seen in the work of some classical philosophers – for example, Aristotle, and implicitly in the work of Plato – natural law was developed in its fullest form during the scholastic era in the twelfth and thirteenth centuries, through the work of theologians such as Thomas Aquinas (Pope, 2012). Aquinas developed a detailed and systematic theological account of natural law, drawing on Patristic sources, Aristotle, Stoicism and Roman legalists. The objective of natural law was to develop a comprehensive Christian legal and ethical framework to enable the church to respond to new situations and new forms of learning that were arising in the rapidly changing society of the high Middle Ages.

The basic tenet of natural law, derived from Aristotle, is that "the good of every organism is to attain fully its natural activity (Pope, 2012, p. 67). In other words, all creatures are directed towards good ends by virtue of their nature. Consequently, any phenomenon that prevents a creature fulfilling its nature will frustrate the good ends of that creature's nature. Aquinas expressed his natural law theory in Q90–94 of *Summa Theologica* (Aquinas, 2010 edition).

The key principles were as follows:

- There are four laws – eternal law, natural law, divine law and human law (Q90, Art 1).
- Natural law is reasonable and arises from the wisdom of God. Humans are therefore rational creatures (Q90, Art 3; Q91, Art 2).
- Natural law is directed towards flourishing, the common good and virtue of all creatures (Q90, Art 2, 3; Q94, Art 3).
- Natural law is the means by which subjects are directed to their good ends (or "proper virtue") (Q92, Art 2).
- General principles of truth and morality apply to all people, and are equally known by all people (Q94, Art 3).

Thomistic natural law therefore has a teleological element – natural law is directed towards the goal of human flourishing, the exercise of virtue (which Aquinas defines as "that which makes something good") and the common good of all people. Thomistic natural law emphasises the importance of reason in moral decision-making, as a reflection of the divine wisdom of God. Aquinas considered the good of human flourishing to be life, procreation,[9] social life, knowledge and rational conduct (Murphy, 2019). Furthermore, natural law does not regard things that are artificial as intrinsically evil, a factor that is significant in this discussion about the applicability of natural law to the ethical evaluation of biomedical technologies.

Thomistic natural law in the Roman Catholic church was revived in the nineteenth century, following the publication of *Aeterni Patris* by Pope Leo

XIII in 1879. This re-emergence of natural law was also in response to rapidly changing conditions in European society, and this publication addressed workers' rights and associated pastoral issues in the increasingly developed industrial society of the Victorian era (Pope, 2012, pp. 77–78). This laid the foundations for the use of Thomistic natural law in Roman Catholic moral deliberation on hormonal contraception in the twentieth century, which I will explore in Chapter 3.

Since Aquinas, there have been various other natural law theorists. These included, in the early modern era, Hugo Grotius and Thomas Hobbes, both of whom downplayed any theological basis for natural law, and also the teleological aspect of natural law (Pope, 2012, pp. 74–77). Grotius sought to develop a framework of natural rights, as opposed to natural law, attempting to develop natural law as a universal political system. Hobbes, on the other hand, interpreted natural law in radically individualist, subjectivist terms, where the central good of human life was self-preservation. The retreat from teleology in natural law in the modern era led to the naturalism of modernity, where moral conclusions were drawn from observations from nature. David Hume criticised this approach, arguing that it is not possible to derive moral precepts from non-moral phenomena (i.e. natural attributes), an argument known as the "is-ought" problem (Hume, 1978 edition, p. 469).

In the twentieth century, the so-called "New Natural Law theorists", such as Germain Grisez and John Finnis, expressed natural law in a way that was independent from theology and any notion of virtue, individualistic rather than emphasising the common good, and which described the goods of humanity in personalist terms (Pope, 2012, pp. 78–79).

As I implied above, there is therefore a major distinction between Thomistic natural law, to which teleology is intrinsic, and the naturalism of modernity, from which biological teleology has been eliminated. In my discussion of natural law in relation to biomedical technologies - both previous biomedical technologies in Chapters 3 and 4 and future biomedical technologies in Chapter 5 – I shall be referring to the Thomistic model of natural law, rather than more modern approaches. This is for three reasons. First, natural law ethical engagement with medicine by the Roman Catholic church to date has been from a Thomist perspective. Second, the Thomist approach is very clearly rooted in theology, and so is most appropriate for a Christian ethical evaluation. Third, the Thomist approach seems to be clearly committed to the common good, which is important given the social, public and political aspects of biotechnology development which I will discuss in Chapter 5.

The main advantage of natural law as a foundation for ethical reflection is that, because it is based on human reason, it claims to be universally applicable to all cultures and it affirms the innate moral capacity of every person. Morality grounded in human nature should, in theory, be the same in all societies and for all people.

There are, however, problems with natural law as a source of ethics. Natural law has been criticised theologically for three main reasons. First, at the Reformation, Martin Luther claimed that, because of its emphasis on human reason, natural law could not be salvific; humans were completely unable to determine morality by reasoning because human reason itself is contaminated by original sin. Second, natural law downplays the role of revelation in the Christian moral life; for this reason, natural law was criticised by the Reformers in the sixteenth century, and by Karl Barth in the twentieth century. Third, because natural law is focused on the reasoning of the individual, it does not account for the supernatural transformative power of the Holy Spirit, nor does it acknowledge the Christian community as an arbiter of morality. In addition, natural law has also been criticised from a scientific basis, because its key concepts appear to be undermined by the findings of evolutionary biology (Pope, 2014). The idea of a fixed and unchanging order of nature is challenged by the evolutionary principle that nature is changing and evolving. This debate questions the ability of natural law to be an adequate foundation for ethics of medicine and biotechnology in the twenty-first century when many of these technologies can manipulate nature itself. This question, in relation to past therapeutic discoveries and proposed future biomedical technologies, will be discussed in Chapter 5.

There may be a parallel between transhumanism and Christian belief in terms of teleology, in that both are concerned with changing humanity to escape corruption and improve the human experience. However, there seems to be a tension between transhumanism and natural law concerning the fixity of human and animal nature that natural law appears to suggest. Inherent in transhumanism – for example, in F.M. Esfandiary's description of the transhumanist as a "transitional human" constituting "an evolutionary link with the coming era of post-humanity" (Esfandiary and FM-2030, 1989, p. 149), and in the evolutionary understanding of transhumanism shown by Kurzweil and Moravec – is the idea that human nature is eminently malleable and changeable. This, however, seems to be in contradiction to the notion of a fixed order of creation and of human nature that natural law suggests.

In any case, there are some goods of life that may not be aligned to the natural world. Hopkins quotes Thomas Aquinas as saying that happiness is the ultimate human goal, but argues that this cannot be fulfilled in a flawed material world (Hopkins, 2013). Conversely, he states that, while advocates of technology might wish to argue that greater knowledge of, and control over, the natural world is desirable, this knowledge and control can be exercised in an arrogant and hubristic way, and thus be immoral. Bailey, a supporter of transhumanism, points out that the application of biomedical technology does not preclude virtuous moral behaviour on the part of the users (Bailey, 2013). He argues that people are not necessarily less moral or loving in a technological age, pointing out that parental love has not been affected by *in vitro* fertilisation (IVF) to aid conception. The argument that the use of supposedly unnatural biomedical technology does not undermine virtue is significant, because natural law theory has historically been the basis for the Roman Catholic church's moral pronouncements about biomedical technologies, such as the contraceptive pill, as I will discuss in Chapter 3.

In an analogous way, some theologians have pointed out that the effects of medical technologies on the nature of the human person do not necessarily constitute a violation of spiritual life. In her review of the theological implications of transhumanist technologies, Elaine Graham has argued that the effects of a medical technology on human nature do not preclude spiritual life (Graham, 2006). Ronald Cole-Turner has argued that medical technology is imposing a new metaphysics on human nature – what could be described as a "meta-technology" (Cole-Turner, 2001). He examines Peter Kramer's controversial book "Listening to Prozac" and argues that reductionist biological arguments have caused humanity to conflate natural and spiritual considerations, and that human society is now trying inappropriately to solve spiritual problems with pharmacological solutions. Both Graham and Cole-Turner envisage a distinctively spiritual component of human life, which the use of biomedical technology does not necessarily undermine.

Consequently, distinctions between what is natural and unnatural are relatively unhelpful in the technological world, although the natural/unnatural distinction may provide a useful starting point. Rather than thinking of nature and natural law as a *yardstick* against which new technologies can be measured, it might be better to think of nature as a *scalpel* with which new technologies can be dissected, to evaluate them and understand what is important about them. The limitations of natural law as a means of ethical evaluation of future biomedical technologies, in the light of past experience, will be developed and explored in detail in Chapter 5.

2.7.4 Embodiment

In the Judaeo-Christian tradition, the human body has an innate moral value, as indicated by Old Testament scriptural emphasis on the sanctity of life (for example, seen in Genesis 9v6, Exodus 20v13). In addition, there are various strands of Christian thought that come together to support the Christian significance of embodied life.

First, there is the goodness of created humanity (Genesis 1v31). Second, there is the incarnation, the belief that God himself assumed the human form as Jesus Christ (Philippians 2v5–7). Third, there is the compassion of Jesus towards the bodily needs of those around him during his earthly life, for example, with his healing miracles (see, for example, the woman with a bleed (Mark 6v25–34), blind Bartimaeus (Mark 10v46–52), and the crippled man by the pool (John 5v1–15)). Fourth, and most obviously connected with a Christian evaluation of life-extending medical technologies in future because of its eschatological dimension, is the resurrection of Jesus and the New Testament concept of the resurrection body – both Christ's resurrection body, and the resurrection bodies that Christian believers will ultimately inherit (Morris, 1996). The concept of the resurrection body emphasises the fact that bodily identity remains significant after death, from a perspective of Christian eschatology, and therefore implies that the body is significant in Christian terms during life.

This contrasts with the dualism of Platonism, which was a key feature of the Greco-Roman thought-world during the New Testament era (Burkett, 2019, p. 85). This dualism maintained that the mortal body has an immortal soul within it and, when the mortal body dies, the immortal soul is released from the "envelope" of the body. Indeed, this idea of the immortal soul living forever after bodily life has found its way into popular belief about the resurrection (Cullmann, 1958, pp. 15–20). The conflict between the importance of embodied life and the significance of the resurrection body in early Christianity on one hand, and the prevailing body-soul dualism of Platonist thought in wider society at that time on the other, stimulated significant teaching about the issue in the Corinthian church (1 Corinthians 15).

Nevertheless, despite this sharp contrast between Christian and Platonic accounts of the body, Christian attitudes to the body have been ambivalent and by no means wholly positive about human bodily experience (Moltmann-Wendel, 1994, pp. 1–4). First, Platonist thought may have exerted a negative influence on the early Christians and their attitudes to the body (hence the need for Paul's teaching on body-related issues – for example, on sex in 1 Corinthians 5–7). Second, Moltmann-Wendel suggests that, in the early church, some Christians may have embraced the Stoic principle of the body as "a necessary evil", as a compromise which enabled them to reject Platonism, but remain coherent and intelligible to the philosophical thought forms of the world around them (Moltmann-Wendel, 1994, p. 42). Third, the value of human life in that era, together with the Christian hope of resurrection, may have meant that the early Christians held lightly to bodily life, and were less troubled by the prospect of death and martyrdom. As Paul said to the Philippian church, "To live is Christ, and to die is gain" (Philippians 1v21). However, Paul has also upheld the value of the body in his rebuttal of the consequences of dualism, because of the spiritual significance of the body (e.g., in 1 Corinthians 6,19, against sexual licence, "do you not know that your body is a temple of the Holy Spirit?").

Some theologians – for example, Origen and Augustine – have, in fact, taken a dualistic approach to theological anthropology and have emphasised the importance of spiritual things in the Christian life over the significance of the physical body, and this dualistic approach has had a significant place in the history of Christian thought. Because of this, it is all the more remarkable that such a positive view of the body is seen in the

Bible and in the early church, especially in a pre-modern age when diseases were not treatable and human life was not valued in the same way as it is in the early twenty-first century. As well as arising from the Christian doctrines of the incarnation and the bodily resurrection of Christ, this emphasis on the significance of the material body may be also related to the idea of *shalom* as human wholeness, wellness and flourishing in the material sense (Landa, 2014).

In any case, because of this strand of Christian thought emphasising the somatic significance of human existence, Christian critiques of transhumanist medical technologies are right to be suspicious of those technologies – for example, mind-uploading and cybernetics – which deprecate the body, and undermine the goods of bodily human life. What might be the problems of a non-embodied existence from a Christian perspective? After all, it could be argued that transformation is transformation, and that transformation of the human body with radical medical technology is no different, in ethical terms, to transformation of the human body from an earthly body to a resurrection body by the power of the risen Christ, as envisaged by New Testament resurrection doctrine (1 Corinthians 15v51: "we shall all be changed").

Brent Waters has extensively critiqued the aims of transhumanism from the perspective of transhumanist attitudes to the body (Waters, 2009, pp. 149–183). He notes that, although transhumanists are seeking the perfection of humanity, this perfection comes at a high price. "The price of perfection for humanity is its deconstruction", he claims (Waters, 2009, p. 150). Drawing on two short stories by Nathaniel Hawthorne, he notes – wisely in my view – that, with some technological interventions, there is no going back, and that the consequences of human invulnerability are uncertain. Along with nihilism and Pelagianism, Waters points to Manichaeism as a key theological influence on transhumanists. The Manichaeists of St Augustine's time wanted to be rescued from the imperfections of their bodies, and the prospect of transhumanist technologies does just this, Waters claims. I would argue, however, that Waters possibly overstates his case. Divestiture of the body is not a central motivation for all transhumanists; for example, Bostrom is primarily seeking a better society (Bostrom, 2005a), and More a better body (More, 2013). Nevertheless, embodied life is important from a perspective of Christian doctrine, as I have shown, and Waters is right to point to the embodied aspects of the life of Jesus as counter-arguments to transhumanist technologies which deprecate the body. In the incarnation of Christ, the necessity of human finitude and mortality of the body are affirmed, Waters claims (Waters, 2009, p159). Furthermore, the resurrection of Christ makes possible the resurrection body of the believer, and the renewal of creation. Drawing on the work of Oliver O'Donovan, Waters argues that moral life is constituted in the ordering of the new creation; he argues, correctly in my view, that an embodied nature is vital to obtain the proper goods of marriage, because people can only love each other meaningfully as embodied creatures (Waters, 2009, pp. 160–161).

There are two specific areas where the concept of embodiment is important to sustain a Christian account of authentic human life, and where Christian theologians are justified in their criticism of biomedical technologies which negate the body. The first of these is in relation to bodily experiences. Some experiences central to human life – for example, sex and eating – are inextricably linked to having a body, and existing as a body, as admitted by Kurzweil, despite his advocacy of radical transhumanist technology (Kurzweil, 1999, pp. 133–134). This is reflected in Christian marriage, which is traditionally predicated, to a greater or lesser extent, on the physical union of the husband and wife. This also reflected in the consumption of the eucharistic sacrament, which is an essential part of religious observance for many Christian traditions.

Being an uploaded mind, rather than living an embodied life, would eliminate, or at the very least seriously undermine, these physical aspects of human life, both of which are "sacramental" in the broadest Christian terms, and are important in a Christian way of life in any culture, in a way which might transcend denominational affiliation.[10] Any attempt to recreate these experiences artificially in an *in silico* world (and indeed Kurzweil discusses the use of, for example, artificial interfaces to simulate sexual experience (Kurzweil, 1999, pp. 133–134)) would be, at best, contrived and, at worst, meaningless. With the development of sophisticated artificial intelligence in the future, it is possible that an uploaded person's virtual world could be made to be indistinguishable from physical reality. However, the fact remains that, however realistic the experience was, it would not actually be physical reality, and the material importance of bodily life would be undermined.

The Christian believer, living life as an uploaded mind, bereft of his or her body, would be deprived of both bodily union with a spouse, and spiritual union with Christ in the Eucharist. These important material things in the Christian life would be robbed of their power in a non-embodied world. This would be detrimental for the body of the individual Christian believer, and also for the body of the church, given the centrality of the sacraments in the ministry of Christ and the role of the sacraments, and their implications for ecclesial communion, in the life of the church on earth.

The second area is in relation to personal identity. The existence of the eschatological resurrection body (1 Corinthians 15v35ff) is linked with personal post-mortem identity. The risen Jesus retained his identity in his resurrection body, and he was recognisable by the disciples, even though his body was different (John 20v10–20). In his discussion of anthropology of identity and the resurrection of the body, Fernando Vidal states that "According to established doctrine, the bodily and psychological identity of resurrected individuals will be the same as that of the persons they were while alive" (Vidal, 2002, p. 940). In other words, a person's physical body corresponds to their resurrection body – although Vidal rightly warns that the current notion of "identity", characterised by "radical reflexivity, a first-person standpoint and disengagement from the body, is essentially a modern concept, and would not have been recognised and understood as such by the early church (Vidal, 2002, p. 937). Nevertheless, in both cases, bodily attributes are linked somehow with personal identity, although the identity of the resurrection body is linked with that of Christ (see 1 Corinthians 15v49).

This contrasts with transhumanist views which suggest that bodily identity is not necessary at all, and that personal identity can be established purely as pattern identity – the thought forms and world of the mind alone (Kurzweil, 1999, pp. 51–55; Moravec, 1988, p. 116). As discussed earlier in this chapter, Ray Kurzweil and Hans Moravec have both appealed to pattern identity as a way of safeguarding personal identity in the possible future scenario of mind-uploading, where an individual's mind could be uploaded onto a computer.

In any case, even if the individual whose mind has been uploaded onto a computer could assert their personal identity in that state, as Moravec supposes, they would not be able to escape their history of previous embodiment. This is because they will have memories and reflections related to their previous bodily existence, which may be significant for personal identity formation. This seemingly inextricable link between consciousness and embodiment is one of the reasons why Katherine Hayles rightly asserts the importance of bodily life and rebuts Moravec's arguments for mind-uploading (Hayles, 1999, p. 1). To quote Hayles, "Embodiment has a history" (Hayles, 1999, p. 284). Also, the claim by Nick Bostrom that intellectual capacity is more significant for a person than species membership is problematic for the idea of human embodiment because it undermines the distinctiveness of human bodily form, as distinct from non-human creatures (Bostrom, 2004).

Embodiment is not only important for human experience and personal identity, in terms of self-understanding, it is also important to enable humans to understand themselves in relation to the created world. The specifically embodied nature of a human being is highly significant for human engagement with the material concerns of the world's environment – for example, maintaining good natural habitats free from pollution, and using the earth's resources in a sustainable manner – because of the specific role of embodied human beings as producers and consumers of the earth's resources.

These considerations emphasise the dualistic – and, in my view, deficient – nature of pattern identity in the non-embodied person. With pattern identity, the individual, disembodied essence of a person is emphasised over, and at the expense of, the rest of the material world. The individual, disembodied essence of a person could possibly be classed as a material entity, in that it is comprised of data units expressed in the state of silicon, but few would regard such an essence as embodied, in that it bears any resemblance to any current realistic understanding of human life and experience. One is left wondering whether the morphological freedom which some transhumanists advocate is at all compatible with the many features and goods of human life, which are grounded in human bodily experience.

On the question of identity, Celia Deane-Drummond argues that the Christian vocation of "fusion" with God is about the discovery of one's true identity, whereas the transhumanist project is about changing and eliminating identity, through biomedical manipulation of functional and cognitive attributes (Deane-Drummond, 2006). Miccoli's critique of the potential consequences of the transhumanist project also touches on the issue of identity (Miccoli, 2010). He argues that transhumanists do not acknowledge their real motivations for using technology to transform human society; transhumanists want to embrace technology to expand themselves – to enhance their identity – but in fact the technology embraces them and changes them instead, thus diminishing their identity. He argues that, with technology, humans believe that they can master the world whereas, by using radical technology, humans sacrifice the opportunity of experiencing the world, and instead objectify the means through which the world should be experienced – the human body itself. Using radical biomedical technology denigrates the body by rendering it an object to be manipulated, rather than a personal subject.

I conclude here that, from a Christian ethical perspective, embodiment is an important, and probably necessary, prerequisite for human flourishing, because it is the ground for authentic human experience and identity. I would argue that material aspects of the Christian faith – particularly the eucharist and marriage – and their significance, to a greater or lesser extent, in Christian life and observance – would be undermined by technologies that negate human bodily life, for example, mind-uploading. As well as undermining the qualities of human life from a perspective of Christian praxis, technologies that negate the body will also have profound effects on the ethics of medical treatment. I will explore this further in the light of the two therapeutic case studies in Chapter 5.

2.7.5 Imago Dei

The Christian doctrine of the image of God – that humanity is made in the image and likeness of God (Genesis 1v26) – has important implications for understanding human nature, and the relationship of human beings to God, and to each other. Before a discussion of the implications of transhumanism for the doctrine of *imago Dei*, a background discussion of the *imago Dei* is necessary.

The doctrine of *imago Dei* is derived from various Biblical texts in the Old Testament (Genesis 1v26–27, 5v1–3 and 9v5–6) and in the New Testament (for example, Colossians 1v15, 2 Corinthians 4v4, Ephesians 4v24). However, the meaning of *imago Dei*, as derived from Biblical exegesis, has been hotly debated.[11] In the history of Christian thought, four main approaches to *imago Dei* theology have been proposed – the substantive, functional, relational and eschatological approaches (summarised by Herzfeld, 2002, pp. 10–32).

The substantive approach attempted to determine which attributes of substance are responsible for the *imago Dei* in human beings and was largely the approach taken in the development of the doctrine by theologians such as Augustine and Aquinas. Traditionally, the substantive attribute that was most commonly thought to represent the *imago Dei* in humans was rationality or reason. However, the substantive approach has various flaws (Herzfeld, 2002, pp. 25–27). First, it has the potential to be dualistic, in that a divinely given substantive attribute, such as rationality, is contrasted with material bodily life, and this can lead to human embodiment being downplayed. Second, because it takes a "bottom-up" approach, which seeks the divine attribute in humans, it is often individualistic and does not accord well with a social world and the corporate dimension of faith and salvation envisaged in the biblical revelation. Third, an emphasis on specific substantive attributes as the *imago Dei* can lead to reductionism, as attributes that are supposedly distinctive of humans are then explained in biological terms and identified in other species in animal behavioural experiments (Deane-Drummond, 2014). A key criticism of the substantive *imago Dei*, however, is that it has a static view of human nature, rather than a dynamic view, and this is particularly important when considering the expected effects of a biomedical intervention on a person from a Christian perspective, in terms of human destiny.

The functional approach takes the view that the *imago Dei* is not about the attributes of substance that human beings have, but about the role, task or vocation they have in the world. The functional approach focuses on a "royal representative" exegesis of Genesis 1v26 concerning humankind ruling over the created world, and sees humanity as representative of God, in their task or office in the world (Middleton, 2005, pp. 88–89).[12] However, the functional view has been criticised because it is often associated with the domination of humans over the non-human creative world, and the consequent anthropocentrism with which the world might be viewed. It is also problematic when considering the humanity of people who are seriously disabled or ill, and who may not have the authority of purposive function in the world. Herein lies another issue with the functional approach; it implicitly assumes some substantive attributes on the part of a person, in order that they might be able to function in the world. For example, one could argue that functioning in the world requires a human person to have attributes such as rational thought or moral capacity.

The functional approach to the *imago Dei* has been expressed in the idea of stewardship, that humanity images God by exercising a vocation to look after world that God created, on his behalf. Southgate has discussed the concept of stewardship as a model for the relationship between humans and the non-human creative world and has summarised its problems (Southgate, 2006). One criticism of the idea of stewardship is that it can be exploitative and treat the earth as a commodity. Another is that stewardship is anthropocentric, focusing on the role and ability of humans to act as stewards, and does not sufficiently account for the "wildness" of the world. However, for Southgate, a key critique of stewardship – and one I endorse – is that it is ethically cautious and not sufficiently future-oriented, in that the goal of stewardship is to leave the world in no worse a state than it was before. A stewardship approach to the exercise of human vocation in the world is therefore probably less applicable in the assessment of the adoption of future technologies in the world because it is insufficiently future-oriented.

A better approach to the exercise of human ethical responsibility in the care of the natural world in a technological world is the idea of humanity as created co-creator. Philip Hefner's concept of the "created co-creator", states that the purpose of human beings is to be "the agency, acting in freedom, to birth the future that is most wholesome for the nature that has birthed us" and that "exercising this agency is said to be God's will for humans" (Hefner, 1993, p. 27). On this basis, scientists have a moral and theological mandate to exercise their vocation to understand the created order by alleviating human suffering and enhancing human life, so long as it is consistent with ethical principles, such as justice and respect.

Ted Peters argues that, as created co-creator, humanity has a moral obligation to use science to transform the world so that it conforms more closely to the vision of God's new creation (Peters, 2005). For Peters, created cocreator-ship is an inherently ethical task, as it is directed towards the human destiny of the renewal of creation, and this, in my view, is its strength. Nevertheless, Peters acknowledges a key criticism of the created co-creator concept, that humanity must be cautious in their co-creativity, to avoid utopian idealism.

Michael Northcott has made a sustained Christian critique of the idea of the created co-creator (Northcott, 2005). Drawing on two examples, a work of concept art by Damien Hirst and the cloned sheep, Dolly, Northcott argues that, in different ways, both modern art and cloning are a denial of the beauty of life, and that not all things made by human hand have aesthetic appeal. He states correctly that all human technology is influenced in some way or other by economic or social factors, and therefore careful attention should be paid to the purpose of the technology, an area that will be central to my discussion in Chapter 5. He argues that the morality of human making depends on an ability to frame that making in the God-given purposes of the original creator and, following Ricoeur, argues that modern art is an "idolatrous expression of the volitional self". In my view, this criticism does not obviate the need for humanity to exercise the role of created co-creator in the use of technology, because the ethical imperative to harness inevitable technology adoption for good ends, consistent with the new creation, is still there. However, this ethical imperative does place a considerable burden of responsibility on humanity in its created co-creator role; in particular, on scientists and therapists as they develop and evaluate new biomedical technologies.

The relational approach proposes that the *imago Dei* is not about what a person is, or what they do, but is about the person's relationship with God and with others. It has its roots in the Reformation, but was developed in its fullest form in the twentieth century by Karl Barth (Barth, 1957, III (2), pp. 76–77, pp. 323–324). The relational approach to *imago Dei* has much to commend it, and has important implications for interpersonal relationships, the development of personhood and social and political theology. For example, Alistair McFadyen has examined the horizontal relationships between fellow humans, in relation to the vertical, dialogical relationship that humans should have with God (McFadyen, 1990, pp. 17–44). However, the relational approach has been criticised for not being sufficiently grounded on biblical exegesis, and also for focusing on certain human relationships at the expense of others (Oberdorfer, 2014).

Both Scott Midson and Matthew Zaro Fisher have attempted to develop a transhumanist theological anthropology, based on an appeal to the relational aspect of the *imago Dei*. In his recent publication, *Cyborg Theology*, Scott Midson has explored whether theological anthropology can accommodate the challenges to human/machinic boundaries presented by the cyborg (Midson, 2018, pp. 5–9). Midson acknowledges the problems of the human-machine boundary that the cyborg presents, as identified previously by Haraway, and examines the different approaches to the *imago Dei,* to determine whether the cyborg can, in any sense, share the *imago Dei* with humanity (Midson, 2018, pp. 19–44). He quickly dismisses the substantive approach – rightly so, in my view – as a point of contact with the cyborg because it emphasises exclusive human characteristics and has been associated with human domination, as described above. He is also critical of a functional approach to the *imago Dei* as a means of developing a cyborg anthropology. He argues, reasonably, that the exercise of human function in the world can also assert human dominance and that, because it assumes human attributes, function is merely an extension of the substantive approach. However, in my view, Midson does not adequately describe the vocational element of the functional approach, the idea that function is concerned with the God-given human vocation to care for the world, which has an important ethical dimension. Midson favours a relational approach to the *imago Dei* as the basis of a cyborg theology. He argues that the relational approach is concerned with relational capacity, rather than human distinctiveness, and this downplays the boundary between the human and the cyborg. Furthermore, noting Anna Case Winters' observation that humans are co-constituted by their relationships, Midson argues that the dynamic understanding of identity that the relational *imago Dei* posits is helpful in accommodating the ontological ambiguity of the cyborg. He therefore concludes that the actor in a relationship need not be human, but could be a cyborg or an artificial intelligence, and in that sense a non-humanoid intelligence could bear the *imago Dei* (Midson, 2018, pp. 44–47). However, in my view, this relational argument does not account for the importance of embodiment. As discussed in the previous section, there are some aspects of life that do not make sense without a body and, from a Christian perspective, the body plays an important part in human identity.

Inspired by Thweatt Bates' work on the cyborg, Matthew Zaro Fisher contends that the uploaded mind, as a relational entity, bears the *imago Dei*, according to the relational approach to *imago Dei* (Zaro Fisher, 2015). He argues that the uploaded mind is not truly disembodied because it still needs a material element to exist, even if that is a computer, rather than a biological body. He then claims that a relational theological anthropology could still accommodate the uploaded mind as a relational entity. He appeals to Karl Rahner's idea of *Vorgriff* (Rahner, 2004). This is the approach to self-transcendence in which matter and spirit in the human person are not separate entities but are mutually constitutive, and the spirit is not a separate substance, but consists in matter's self-realisation. Zaro Fisher argues that, because of *Vorgriff*, a person can encounter God, others and themselves in a relational way, and the encounter is agnostic of the material nature of the person, which could equally be a biological body or a computer. From this, he concludes that the uploaded mind, or an artificial intelligence, could have the self-presence of personhood and, in that sense, bear the relational *imago Dei*.

I am unconvinced by this argument. Rahner's concept of *Vorgriff* is certainly helpful for understanding human personhood. However, if self-transcendence is material self-realisation, according to the Rahnerian account, then the material self-realisation of the embodied human and that of the uploaded mind will be different precisely because the materials involved are different in each case.

Following from New Testament passages describing Christ as the visible image of God (Colossians 1v15), the eschatological approach asserts that the *imago Dei* in human beings is perfected in relation to Christ, as the believer is conformed to Christ. However, the eschatological approach proposes that the *imago Dei* is still developing and will be ultimately perfected in humanity in perfect relationship with God at the eschaton. The German theologian, Wolfhart Pannenberg, was a key proponent of the eschatological approach and described human nature, and its natural dynamic movements to its destiny of life with God using the term *exocentricity* (*Weltoffenheit*) – an openness to the world, to each other and to our self-consciousness (Pannenberg, 1970, pp. 1–13). The eschatological approach therefore takes seriously the dynamic nature of the *imago Dei*, as emphasised by the New Testament texts, and the concept of "human becoming" that has been proposed by theologians such as Arthur Peacocke (Peacocke, 1990, p. 312). Pannenberg's eschatological approach to the *imago Dei*, with its emphasis on openness to the world and freedom to enquire into the world is also consistent with the idea of autonomy, defined as self-determination, in response to the world, as discussed earlier. A key problem with the eschatological approach to the *imago Dei* is that the *imago Dei* motif in Genesis 1v27 is introduced in the context of the creation account, and its significance seems more likely to be protological than eschatological. In addition, the eschatological approach has also been criticised for being individualistic, with insufficient emphasis on social structures and ethical action in the world, and potentially deterministic (Stewart, 2000, pp. 151–152). However, although there is the potential for the Christological dimension of the *imago Dei* to be individualistic, because it is about the individual's relationship with God in Christ, conformation to Christ ("the image of the invisible God" (Colossians 1v15)) as the eschatological goal (*telos*) for humanity is ultimately not an individual and private matter, but a corporate matter, in line with the New Testament idea of the body of Christ (1 Corinthians 12v12–27) and of the city of God (Revelation 21) (Weng, 2001, pp. 13–14).

An important aspect of an eschatological understanding of the *imago Dei* is the Christian aspiration of *theosis*, or participation in the divine nature.[13] The destiny of the believer is to become more like God. The *imago Dei* is perfected in the believer when they transcend themselves, and the distance between them and God is reduced. Interestingly, various scholars have noted recently that *theosis* provides a point of dialogue between Christianity and transhumanism, enabling Christian eschatology and the secular eschatology of transhumanism to be compared (Hupala, 2020; Torrance, 2019; Lipps, 2020; Peters, 2018).

The idea of *theosis* is particularly prominent in the theology of Maximus the Confessor, which is discussed in detail by Eugenia Torrance (Torrance, 2019). There are some similarities between the goals of transhumanism and the *telos* of theosis – union with God. Torrance quotes Todd Daley, saying that the monastic traditions have three ideas in common with transhumanism: 1) that death is our greatest enemy, 2) that bodily decay is an unnecessary element of our existence and 3) that there are steps we can take now to participate in a life that transcends the human. In my view, however, these three apparent similarities are debatable. First, in the light of the resurrection of Jesus, death may not, in fact, be the greatest enemy; for example, human depravity and indignity are also significant enemies. In the second place, bodily decay is indubitably a thermodynamic necessity in the material world in which we live. Third, while both theologians and transhumanists might believe there are ways in which transcendence might be achieved now, spiritual transcendence and transcendence achieved by technology are two very different prospects.

The similarities between monastic spirituality and transhumanism may therefore not be as close as might first appear. Nevertheless, comparison of the deification by *theosis* in Christian eschatology with the self-deification provided by biomedical technology reveals important details about the nature of transhumanism and how theology might respond to it. Torrance rightly argues that, while *theosis* is concerned with the transcendence of human nature, it does not advocate the abandonment of human nature.

While she overstates her case in terms of a contrast between *theosis* and transhumanism – there are some forms of technology that do not seek the complete abolition of human nature – she is correct to assert that human nature is left intact by participating in the divine nature.

Ted Peters makes a similar point, arguing that *theosis* as a path to deification is, in fact, a restoration of our true humanity, not an abandonment of it (Peters, 2018). He notes that *theosis* is not just concerned with the process of overcoming death, but also overcoming sin. While transhumanism may claim to overcome death, it is generally ineffective against sin as a universal human problem. Peters argues that *theosis*, the process of increasing participation in the divine nature as envisaged by Orthodox theology, is not an arrogant grasp at deity by humanity (in contrast with Christ's self-emptying in Phil 2v5), nor a denial of creaturely finitude by humans. Instead, it is about the person participating in God, by being infused by the Holy Spirit. Peters argues – correctly, in my view – that *theosis* is concerned with participating in God, whereas enhancement constitutes *theopoiesis* – that is, becoming a god.

Jonathan Lipps makes a helpful comparison between human destiny from the perspective of Christian eschatology, and the destiny provided by transhumanism (Lipps, 2020). The Christian perspective is that humans are like God, and should be on a trajectory to be more like God; the *imago Dei* is perfected when a person participates radically in the life of God through Christian belief and spiritual life. For the transhumanist, however, the end goal is the secular eschaton of full technology implementation, which is a triumph of the will to power of the individual. On this account, Lipps argues, the human person is instead in the image of the machine (*imago machinae*), and that image is perfected in them by the technology. Lipps therefore argues that *theosis*, the transcendence of deification, is therefore not a bad thing in itself, but needs to be enacted in a context of dependence on God. Lipps concludes correctly that, since transhumanism will develop organically from current technology adoption, the church must decide proactively what its relationship with technology will be.

Although these four approaches to *imago Dei* have been proposed – the substantive, functional, relational and eschatological approaches – it is unlikely that any one of these alone can provide a definitive description of humanity, in the light of current scientific knowledge about human beings. Human life is, at the same time, dynamic, embodied, relational, functional, and teleological, so actually there would be elements of all four of these approaches in any contemporary theological description of human life.

There are various criticisms of transhumanism that arise from *imago Dei* theology. First, as mentioned earlier, some proponents of transhumanism – for example, Campbell and Walker – cite the *imago Dei* in support of the transhumanist project, arguing that biomedical technologies are somehow needed to perfect the *imago Dei* in humanity (Campbell and Walker, 2005).[14] This approach is problematic, because it suggests that the *imago*

Dei is distorted, and so somehow incomplete, in disabled – or even just unenhanced – people (Kilner, 2015, p. 19). Furthermore, it implies that technology (which may not be realistically available) may be needed to somehow enact the *imago Dei* in the disabled or unenhanced person, to validate that person. It also suggests the *imago Dei* can be completed in human beings by human will, with the application of medical technology, whereas the Christological dimension of the *imago Dei* would suggest that human beings can only be perfected by God's initiative through being in Christ, who is the perfect image of God (Colossians 1v15).

Second, transhumanists tend to focus on the individual as the subject for enhancement, and on individual autonomy in choosing enhancements. This, however, is in tension with functional and relational approaches to the *imago Dei* which are not individualist in nature. The functional approach to the *imago Dei*, based on the "royal representative" exegesis of Genesis 1v26 (Middleton, 2005) states that humans exercise representative authority on behalf of God on earth, and that they have a vocation or office which necessarily brings them into relationship with the world around them. Ng argues that, just as in the Old Testament, the king had a covenantal relationship with God and a duty of ethical and social responsibility to the kingdom, analogously, with the functional view of the *imago Dei*, humans have an ethical and social responsibility for the whole of creation by virtue of being part of creation (Weng, 2001, pp. 11–12). Along similar lines, Brent Waters argues that, whether or not they remain human by biological criteria, those who undergo radical transhumanist enhancements cease to be bearers of the *imago Dei* precisely because they reject their election or calling by God to be co-regents in the world (Waters, 2006a, p. 123). Waters' argument here is that the adoption of radical transhumanist enhancements impairs the eschatological *imago Dei* because it prevents the person from progressing to their eschatological destiny from a Christian perspective – finitude and union with Christ. Set against this, however, is the possibility that a transhumanist enhancement might enable a person to live a better, more moral, life in this world (the prospect of moral enhancement, described earlier). Interference of biomedical technology with Christian eschatological destiny is a key aspect of the debate about the Christian acceptability of radical transhumanist enhancements, which I shall explore further in Chapter 5.

Although adherents of transhumanism may publicly proclaim the benefits of biotechnology for society and human flourishing, a close examination of the literature of the transhumanist movement shows that transhumanism is largely concerned with enhancement of the individual, as opposed to medical treatment, for personal benefit other than the healing of diseases, and is guided by individual human will. Unsurprisingly, this tends to be an individualistic and private endeavour. It is no coincidence that the rejection of traditional family values was one of the criteria for transhumanism proposed by philosopher F.M. 2030 (Bostrom, 2005b).

Third, the transhumanism project is concerned with the attributes of the individual human being, often at the expense of other aspects of human life, such as relationships and culture. While this transhumanist aim is purportedly for good ethical ends – the survival and flourishing of humanity – an approach to humanity and the goods of human life that is focused on human attributes only represents a deficient view of humanity as created in the image of God. As discussed earlier, a substantive approach to the *imago Dei*, which focuses on the attributes of substance of the human being – for example, reason – is only one approach, which alone does not do justice to a comprehensive understanding of humanity as created in God's image, based on the Biblical *imago Dei* texts. A person is more than the sum of their attributes, and cannot simply be reduced to those attributes, so an attribute-based measurement of a human being, such as transhumanists might propose, is a deficient, reductionist view of the human being, similar to that proposed by reductionist, atheist scientists such as Francis Crick (Barbour, 1998, p. 79).

Fourth, transhumanism challenges an eschatological approach to the *imago Dei* because it provides humanity with an alternative eschatology. In her commentary on transhumanism, Elaine Graham argues that the *imago Dei* points to a framework of values by which the proper ends of humanity might be adjudicated, whereas transhumanism provides a realised eschatology of immortality and escape from biological contingency (Graham, 2006). Brent Waters too has examined the implications of biomedical technology for Christian eschatology. He argues that the postmodern view of the world assumes a sharp dichotomy between an open and a deterministic view of the universe (Waters, 2006b, pp. 123–125). He asserts that theology influenced by postmodernity tends to adopt an open view of the universe. This downplays the notion of pre-destination, he contends, but it also undermines human purpose and destiny. Waters goes on to argue that, if there is no eschatological *telos* for humanity, then there is no concept of divine providence, and therefore no purpose to the ordering of creation (Waters, 2006b, p. 123). This argument is compelling given the evident interrelation of the doctrines of creation and providence. This leads to what Waters describes as a "eviscerated eschatology" (Waters, 2006b, p. 124). As he pithily describes it, "the postmodern world is going nowhere, because it's got nowhere to go" (Waters, 2006b, p. 123).

Waters claims that theology is faced with a stark choice if it wishes to embrace the postmodern values that underpin the use of radical technologies: it must either discard eschatology or redefine it in realised terms. In other words, if there is no robust eschatology, then every moral choice is a moment of judgment, where a person may be condemned because of their actions. Waters concludes that, in ethical terms, a postmodern approach to technology, as advocated by transhumanism, leads to slavery rather than freedom. This is consistent with the philosophical reflections by Sparrow on the loss of autonomy in a technology-enabled world (Sparrow, 2014).

While I agree broadly with Waters' eschatological analysis, he does not seem to distinguish adequately between modernity and postmodernity as influences on technology adoption. As discussed earlier in this chapter, transhumanism has its roots in liberal modernity, and a key aspect of the culture of modernity has been the notion of "progress" in society and human living conditions, with the ethical implications this brings. With postmodernism, however, and its emphasis on individual experience, rather than corporate authority or epistemology, this element of progress is absent, and the adoption of technology becomes an individualistic, experiential endeavour. This would lead to a subtly different interpretation of the transhumanist movement as a world-improving philosophy.

Waters identifies a realised eschatology in transhumanism, which contrasts with the Christian eschatological hope. With transhumanist technologies, hope of perfection is realised – or not – when the technology is applied to the human person. From that point onward, hope is diminished because the eschatological destiny has already been realised, and there is nothing more to hope for. The realised eschatology of transhumanism therefore seems to be a human self-restriction of eschatological freedom. Christian soteriology provides a means of transformation and perfectibility, but when human beings restrict themselves to technology as the primary means of transformation, as transhumanists generally do, they foreclose other means of achieving their destiny. It is ironic that transhumanists use the word *extropy,* to denote that humanity is an "open system" – when, in fact, manipulation of the human body to gain biomedical immortality places a limit on humanity, compared with the hope of immortality offered by Christian eschatology.

A fifth area of concern with transhumanism and the *imago Dei* is the Christian prohibition of idolatry. Wenzel Van Huyssteen explores this issue in some detail in his account of the *imago Dei* from the perspective of human distinctiveness (Van Huyssteen, 2006, pp. 116–132). Genesis 1v26 states that human beings are made in the image of God, suggesting a material image (Wenham, 1987, pp. 26–33),[15] but elsewhere in the Old Testament (e.g., Exodus 20), idols are prohibited. Van Huyssteen argues that the *imago Dei* is the one exception to the prohibition, saying that it was God's prerogative to create humans in his image, but this privilege does not extend to human creativity, and humans cannot create God in their image. This raises the question of whether the use of transhumanist technologies to change human nature is an act of idolatry. The perfected *imago Dei* – the visible image of the invisible God (Colossians 1v15) – is Jesus, so it could be argued that transformation that leads to conformation to Christ is the kind of transformation that is seeking and worshipping God, rather than seeking to worship a material idol. This relates also to the idea that application of medical technology treats the body as an artefact to be engineered, rather than a personal subject in relationship with others and with God, an argument which has been advanced by the Anglican ethicist, Oliver O'Donovan

(O'Donovan, 1984, pp. 1–6). In my view, O' Donovan's distinction between person and artefact is helpful from a perspective of a Christian ethical evaluation of biomedical technology because it shows how the application of technology can seek to undermine the uniqueness of God's creative power, in favour of self-creation of the human body by humanity, where the body becomes an idol. Also, the treatment of the body as a "thing" rather than a person shows that indiscriminate application of biomedical technology to the body may be problematic for human dignity, even if not for personal autonomy. Even if a person chooses freely to apply some form of medical technology to themselves, it may undermine their dignity as a human being.

Yet some theologians have argued that the use of biomedical technology in human beings does not necessarily impair the expression of the *imago Dei* in humanity. Elaine Graham states that in a world where there is an evolutionary understanding of human life, concepts of humanity can no longer be fixed and absolute, and she argues that human beings enact the *imago Dei* when they engage in technological innovation (Graham, 2006). Graham reflects that just as humans are created in the image of God, yet are continuous with the animal world, so humans have always been "mixed up" and hybridised with the technologies that they use, which have become a part of them. What is happening in the material world, and what it means to be human, does not detract from human spiritual life, but it is a necessary pre-condition. She argues that, if the aspiration of being in the image of God is the Christian goal of conformation to Christ, then a right response to technology use would be humility, rather than hubris; in other words, technology would be used with care, in a way that respects the sovereignty of God and does not detract from God's ultimate purposes for humanity.

Theologians critical of transhumanism have suggested that the transhumanist view of humanity is characterised by a privatised, individualised attitude to human life, in which personal autonomy and exercise of the will concerning individual lifestyle choices plays a dominant part (see, e.g., Deane-Drummond, 2006). Transhumanism appears to place significant emphasis on the attributes of the individual human being, and the way in which they are used in the individual's interactions with the world. I would argue that this view of humanity is aligned largely with a substantive approach to the *imago Dei*, at the expense of the functional and relational approaches. But, as argued earlier, a human person is more complex than the sum of his or her substantive attributes – and should be, if they are to flourish in a world where they are one creature among many, a world where they must negotiate relationally with other creatures – human or otherwise – to achieve good ends which promote the flourishing of the whole creation.

This discussion shows that the different aspects of the *imago Dei* are important for a comprehensive understanding of how biomedical technologies might affect human flourishing in the future, in terms of valuing all people and the goods of human life for all. I will draw upon this analysis for the ethical evaluation of the case studies in Chapter 5. However, I will be assessing both past and future forms of technology by means of objective criteria. I have already introduced some general criteria for what constitutes a transhumanist technology, as proposed by the literature of the transhumanist movement. However, in the light of these theological criticisms of transhumanism, I will now return to the theological criteria that I briefly introduced in Chapter 1. I will discuss and define the criteria in more detail, giving a rationale for why I chose them.

2.8 Theological Criteria for Transhumanist Developments

To perform an ethical assessment of a proposed biomedical technology, the general criteria for what might constitute a transhumanist technology would need to be overlaid by some specific theological criteria, which would facilitate a Christian ethical evaluation of those technologies.

Earlier, I proposed a list of theological criteria for ethical assessment of future biomedical technologies, namely:

1 Is the project good news for the poor?
2 Is the project an attempt to be "like God" (in respect of Genesis 3v5) or does it conform to the image of God? (Genesis 1v26).
3 What attitude does the project embody towards the material world (including our own bodies)? And how does the technology affect the corporate "body" of society?
4 What attitude does the project embody towards past failures?
5 Does the technology enable unbridled autonomy in a negative manner?
6 Does the technology focus too much on the users' subjective experiences?

As discussed in the introduction, these criteria are a combination of Neil Messer's "diagnostic questions" of a biotechnology project (Messer, 2007, pp. 229–235), and Elaine Graham's theological critiques of transhumanism (Graham, 2006). I will now discuss the usefulness and applicability of these criteria.

The criteria proposed by Messer (1), 2), 3) a) and 4)) are useful because they have been proposed in the context of a study of ethical issues with biotechnology, and how biotechnology relates to the doctrine of creation, which is a good place to start to evaluate scientific interventions as material phenomena. The strengths of these criteria are that they are clearly ethical in nature (concerned with attitudes, justice and the goods of human life), and that they are firmly located in a Christian view of relationships between humanity and God, and within human society. The key weakness of Messer's criteria is that they do not explore the issue of personal autonomy which, as noted earlier on in this chapter, is likely to be a significant factor in an ethical discussion of transhumanist biomedical technologies, and which is an important principle of medical ethics as it has developed to date.

The criteria derived from Graham's work (3b), 5) and 6)) are not comprehensive in their scope but are significant in their impact. One concerns autonomy, which helpfully complements Messer's criteria, and which will be a useful tool to explore the role of autonomy in the use of transhumanist technologies. Another concerns subjectivity, which will be useful for exploring the phenomenon of the objectification of the human body by technology, at the expense of the human as a personal subject. The third, on embodiment, overlaps with Messer's criteria, but introduces the helpful additional concept of corporate "embodiment" as the community.

The next section provides a preliminary evaluation of the proposed transhumanist biomedical technologies listed earlier against these criteria.

2.9 Preliminary Evaluation of Transhumanist Technology

In the Introduction, we briefly considered five future technological interventions that transhumanists have proposed. They are as follows:

1 Medical nanotechnology – the use of microscopic particles, tools and robots to interact with the body for medical applications.
2 Genetic enhancements – including germ-line modifications.
3 Cybernetics – the use of prostheses and robotics to develop and enhance bodily function.
4 Cryonics – placing the human body in suspended animation using cryogenic techniques, so that a person can be revived in the distant future when radical new medical technologies are available.
5 Mind-Uploading – where all the information in the human brain is uploaded onto a computer, in order that a person can live on "in silico" rather than in a biological body.

In previous sections of the chapter, I have argued that approaches to transhumanism – philosophical, technological and ideological – are diverse and, although transhumanism is broadly aligned to secular modernity, the different approaches to transhumanism vary in their metaphysics and their epistemology.

However, the various technologies cited by scholars as transhumanist technologies are different technologically too, and have different effects on, and implications for, the human person. So, for example, the technological resources and processes used to enable genetic enhancements are different from those required for mind-uploading, and the specific implications for human life will be different. This section will evaluate these technologies, using the criteria defined in the previous sections.

In terms of the general criteria for transhumanist technologies, derived from the transhumanist literature, all the transhumanist technologies described – medical nanotechnology, genetic enhancements, cybernetics, cryonics and mind-uploading – fulfil the first two criteria, in that each is a technology (a material means of effecting a task or process) and each is a technology applied to the human person, to make a difference to human experience. Concerning the third criterion, that the technology is applied to the human person to improve human function, increase longevity and promote human flourishing, the situation is less clear. All these transhumanist technologies are certainly intended to have a beneficial effect on human function or longevity. However, because the interventions they propose are radical (some more so than others), it is less clear whether they can or will actually improve human flourishing, for reasons that will be explored in the forthcoming section. However, that the transhumanist technologies cited here fulfil these three criteria for a transhumanist technology is largely unremarkable, as these criteria are themselves derived from the transhumanist literature.

However, whether the fourth criterion applies – that the human subject has autonomy in the use of the technology, and that the technology is not applied in a coercive manner – is debatable. Individual users of these technologies may have the autonomy to choose to use these technologies at the outset, with an informed understanding of the risks involved. This is no different to informed consent to established medical treatments and procedures in the current healthcare system. However, as discussed by Michael Burdett, transhumanist technologies have the potential to effect radical changes to the human person at will, which elevates personal choice to a level of significance that it has not previously had in healthcare (Burdett, 2014, p. 5). The expansion of personal choice in the application of future radical technologies clearly has implications for the exercise of autonomy.

Consequently, if the consequences of the transhumanist technologies here are considered in more detail, concerns about autonomy and choice emerge. Medical nanotechnology is relatively unproblematic, although, as with all medical technologies that are highly specific in their biological actions, there may be unintended consequences, which may raise questions about the ongoing autonomy of the subject. However, genetic enhancements may well be chosen freely by a person but, if they are germ cell modifications which affect the genetic profile of that person's offspring, then the person's children and subsequent generations will be affected. These offspring cannot exercise autonomy because they did not choose the enhancement, and the enhancement is therefore applied to them in a coercive way. Cybernetics raises the issue of whether the person has full control over their cybernetic components; if an in-grafted robotic arm was used to commit an offence, would it be the responsibility of the person, or a fault with the prosthesis? Lawyers might attempt to argue the latter, in the person's defence. With cryonics, a person might freely consent to being cryogenically frozen so that they could avoid death from an incurable disease and remain in suspended animation until a cure was discovered. However, their life in suspended animation would then be in the hands of others and they would have no power of choice concerning the time and circumstances of their revival, even if it happened at all. With mind-uploading, a person might freely choose the procedure, but the procedure is radical and irreversible, and may lead to unintended consequences because the person has a disembodied existence, and these could have serious repercussions for life choices and personal autonomy, as highlighted in the previous section on autonomy in this chapter. These concerns with autonomy on the application of transhumanist technologies align well with Sparrow's comments about the deficiency of biomedical technology as a means of developing moral agency and reasoning, in comparison with education and culture.

The use of medical enhancements in the wider social and cultural context also has implications for personal autonomy. Societal trends and peer pressure may coerce an individual to have an enhancement that they might not be happy with personally. If the use of a certain enhancement is almost universal in society and the government recommends that enhancement because of its purported benefits for personal security, well-being and access to public services, it would be hard for an individual to choose not to have the enhancement, without good reason. This is analogous to, for example, the almost universal use of mobile phones in current society. In this situation, the use of medical enhancements by some individuals in the population may restrict the personal choices of other individuals. For example, if it was routine for all jockeys to have genetic enhancements that enabled them to have a small body size, significantly faster reactions and longevity and physical durability to enable them to have a racing career of over one hundred years, this would effectively restrict a career in horse racing to those who were thus enhanced, and would exclude those who were not.

Further ethical concerns about transhumanism become apparent if transhumanist technologies are assessed using the specific, ethical criteria (Messer, 2007, pp. 229–235; Graham, 2006).

First, is the project good news for the poor? All the technologies described above – nanotechnology, genetic enhancements, cybernetics, cryonics and mind-uploading – would be potentially resource-intensive, both in terms of materials and technical expertise. Even if they were all technically feasible at present, they would be very costly and would not be realistically available to citizens all over the world, but only to the wealthiest citizens of Europe and North America. For example, cryogenic preservation is still at an experimental stage and the Alcor Life Extension Foundation of Scottsdale, Arizona, offers this service for a minimum of $200,000 life insurance cover (Alcor, 2022). Even relatively modest biotechnological interventions that are routinely available now are relatively expensive, compared to the small molecule medicines of the "therapeutic revolution" era of the twentieth century, and therefore realistically available only through the health services of first world countries. Swindells argues that neither government prohibition nor an unfettered free market for biotechnology will support equity of access to these technologies, but some form of compromise is needed, in terms of government funding support

(Swindells, 2014). He also makes the important point that, like "hi-tech" medicines and biotechnology at present, future transhumanist technologies will need to be distributed at scale for costs of the technology to decrease.

Furthermore, when considering the impact of biomedical technology on the poor, various other ethical factors come into play, in addition to the basic affordability of the technology. If biomedical enhancements were used to support personal and societal well-being, then they may be good news for the poor, but if they were deployed by those in power for exploitation of vulnerable sectors of society or for social engineering, they would not be good news for the poor. Biomedical enhancements would be good news for the poor if regulation and health service resource allocation were such that the same enhancements could be offered to all in a society on an equal basis, so that all had the same socio-political opportunities.

Second, is the project an attempt to be "like God" (referring to Genesis 3v5) or does it conform to the image of God? (Genesis 1v26). As previously discussed, the *imago Dei* may be described substantively, functionally, relationally or eschatologically, and has a dynamic dimension. However, the vision of human life promoted by transhumanism, with its focus on the individual attributes of the human being, is consistent with an approach to the *imago Dei* that is largely substantive, and which does not reflect other approaches to the *imago Dei*, and so provides a distorted view of the human being. Indeed, it is ironic that the transhumanism movement, which is in part predicated on the evolution of humanity, reflects a substantive approach to the *imago Dei*, bearing in mind that such substantive approaches to the *imago Dei* are of less contemporary value, in part because of the insights of evolutionary biology.

As mentioned previously, the problems with transhumanism are: a) it is individualistic because it is concerned primarily with the attributes of the individual person (a similar criticism can be made of the substantive *imago Dei*); b) it focuses on human attributes, at the expense of other aspects of human life, such as relationships, culture and corporate identity and values, which are not simply based on individual attributes, and c) it provides an alternative, over-realised eschatology, which is excessively inward-looking and privatised and provides immortality now, but which does not deal with the reality of sin and human moral responsibility.

Moreover, Peters has argued that a major criticism of transhumanism is that it assumes that human nature is infinitely malleable and that the human being can be absolutely manipulated by technologies applied by humanity, to achieve the functional objectives of enhancement (Peters, 2006). This would suggest that, according to Messer's criteria, these transhumanist technologies are indeed an attempt to be like God, rather than to enable humanity to conform to the image of God. Some of the technologies described – for example, mind-uploading or cybernetics – represent highly visible and tangible attempts to manipulate human bodily life and to remake human beings in their own image, rather than God's image.

Third, what attitude does the project embody towards the material world, including our own bodies? Earlier in this chapter, I outlined the significance of the body and bodily life in Christian theology and referred to the material connotations of the *imago Dei* in Genesis 1v26. I have previously noted that transhumanists have differing attitudes to the material world (More, 2013). Some transhumanists are materialists in that they see the functions of the physical human body as the sum of all reality. However, some transhumanists are also functionalists, who believe that human mental function constitutes the person, and must be instantiated in a physical, material medium, but not necessarily a biological one. Some transhumanist scholars, such as Hans Moravec (Moravec, 1988, pp. 116–118), are unconcerned by the prospect of disembodiment, and are happy to rely on thought for identity (pattern identity) whereas others, such as Katherine Hayles (Hayles, 1999, p. 1), see embodiment as an essential prerequisite of humanity, regardless of what other technologies might be employed for human enhancement.

The transhumanist technologies described here demonstrate this variation of views concerning embodiment. Medical nanotechnology and genetic enhancement are both technologies that elicit beneficial effects in and through the functioning of the human body and may be considered affirming of human embodiment. In fact, cryogenic preservation is concerned with preserving the human body at any cost, even when the body is threatened with incurable disease or apparently irreversible degeneration. On the contrary, however, cybernetics appears to be a technology that does not affirm the human body. The premise of cybernetics is that parts of the human body can be replaced by prostheses and robotic enhancements that will function better than – or differently to – the original biological body parts. For some transhumanism advocates, for whom personhood is largely related to functional ability, the concept of the cyborg – the human/robot hybrid – would be seen positively and would present no specific problems. Nevertheless, as Hayles observes, the concept of the cyborg destabilises established ways of understanding human ontology (Hayles, 1999, p. 21), so might prompt some objections from Christian and other religious commentators on the grounds of natural law.

At the far end of the anti-embodiment spectrum is the proposed transhumanist technology of mind-uploading, where the information in a person's mind is uploaded onto a computer, so they can live life *in silico*, without a human body. With this technology, the human body is totally deprecated, and morphological freedom is prioritised over human embodiment. As noted above, transhumanists who advocate mind-uploading, such as Ray Kurzweil and Hans Moravec, deal with the problem of maintaining personal identity in a disembodied existence by appealing to a distinction between *body identity*, where the person is defined by the material matter of their human body, and *pattern identity*, where a person is defined by their thought patterns and processes. However, Kurzweil admits that disembodiment is problematic for human existence, given that many human experiences are essentially bodily experiences – for example, eating, sex and sport – and are meaningless without a body. Furthermore, as argued previously, his proposals for complex sensory interfaces to mediate these experiences to a disembodied mind are aspirational and overly optimistic.

Elaine Graham notes that the problem with transhumanist technologies which interfere with the integrity of the individual body is that they therefore have a disruptive effect on the corporate body – the community. In relating changes to the individual body to changes in the corporate body of the community, Graham wisely roots this discussion in the concept of the church as the body of Christ, as found for example in Romans 12v4–8, 1 Corinthians 12 or Ephesians 4v4–13. I would argue that her theological concern here is warranted with the transhumanist technologies being considered. Regardless of their specific objectives, all the transhumanist technologies described here – nanotechnology, genetic enhancements, cybernetics, cryonics and mind-uploading – affect the structure and functioning of the human body in one way or another, and bring about significant changes in human life because of this – in terms of longevity, freedom from disease, but also in terms of motor and cognitive function. Although these are mainly effects on the individual human body, they also have an impact on the corporate body of society, as the previous discussion in this chapter on the social ethical implications of enhancement have shown – for example, the implications of biomedical enhancement for health and welfare provision, for working patterns, and for marriage as an important institution in human society. Given the discussion about embodiment earlier in this chapter, Graham's concerns about the implications of transhumanist technologies on both individual and corporate bodily life are therefore justified.

Fourth, what attitude does the project embody towards past failures? From a Christian perspective, the most appropriate way for scientists and technologists to view past failures, especially those that have been exploitative or at great human cost, would be an attitude of humility to future endeavours. At first sight, this question seems to be pitching transhumanist hubris against Christian humility but a close inspection of the meaning and scope of humility as a Christian grace suggests that this issue is more complex. In her definition of humility, Helen Oppenheimer notes that pride is a sin, but humility is not so much a virtue as a grace (a gift from God) (Oppenheimer, 1986, p. 284). She highlights the ambivalence of humility, drawing on Aquinas's assertion that it is possible to be proud of being humble, and she asks whether humility might be ruined by its attainment. She also notes the strange situation that, according to Matthew 23v12, the reward for humility seems to be exaltation, which suggests that humility might be a means to a non-humble objective, rather than a virtue in itself. Consequently, she wonders whether humility can ever be a lasting moral good of human life. Helpfully, however, she identifies five important components of humility:

1 It should not be false,
2 It should not be about self-loathing,
3 It should be an objective lowliness – acknowledging one's unimportance as an individual, which paradoxically is important to God,
4 It should concern reverence in acknowledging glory not one's own (1 Corinthians 4v7),
5 It should be ultimately about agape – self-emptying for the sake of others (Philippians 2v5–11). There is a paradoxical self-confidence in this kind of humility, in that the individual can afford to take delight in attending to the needs of others (which would be a good motive for using biotechnology well according to Messer's fourth criterion).

I would argue that these components are helpful in describing the kind of humility needed to act responsibly in a technological world. Of prime importance is Oppenheimer's fourth element – humility is reverence in acknowledging a glory that is not our own – in other words, the detailed scientific processes underpinning the natural world, a world that was ultimately created by God, not humanity. A common theme in the Psalms is that a natural response of humanity to the created world is one of wonder and awe – as illustrated, for example, in Psalm 8 and Psalm 19. From this sense of awe would develop the response: of knowing one's limitations when faced with the glory and mystery of the universe and also living – and making biomedical decisions – as part of a community, rather than as an individual. This kind of humility can be set in an explicitly Christian framework; Elaine Graham argues that, if the aspiration of being in the image of God is the Christian goal of conformation to Christ, then a right response to technology use would be humility, rather than hubris (Graham, 2006).

However, a study of the various strands of transhumanism suggests that many of these aspects of humility are absent. On the contrary, main advocates of transhumanism speak in terms of throwing off the shackles of human limitation. More's famous "No more gods, no more faith ... the future belongs to post-humanity", epitomises a human-centredness that allows no wonder or awe in response to a greater glory. Individualism and individualistic autonomy are an important part of the transhumanist endeavour, and these negate the humility of community living – and community bioethical decision-making. All the transhumanist technologies mentioned above could, depending on how they are used, represent the human Promethean desire to rebel against "given" human nature.

Fifth, do transhumanist medical technologies enable unbridled autonomy in a negative manner? This is partly true in that the radical nature of transhumanist technologies and their ability to make profound changes to the human experience makes personal choice a far more significant factor in decision-making about enhancements than it has been previously in healthcare. However, as argued earlier in this chapter, it is debatable whether personal autonomy can be maintained during all stages of technology use due to the nature of the technologies and their unintended consequences. It is not true, therefore, to say that transhumanist technologies enable "unbridled autonomy" Furthermore, transhumanist technologies need not be chosen in a "negative manner". A person's attitude to the use of technology is important, as seen above; an attitude of humility, rather than hubris, is more in keeping with scriptural descriptions of the wonder of creation (Psalm 8, Psalm 19), and the limits of human wisdom (Isaiah 55v8–9). Furthermore, there are many instances in medicine at present where biomedical technology can be intentionally adopted and used in a positive way, so this could equally apply to future technologies.

Sixth, does the technology focus too much on the users' subjective experiences? This seems to be a valid criticism of transhumanist technologies – these technologies may be applied according to the individual's will, to render the body an object and to enhance the subjective human experience. As previously discussed, absolute personal choice and autonomy in choosing enhancements is a major component of transhumanist thought (World Transhumanist Association, 2013), and this has been strongly criticised by opponents of transhumanism, because of the potentially detrimental effects of the technologies on society, due to the self-centred – and subjective – choices of individuals (McNamee and Edwards, 2006)

However, the irony is that, although transhumanist technologies enhance the personal, subjective experience, they are ultimately problematic because they objectify the human body, so that the body is in danger of becoming an artefact to be engineered and manipulated at will, rather than a human person (Miccoli, 2010, pp. 123–133). Anglican theologian, Oliver O'Donovan highlights this issue in his exploration of the distinction between person and artifice in the application of reproductive technologies (O'Donovan, 1984, pp. 1–6). By rendering a human person as a product or artifice to be engineered, rather than someone who is in relationship with a personal God, they are depersonalised, and their body is objectified, instead of having true personhood, as a personal subject.

In this chapter, I have reviewed the various approaches to transhumanism, and outlined the major religious and ethical critiques of them. I have outlined general and specific (theological) criteria with which to assess transhumanist developments. I have shown, in a preliminary evaluation of various transhumanist proposals, that transhumanism is mixed – both in terms of its metaphysical and epistemological claims, and in terms of its ethical goods for humanity. Transhumanist technologies may ostensibly provide some benefits, in terms of improvement of human function and longevity, and these benefits may be proposed and applied with good intentions. However, on application of the criteria, various problems and complexities emerge, and it is questionable whether these technologies truly enable human flourishing from a perspective of Christian social and medical ethics.

The next two chapters will describe the development of two important areas of therapeutics over the last 60 years during the "therapeutic revolution" era – the oral contraceptive pill and selective serotonin reuptake inhibitor (SSRI) antidepressants. Each chapter will evaluate these developments against the criteria for a transhumanist technology, as outlined above, and will consider the ethical issues presented by the therapeutic case and the extent to which it is a transhumanist development of its time, according to the criteria. The findings of the case studies will then inform an ethical re-evaluation of transhumanism.

Notes

1 This aligns with the holistic view of health associated with Christian healing (see Lawrence W. Althouse, "Healing and Health in the Judaic-Christian Experience: A Return to Holism", *Journal of Holistic Nursing*, 3 (1985), pp. 19–24.
2 The idea of correction of creation is problematic theologically in that it calls into question the perfection of creation and the workmanship of God, and it implies that humanity can make decisions about what is "correct" in humanity.
3 As envisaged by the corporate element of the Jewish idea of *shalom*.
4 See the discussion of *theosis*, in relation to the *imago Dei*, later in this chapter.
5 The problems of bio-conservatism, compared to biotechnological libertarianism, are explored in Chapters 5 and 6.
6 Philosopher, Bernard Williams has argued from human experience and desire that, even if immortality were conceivable, it would be intolerable. See Bernard Williams, "The Makropulos Case: Reflections on the Tedium of Immortality", in *Problems of the Self: Philosophical Papers – 1956–1972* (Cambridge: Cambridge University Press, 1973), pp. 82–100.
7 See, for example, Alfred Tauber, "Sick autonomy", *Perspectives in Biology and Medicine*, 46 (2003), pp. 484–495, and Natalie Stoljar. "Informed consent and relational conceptions of autonomy", *Journal of Medicine and Philosophy*, 36 (2011), pp. 375–384.
8 For example, Savulescu, *The Human Prejudice*, pp. 211–250.
9 This is significant for the Roman Catholic church's opposition to hormonal contraception, as discussed in Chapter 3.
10 With Baptism, the Eucharist is one of the two dominical sacraments (the sacraments instituted by Christ), and marriage is a sacrament of the Roman Catholic church.
11 Westermann has given an overview of the exegetical issues with the Gen 1v26–28 text in an excursus in his commentary of Genesis (Claus Westermann, *Genesis 1–11: A Continental Commentary*, translated by J.J. Scullion (Minneapolis: Fortress, 1994), p. 144.
12 Middleton draws on Von Rad's exegesis of *imago Dei* in Genesis 1; the *imago Dei* in humanity expresses the authority and purpose of God in the world, in the same way as the statue of the king in a town would represent the rule and authority of the king in that place in the societies of the Ancient Near East.
13 The idea of *theosis* has been developed in the Orthodox tradition.
14 The theologian, Ruth Page, makes a similar argument (Ruth Page, "The Human Genome and the Image of God", in *Brave New World? Theology, Ethics and the Human Genome*, edited by Celia Deane-Drummond (London: T and T Clark, 2003), pp. 68–85).
15 Wenham notes that possible roots of the word *tselem* (image) include "to cut or hew" (from Arabic), which fits well with the idea of the image of God as a material representation.

References

Alfred Archer, "Moral Enhancement and Those Left Behind", *Bioethics*, 30 (2016), pp. 500–10.
Anke Bouzenita, "The Most Dangerous Idea: Islamic Deliberations on Transhumanism", *Danilfunun Ilahiyat*, 29 (2018), pp. 201–228.
Apolos Landa, "Shalom and Eirene: The Full Framework for Health Care", *Christian Journal for Global Health*, 1 (2014), pp. 57–59.
Alistair McFadyen, *The Call to Personhood: A Christian Theory of the Individual in Social Relationships* (Cambridge: Cambridge University Press, 1990).
Alcor Marketing Information, http://www.alcor.org/BecomeMember/scheduleA.html, (accessed October 2022).
Anthony Miccoli, *Post-human Suffering and the Technological Embrace* (Lanham: Lexington, 2010).
Arthur Peacocke, *Theology for a Scientific Age* (London: SCM, 1990).
Alfred Tauber, "Sick Autonomy", *Perspectives in Biology and Medicine*, 46 (2003), pp. 484–495.
Adriana Warmbier, "Moral Enhancement: Enhancing Motivational Processes and Agent-Based Ethics", in *The Idea of Excellence and Human Enhancement: Reconsidering the Debate on Transhumanism in Light of Moral Philosophy and Science*, edited by Adriana Warmbier (Berlin: Peter Long, 2018), pp. 177–198.
Adam Willows, "Supplementing Virtue: The Case for a Limited Theological Transhumanism", *Theology and Science*, 15 (2017), pp. 177–187.
Brian Earp, "Psychedelic Moral Enhancement", *Royal Institute of Philosophy Supplement*, 83 (2018), pp. 415–439.
Benedikt Paul Göcke, "Christian Cyborgs: A Plea for Moderate Transhumanism", *Faith and Philosophy*, 34 (2017): 347–364.
Benedikt Ley, Corinna Ogonowski, Jan Hess, Tim Reichling, Lin Wan and Volker Wulf, "Impacts of New Technologies on Media Usage and Social Behaviour in Domestic Environments", *Behaviour and Information Technology*, 33 (2014), pp. 815–828.
Bernd Oberdorfer, "The Dignity of Human Personhood and the Concept of the Image of God", in *The Depth of the Human Person: A Multidisciplinary Approach*, edited by Michael Welker (Grand Rapids: Eerdmans, 2014), pp. 265–272.
Brent Waters, "Saving Us from Ourselves: Christology, Anthropology and the Seduction of Posthuman Medicine", in *Future Perfect?: God, Medicine and Human Identity*, edited by Celia Deane-Drummond and Peter Manley Scott (London: T and T Clark International, 2006a), pp. 183–195.
Brent Waters, *From Human to Posthuman: Christian Theology and Technology in a Postmodern World* (Farnham: Ashgate, 2006b).
Brent Waters, *This Mortal Flesh: Incarnation and Bioethics* (Grand Rapids: Brazos Press, 2009).
Bernard Williams, "The Makropulos Case: Reflections on the Tedium of Immortality", in *Problems of the Self: Philosophical Papers – 1956–1972* (Cambridge: Cambridge University Press, 1973), pp. 82–100.
Celia Deane-Drummond, "Future Perfect? God, the Transhuman Future and the Quest for Immortality", in *Future Perfect? God, Medicine and Human Identity*, edited by Celia Deane-Drummond and Peter Manley Scott (London: T and T Clark International, 2006), pp. 168–182.

Celia Deane-Drummond, "In God's Image and Likeness: From Reason to Revelation in Humans and Other Animals", in *Questioning the Human: Toward a Theological Anthropology for the Twenty-first Century*, edited by Lieven Boeve, Yves De Maeseneer and Ellen Van Stichel (Oxford: Oxford University Press, 2014), pp. 74–75.

Carl Elliot, "The Tyranny of Happiness: Ethics and Cosmetic Psychopharmacology", in *Enhancing Human Traits: Ethical and Social Implications*, edited by Erik Parens (Washington DC: Georgetown University Press, 2000).

Christopher Southgate, "Stewardship and its Competitors: A Spectrum of Relationships Between Humans and the Non-Human Creation", in *Environmental Stewardship: Critical Perspectives – Past and Present*, edited by R.J. Berry (London: T and T Clark, 2006), pp. 185–195.

Claus Westermann, *Genesis 1–11: A Continental Commentary*, translated by J.J. Scullion (Minneapolis: Fortress, 1994).

Delbert Burkett, *An Introduction to the New Testament and the Origins of Christianity* (Cambridge: Cambridge University Press, 2019).

D. David DeGrazia, "Prozac, Enhancement, and Self-Creation", *Hastings Center Report*, 30 (2000), pp. 34–40.

Donna Haraway, *Simians, Cyborgs and Women: The Reinvention of Nature* (New York: Routledge, 1991).

David Hume, *A Treatise of Human Nature*, edited by L.A. Selby-Bigge (Oxford: Clarendon Press, 1978).

Daniel Rizutto and Joshua Frost, "Transhumanism and Cognitive Enhancement", in *The Routledge Companion for Religion and Science*, edited by Haag, Peterson and Spezzo (New York: Routledge, 2012), pp. 569–577.

Elaine Graham, "In Whose Image? Representations of Technology and the Ends of Humanity", in *Future Perfect? God, Medicine and Human Identity*, edited by Celia Deane-Drummond and Peter Manley Scott (London: T and T Clark International, 2006), pp. 56–69.

Elizabeth Moltmann-Wendel, *I am my Body: New Ways of Embodiment*, translated by John Bowden (London: SCM, 1994).

Eugenia Torrance, "Acquiring Incorruption: Maximian *Theosis* and Scientific Transhumanism", *Studies in Christian Ethics*, 32 (2019), pp. 177–186.

Fereidoun M. Esfandiary and FM-2030, *Are You a Transhuman? Monitoring and Stimulating Your Personal Rate of Growth in a Rapidly Changing World* (New York: Warner, 1989).

Francis Fukuyama, *Our Posthuman Future: Consequences of the Biotechnology Revolution* (New York: Farrar, Strauss and Giroux, 2002).

Fox Swindells, "Economic Inequality and Human Enhancement Technology", *Humana Mente Journal of Philosophical Studies*, 26 (2014), pp. 213–222.

Fernando Vidal, "Brains, Bodies, Selves, and Science: Anthropologies of Identity and the Resurrection of the Body", *Critical Inquiry*, 28 (2002), p. 940.

George Ghergikov, "Transhumanism and the Western Monotheistic Religions", *Balkan Journal of Philosophy*, 12 (2020), pp. 37–50.

Guy Kahane and Julian Savulescu, "Normal Human Variation: Refocussing the Enhancement Debate", *Bioethics*, 29 (2015), pp. 133–143.

Geoffrey Redmond, "Extreme Longevity: Insights from Three Chinese Spiritual Traditions", in *Religion and Transhumanism: The Unknown Future of Human*

Enhancement, edited by Calvin Mercer and Tracy Trothen (Santa Barbara: Praeger, 2015), pp. 149–160.

Gregory Stock and Daniel Callahan, "Debates: Point-Counterpoint: Would Doubling the Human Life Span Be a Net Positive?" *Journals of Gerontology Series A: Biological Sciences and Medical Sciences*, 59 (2004), pp. B554–B559.

Gordon Wenham, *World Biblical Commentary: Genesis - Volume 1* (Waco: Word Books, 1987).

Gregor Wolbring, "Nanotechnology and the Transhumanization of Health, Medicine, and Rehabilitation", *Controversies in Science and Technology*, 3 (2010), pp. 290–303.

Heidi Campbell and Mark Walker, "Religion and Transhumanism: Introducing a Conversation", *Journal of Evolution and Technology*, 14 (2005), pp. i–xv.

Hannah Maslen, Nadira Faulmüller and Julian Savulescu, "Pharmacological Cognitive Enhancement—How Neuroscientific Research Could Advance Ethical Debate", *Frontiers in Systems Neuroscience*, 8 (2014), p. 107.

Hans Moravec, *Mind Children: The Future of Robot and Human Intelligence* (Cambridge: Harvard University Press, 1988).

Helen Oppenheimer, "Humility", in *A New Dictionary of Christian Ethics*, edited by John MacQuarrie and James Childress (London: SCM, 1986), p. 284.

Hava Tirosh-Samuelson, "Utopianism and Eschatology: Judaism Engages Transhumanism", in *Religion and Transhumanism: The Unknown Future of Human Enhancement*, edited by Calvin Mercer and Tracy Trothen (Santa Barbara: Praeger, 2015), pp. 261–280.

Ian G. Barbour, *Religion and Science: Historical and Contemporary Issues* (London: SCM, 1998).

Ingmar Persson and Julian Savulescu, "Moral Hardwiring and Moral Enhancement", *Bioethics*, 31 (2017), pp. 286–295.

Jan Christoph Bublitz and Reinhard Merkel, "Autonomy and Authenticity of Enhanced Personality Traits", *Bioethics*, 23 (2009), pp. 360–374.

John Christman, "Autonomy in Moral and Political Philosophy", *Stanford Encyclopaedia of Philosophy*, 2015, https://plato.stanford.edu/entries/autonomy-moral/ (accessed April 2019).

James Hughes, "The Compatibility of Religious and Transhumanist Views of Metaphysics, Suffering, Virtue and Transcendence in an Enhanced Future", *Director*, 860 (2007), pp. 297–2376.

J. Wentzel Van Huyssteen, *Alone in the World? Human Uniqueness in Science and Theology* (Grand Rapids: Eerdmans, 2006).

John Kilner, *Dignity and Destiny: Humanity in the Image of God* (Grand Rapids: Eerdmans, 2015).

Jonathan Lipps, "The *Imago Dei* vs The *Imago Machinae*" (Vancouver: Regent College Students Association, 2020).

John Stuart Mill, "On Liberty", in *John Stuart Mill: A Selection of his Works* (London: Palgrave, 1966).

Julian Savulescu, "Procreative Beneficence: Why We Should Select the Best Children", *Bioethics*, 15 (2001), pp. 413–426.

Julian Savulescu, "The Human Prejudice and the Moral Status of Enhanced Beings: What Do We Owe the Gods?", in *Human Enhancement*, edited by Julian Savulescu and Nick Bostrom (Oxford: Oxford University Press, 2009), pp. 211–250.

Julian Savulescu and Ingmar Persson, "Moral Enhancement, Freedom and the God Machine", *The Monist*, 95 (2012), pp. 399–421.

Jacqui Stewart, *Reconstructing Science and Theology in Postmodernity* (Aldershot: Ashgate, 2000).

Jeanine Thweatt Bates, *Cyborg Selves: A Theological Anthropology of the Post Human* (Burlington: Ashgate, 2012).

Karl Barth, *Church Dogmatics* (Edinburgh: T and T Clark, 1957), Vol. III, Part 2.

Karl Rahner, "Natural Science and Reasonable Faith", *Theological Investigations*, 21 (2004), pp. 2–3.

Lawrence W. Althouse, "Healing and Health in the Judaic-Christian Experience: A Return to Holism", *Journal of Holistic Nursing*, 3 (1985), pp. 19–24.

Leon Kass, "L'Chaim and Its Limits: Why Not Immortality?", *First Things*, May (2001), pp. 17–24.

Leon Morris, "Resurrection", in *New Bible Dictionary*, edited by Iain Marshall, Alan Millard, James Packer and Donald Wiseman (Leicester: IVP, 1996), pp. 1011–1012.

Michael Burdett, *Technology and the Rise of Transhumanism* (Cambridge: Grove, 2014).

Mariia Hupala, "Motion of Human Nature towards *imago Dei* in the thought of Maximus the Confessor", *Vox Patrum*, 75 (2020), pp. 201–228.

Michael LaTorra, "What Is Buddhist Transhumanism?", *Theology and Science*, 13 (2015), pp. 219–229.

Markus Lipowicz, "Transhumanism and Christianity: A Ratzingerian Approach to the Concept of Biotechnological Human Enhancement", *Religion and Theology*, 27 (2020), pp. 47–73.

M.J. McNamee and S.D. Edwards, "Transhumanism, Medical Technology and Slippery Slopes", *Journal of Medical Ethics*, 32 (2006), pp. 513–518.

Max More, "The Philosophy of Transhumanism", in *The Transhumanist Reader: Classical and Contemporary Essays on the Science, Technology and Philosophy of the Post-Human Future*, edited by Max More and Natasha Vita-More (Chichester: Wiley Blackwell, 2013), pp. 1–17.

Mark Murphy, "The Natural Law Tradition in Ethics", in *Stanford Encyclopaedia of Philosophy* (2019), https://plato.stanford.edu/entries/natural-law-ethics/ (Accessed September 2020).

Michael Northcott, "Concept Art, Clones and Co-Creators: The Theology of Making", *Modern Theology*, 21 (2005), pp. 219–236.

Michael Shapiro, "Performance Enhancement and Legal Theory", in *The Transhumanist Reader: Classical and Contemporary Essays on the Science, Technology and Philosophy of the Post-Human Future*, edited by Max More and Natasha Vita-More (Chichester: Wiley-Blackwell, 2013), pp. 281–283.

Michael Tennison, "Moral Transhumanism: The Next Step", *Journal of Medicine and Philosophy*, 37 (2012), pp. 405–416.

Matthew Zaro Fisher, "More Human than the Human? Towards a "Transhumanist" Christian Theological Anthropology", in *Religion and Transhumanism: The Unknown Future of Human Enhancement*, edited by Calvin Mercer and Tracy Trothen (Santa Barbara: Praeger, 2015), pp. 23–38.

Nick Bostrom, "Human Genetic Enhancements: A Transhumanist Perspective", *Journal of Value Inquiry*, 37 (2004), pp. 493–506.

Nick Bostrom, "Transhumanist Values", *Journal of Philosophical Research*, 30 (Supplement) (2005a), pp. 3–14.
Nick Bostrom, "A History of Transhumanist Thought", *Journal of Evolution and Technology*, 14 (2005b), pp. 1–25.
N. Katherine Hayles, *How We Became Posthuman: Virtual Bodies in Cybernetics, Literature and Informatics* (Chicago and London: University of Chicago Press, 1999).
Noreen Herzfeld, *In Our Image: Artificial Intelligence and the Human Spirit* (Minneapolis: Fortress, 2002).
Neil Levy, Thomas Douglas, Guy Kahane, Sylvia Terbeck, Philip J. Cowen, Miles Hewstone and Julian Savulescu, "Are You Morally Modified? The Moral Effects of Widely Used Pharmaceuticals", *Philosophy, Psychiatry and Psychology*, 21 (2014), pp. 111–125.
Neil Messer, *Selfish Genes and Christian Ethics: Theological and Ethical Reflections on Evolutionary Biology* (London: SCM, 2007).
Neil Messer, "Bioethics and Practical Theology: The Example of Reproductive Medicine", *International Journal of Practical Theology*, 21 (2017), pp. 291–314.
Natalie Stoljar. "Informed Consent and Relational Conceptions of Autonomy", *Journal of Medicine and Philosophy*, 36 (2011), pp. 375–384.
Ng Kam Weng, "The Image of God, Human Dignity, and Vocation", in *Humanity – Texts and Contexts: Christian and Muslim Perspectives*, edited by Michael Ipgrave and David Marshall (Washington, DC: Georgetown University Press, 2001), pp. 11–12.
Oscar Cullmann, *Immortality of the Soul or Resurrection of the Dead* (London: Epworth, 1958).
Oliver O'Donovan, *Begotten, or Made?* (Oxford: Clarendon, 1984).
Onora O'Neill, *Autonomy and Trust in Bioethics* (Cambridge: Cambridge University Press, 2002).
Philip Hefner, *The Human Factor: Evolution, Culture, and Religion* (Minneapolis: Fortress, 1993), pp. 255–277.
Patrick Hopkins, "Is Enhancement Worthy of Being a Right?", in *The Transhumanist Reader: Classical and Contemporary Essays on the Science, Technology and Philosophy of the Post-Human Future*, edited by Max More and Natasha Vita-More (Chichester: Wiley-Blackwell, 2013), p. 351.
Paul Ramsey, *The Patient as Person* (Newhaven: Yale University Press, 1970).
Pei-hua Huang, "Authenticity, Autonomy and Enhancement", *Desiderata*, 7 (2015), pp. 39–52.
Ronald Bailey, "For Enhancing People", in *The Transhumanist Reader: Classical and Contemporary Essays on the Science, Technology and Philosophy of the Post-Human Future*, edited by Max More and Natasha Vita-More (Chichester: Wiley-Blackwell, 2013) pp. 327–344.
Ronald Cole-Turner, "Towards a Theology for the Age of Biotechnology", in *Beyond Cloning: Religion and the Remaking of Humanity*, edited by Ronald Cole-Turner (Harrisburg PA: Trinity Press International, 2001).
Robert Freitas, "Welcome to the Future of Medicine", in *The Transhumanist Reader: Classical and Contemporary Essays on the Science, Technology and Philosophy of the Post-Human Future*, edited by Max More and Natasha Vita-More (Chichester: Wiley-Blackwell, 2013), pp. 67–72.

Raanan Gillon, "Autonomy and the Principle of Respect for Autonomy", *British Medical Journal*, 209 (1985), pp. 1806–1808.
Ray Kurzweil, *The Age of Spiritual Machines: When Computers Exceed Human Intelligence* (New York: Penguin, 1999).
Ruud ter Meulen, "Human Enhancement: A Policy Perspective for the European Union", in *Human Enhancement: Scientific, Ethical and Theological Aspects from a European Perspective*, edited by Theo Boer and Richard Fischer. Church and Society Commission of CEC (2013), pp. 9–12.
Richard J. Middleton, *The Liberating Image: The Imago Dei in Genesis 1* (Grand Rapids: Brazos Press, 2005).
Ruth Page, "The Human Genome and the Image of God", in *Brave New World? Theology, Ethics and the Human Genome*, edited by Celia Deane-Drummond (London: T and T Clark, 2003), pp. 68–85.
Robert Sparrow, "Better Living through Chemistry? A Reply to Savulescu and Persson on Moral Enhancement", *Journal of Applied Philosophy*, 31 (2014), pp. 23–32.
Sarah Ahamad, Palak Madan and Avinash Kumar Singh, "Transhumanism in India: Past, Present and Future", in *The Transhumanism Handbook*, edited by Newton Lee (Cham: Springer, 2019), pp. 701–714.
Sarah Buss, "Personal Autonomy", *Stanford Encyclopaedia of Philosophy*, 2018, https://plato.stanford.edu/entries/personal-autonomy/ (accessed April 2018).
Steve Fuller and Veronika Lipinska, "Proactionary Theology: Discovering the Art of "God-playing"", in *The Proactionary Imperative: A Foundation for Transhumanism* (Basingstoke: Palgrave MacMillan, 2014), 44–62.
Stephen Garner, "Transhumanism and Christian Social Concern", *Journal of Evolution and Technology*, 14 (2005), pp. 29–43.
Sarah Hejazi, "Humankind, the Best of Molds: Islam Confronting Transhumanism", *Sophia*, 58 (2019), pp. 677–688.
Scott Midson, *Cyborg Theology: Humans, Technology and God* (London/New York: I.B. Tauris, 2018).
Stephen Pope, "Natural Law and Christian Ethics", in *Cambridge Companion to Christian Ethics*, edited by Robin Gill (Cambridge: Cambridge University Press, 2012), pp. 67–86.
Stephen Pope, "Theological Anthropology: Science and Human Flourishing", in *Questioning the Human: Toward a Theological Anthropology for the Twenty-First Century*, edited by Lieven Boeve, Yves De Maeseneer and Ellen Van Stichel (Oxford: Oxford University Press, 2014), pp. 16–17.
Stuart Ray Sarbacker, "Buddhist Medication and the Ethics of Human Augmentation", *Journal of the Japanese Association of Digital Humanities*, 5 (2020), pp. 61–83.
Steven Woolf, "Evidence-Based Medicine: A Historical and International Overview", *Proceedings of the Royal College of Physicians of Edinburgh*, 31 (2001), pp. 39–41.
Thomas Aquinas, "Summa Theologica Q90–94", 2010, https://www.documentacatholicaomnia.eu/03d/1225–1274,_Thomas_Aquinas,_Summa_Theologiae_%5B1%5D,_EN.pdf. (accessed September 2020).
Thomas Beauchamp, "The 'Four Principles' Approach to Health Care Ethics", in *Principles of Health Care Ethics*, edited by Richard Ashcroft, Angus Dawson, Heather Draper and John McMillan (Chichester: Wiley, 2007), pp. 3–10.

Thomas Douglas, "Moral Enhancement", *Journal of Applied Philosophy*, 25 (2008), pp. 228–245.
Ted Peters, "Techno-secularism, Religion, and the Created Co-creator", *Zygon*, 40 (2005), pp. 845–862.
Ted Peters, "Perfect Humans or Trans-Humans?", in *Future Perfect?: God, Medicine and Human Identity*, edited by Celia Deane-Drummond and Peter Manley Scott (London: T and T Clark International, 2006), pp. 15–32.
Ted Peters, "Imago Dei, DNA and the Transhumanist Way", *Theology and Science*, 16 (2018), pp. 353–362.
Toni Saad, "The History of Autonomy in Medicine from Antiquity to Principlism", *Medicine, Health Care and Philosophy*, 21 (2018), pp. 125–137.
Woody Evans, "If you see a cyborg in the road, kill the Buddha", *Journal of Evolution and Technology*, 24 (2014), pp. 92–97.
Wolfhart Pannenberg, *What is Man? Contemporary Anthropology in Theological Perspective*, translated by D.A. Priebe (Philadelphia: Fortress, 1970).
World Transhumanist Association, "The Transhumanist FAQ, v2.1", 2003, http://www.transhumanism.org/index.php/wta/faq21/81/ (Accessed August 2016).
World Transhumanist Association, "Transhumanist Declaration", in *The Transhumanist Reader: Classical and Contemporary Essays on the Science, Technology and Philosophy of the Post-Human Future*, edited by Max More and Natasha Vita-More (Chichester: Wiley-Blackwell, 2013), pp. 54–55.

3 New World, New People
The Contraceptive Pill

3.1 The Birth of the Contraceptive Pill

Previously, I have discussed the origins, claims and ideas of the transhumanism movement and developed a taxonomy of the transhumanism movement to illustrate the differing approaches and emphases of transhumanist scholars. I have also discussed social and theological ethical critiques of transhumanist technologies. Transhumanist technologies may be evaluated by objective criteria; general criteria, developed from the transhumanist literature, to determine whether a technology could be classified as transhumanist, but also specific, theological criteria, which Christian ethicists might use to evaluate a transhumanist technology, drawing on the work of Neil Messer and Elaine Graham. I have also made a preliminary ethical analysis of some specific transhumanist proposals to date using these objective criteria.

In the previous chapter, I found that although transhumanist technologies were applied to human beings with the stated aim of improving human flourishing, the use of these technologies was in some tension with Christian theological ethics. This is because their effects on personal autonomy are ambivalent, they have a variable attitude to embodiment, and they reflect a substantive approach to the *imago Dei,* at the expense of other approaches to the *imago Dei* which would define humanity more fully. While transhumanist technologies have the capacity to enhance a person's subjective experience, they also have the potential to objectify the human body. Furthermore, although the transhumanist movement maintains that users of these technologies have autonomy in choosing and adopting them, there are potential ethical concerns surrounding their equitable use and attitudes to their use in society.

This chapter presents the first of two case studies of previous therapeutic developments, which took place during the "therapeutic revolution" years (1950–1990) – the development of the oral contraceptive pill, which was introduced in 1960. This case study concerns the use of the oral contraceptive pill only, as first launched in 1960 and developed from that time, because this is what has had the greatest initial impact on society, and this is what the

DOI: 10.4324/9781003290421-4

Roman Catholic church significantly reacted to, with the publication of *Humanae Vitae* in 1968. This case study does not include other forms of hormonal contraception, such as depot injections (Depo-Provera) and implants (Norplant, NexPlanon, etc.).[1] In addition, abortion is out of the scope for discussion here. Although abortion, as a procedure, also has eugenic potential, and may be chemically mediated, some of the ethical considerations – for example, the motivations of the user – are quite different, and will not be considered here.

The first section of this chapter will describe the history of the oral contraceptive pill, discussing the events that led to its introduction and widespread use. The second section will discuss the effects of the pill on the lives of women and men, on marriage, and on society. It will then examine the Roman Catholic church's theological and ethical concerns with the pill following its introduction. Finally, the contraceptive pill will be assessed against the objective criteria I have proposed for evaluation of transhumanist technologies to determine the extent to which, in its time, the pill could have been regarded as a transhumanist development, and to evaluate it from the perspective of theological concerns about transhumanist technologies.

Although the practice of contraception has a long history, dating back to classical times (Wood and Suitters, 1970, pp. 202–223; Draper, 1965, pp. 55–66), the development of the oral contraceptive pill in the 1950s was highly significant, and has arguably represented a "contraceptive revolution", for two reasons (McLaren, 1990, p. 2). First, the pill was the first contraceptive technology that enabled the technology for contraception to be separated from the sex act itself, enabling greater romance and spontaneity in sex. Second, with the pill, the method of contraception was controlled by the female partner (McLaren, 1990, p. 2). This has enabled women to control their fertility and plan their families, in a way that had not been possible previously. Consequently, as well as its benefits to women, the contraceptive pill has had a significant impact on marriage, sexual politics and socioeconomic developments in the western world, which will be discussed later in this chapter.

The development of the pill was the result of a detailed understanding of the role of the sex hormones controlling the menstrual cycle – oestrogen and progesterone – following the isolated organ experiments in the nineteenth century, and the popularity of "organotherapy" for sexual disorders in the early twentieth century (Davis et al., 2005). Crucially, though, the development of the contraceptive pill as a marketed pharmaceutical product in the 1950s was only enabled by the ability of pharmaceutical manufacturers to produce these sex hormones synthetically, rather than from natural sources, and therefore to be able to produce them in large quantities (Sneader, 2005), a development that took place in the mid-twentieth century. The pill is significant in pharmaceutical medicine in that it was the first drug affecting the whole body ever to be given to a healthy population on a large scale (Jutte, 2008, pp. 288–290). Given its purpose and its mass distribution, it is therefore not surprising that the oral contraceptive pill has had far-reaching consequences for human society and culture.

However, in the 1950s, research into contraception was seen as a disreputable business, which neither the government nor the pharmaceutical industry would fund, and the public were reluctant to accept contraception research as a legitimate and respectable scientific activity (May, 2010, p. 16). Consequently, the story of how the first oral contraceptive pill reached the market in 1960 is a remarkable one, involving three key protagonists (May, 2010, p. 16). Margaret Sanger was a socialist and feminist from a working-class background, who had imagined the benefits to modern society of a contraceptive pill as long ago as 1912. Sanger's longtime friend, Katharine Dexter McCormick, was, by contrast, from a privileged background and was only the second woman to graduate from the Massachusetts Institute of Technology (MIT), where she studied biology. Sanger and McCormick believed that there was a need for a form of contraception that could be "managed entirely by the women who used it" (May, 2010, p. 22). The third protagonist, Gregory Pincus, was a reproductive biologist. Pincus had previously genetically altered a rabbit embryo in the laboratory and, although this experiment had been a significant scientific advance, he had been reviled by the media as an unscrupulous eugenicist. In 1950, Pincus was famously invited to a dinner party hosted by Margaret Sanger, where she asked him just how much the development of an oral contraceptive might cost (Jutte, 2008, p. 288). Pincus hazarded a guess at $2 million dollars – a substantial sum of money at the time – and Sanger subsequently asked her friend, Katherine McCormick, for the money. Consequently, the contraceptive pill was developed with no state or public funding (Draper, 1965, p. 220), which is remarkable considering the collaboration and investment that would be required for such a medical development at the current time.

To establish clinical trials, Pincus approached John Rock, a Boston gynaecologist and devout Catholic, who had been treating women with oestrogen/progestogen combinations for menstrual disorders. Rock immediately saw that a contraceptive pill had potential benefits for society, and he regarded oral contraception as a "natural" form of contraception, which did not trouble his Catholic conscience, a stance that would eventually bring him into conflict with the Catholic Church. Because of the lack of public support for contraceptive research, Rock was unable to recruit many volunteers for his clinical trials, and so various involuntary subjects were recruited to the trials – including 15 psychiatric inpatients from the Worcester State Hospital (May, 2010, pp. 23–26). Although the use of coerced subjects is not ethically acceptable by twenty-first-century standards of clinical research, it was commonplace in the 1950s. In due course, to enable the recruitment of larger numbers of subjects to the trials to improve their statistical power, Rock and his colleagues looked at recruiting for the trials in countries other than the United States. The island of Puerto Rico was chosen for the contraceptive trials as it had a dense population, living in poverty and disease, and therefore women there were longing for adequate birth control. In addition, there were no local laws against contraception, and birth control clinics had already been established in that country (May, 2010, pp. 23–25).

The first oral contraceptive pill, Enovid, produced by G.D. Searle and Co, was approved by the Food and Drugs Administration (FDA) and introduced to the American market in 1960 (McLaren, 1990, pp. 240–245). However, the oral contraceptive pill was considered too politically and morally sensitive for the British market at that time (May, 2010, pp. 32–33), and Searle's product (branded En*a*vid in the UK) was not introduced into British family planning clinics until 1961 (Szarewski and Guillebaud, 1991).

As might be expected with a hormonal medicine with a range of biological actions, the oral contraceptive pill has been shown to have various non-contraceptive beneficial effects too (Caserta et al., 2014). These include control of the menstrual cycle, alleviation of pre-menstrual tension (PMT), reduced incidences of ovarian, endometrial and colorectal cancer (Bahamondes et al., 2015), and possible beneficial effects on cardiovascular disease and depression (Mendoza and Sanchez-Borrego, 2014).

The contraceptive pill has been widely adopted in human society (Wood and Suitters, 1970, pp. 202–223). In 1962, two years after the pill was launched, 2 million women in the United States were taking it, and by 1964, 6.5 million American women were using oral contraception. Following its introduction in the United States, the pill began to be adopted in other developed countries. By 1966, an estimated 10 million women in the world were taking the oral contraceptive pill. In 2010, it was estimated that 10.6 million women – 28% of all women of reproductive age who were using contraception – were taking the contraceptive pill (Jones et al., 2012). This is despite varying pill use over the years, because of adverse events, and decreasing use of the pill in general over time due to recent development of long-acting injectable forms of hormonal contraception, and a revival of barrier contraception in the last 20 years, due to the risk of HIV and sexually transmitted diseases.

3.2 Flashpoint for Social Transformation – The Social and Cultural Impact of the Pill

Compared to some other medical developments during the therapeutic revolution years of the twentieth century – for example, specific antibiotic therapy or beta-blockers for cardiovascular diseases – widespread use of the contraceptive pill has not led to an appreciable reduction in mortality. Nevertheless, the availability of the oral contraceptive pill has had positive effects on women's health in other respects, due to its multisystemic actions, and it has had far-reaching societal effects beyond the individual user – on sexual practices and politics, relationships and family roles, and laws and policies (Tyrer, 1999). This section will explore these influences.

Social acceptance of oral contraception in western society was for a variety of socio-political and humanitarian reasons. Although Gregory Pincus and his colleagues explored the use of sex steroids for contraception as a scientific endeavour, they were very much a minority. On the contrary, Margaret Sanger and Katherine McCormick saw the pill in terms of its social effects and took a feminist view that oral contraception was a means of liberating women, and enabling women to take control of their contraceptive needs (May, 2010, pp. 1–5). Sanger saw "birth control", as she termed it, as a working-class rebellion, a method of avoiding supplying the capitalist market with the human resources it needed for a workforce (May, 2010, p. 16).[2] In 1950s America, as a result of the post-war baby boom, many were concerned about possible population explosion, and its consequent effects on poverty and social order (May, 2010, pp. 1–5). Although Malthus had brought the issues of excess fertility and over-population into public debate as far back as 1798, this issue took on a new political urgency in post-war America, because of the Cold War. Many US commentators reasoned that, if poverty could be alleviated through population control, then social unrest could be avoided, and the scourge of communism would be kept at bay. Conversely, however, some leading anti-communists in American society – for example, Senator Joseph McCarthy – saw contraception as a communist conspiracy to weaken the country (May, 2010, p. 42). Others, for example, the gynaecologist John Rock, who conducted clinical trials on the pill, advocated the pill for humanitarian reasons (McLaren, 1990, pp. 240–245). As a clinician, Rock had seen first-hand the suffering of women both in childbirth and with debilitating menstrual disorders, and he wanted to do something to alleviate that suffering, and to give women control of their fertility, for their health and well-being. However, despite the health, social and political issues, for many of the women who took the pill, their motivation was purely personal – they simply wanted the convenience of being in control of their own fertility (May, 2010, pp. 50–52).

Women have been the prime beneficiaries of the availability of the contraceptive pill. Louise Tyrer has claimed that being able to control the timing of childbearing has had positive consequences for women in respect of both mental and physical well-being (Tyrer, 1994). The pill is a highly effective contraceptive and is convenient to use. It does not have the unromantic connotations of barrier and spermicidal methods of contraception (Tyrer, 1994), and separates the contraceptive technology from the sex act, and so does not interfere with the intimacy of sex (May, 2010, pp. 1–5).

Most significantly, the pill was the first contraceptive method where the woman had control over the contraceptive process and the man was correspondingly absolved – or sometimes deprived – of this responsibility (McLaren, 1990, pp. 240–245). This is the exact opposite of the era prior to the pill, where the standard method of contraception was condoms, which were sourced and used by the man. Indeed, as it was controlled by the woman, the pill was the "ideal" method of contraception that Margaret

Sanger and Katharine McCormick had envisaged prior to its development (May, 2010, p. 22). Because it could be used by a woman without even the man's knowledge, the pill was liberating for women, and therefore celebrated by feminists (May, 2010, p. 22; Hartmann, 1995, p. 189).

Nevertheless, while the pill has undoubtedly revolutionised women's lives and provided various benefits to women – both medical and non-medical – it has not always been seen in a positive light by women. The pill is a prescribed medicine so, although the woman can take responsibility for using hormonal contraception, she does not have complete autonomy to do so, as the pill must be prescribed for her by a doctor (and, in the early years of marketing the pill, this would most likely have been a male doctor). Consequently, feminists (ironically) have also criticised the pill, claiming that it has been used as a means of objectifying and medicalising the female body, and that use of the pill has led to the disembodiment of women (Jutte, 2008, p. 111). Furthermore, it has been suggested that, far from emancipating women, the pill has, in fact, increased the extent to which women are exploited by men. With the arrival of the pill came what is referred to as the *coital imperative* – with the risk of unwanted pregnancy removed, there was no reason for a woman to withhold sex (Thatcher, 2011, p. 221). Consequently, in recent years, there has been considerable social pressure for young women to have penetrative sex with their partners in a way that was not expected in previous centuries (Thatcher, 2011, p. 214; Cook, 2004, pp. 1–3).

The development of the pill has also had a significant impact on the lives of men. May has pointed out that, for every woman taking the pill, there is at least one man involved too (May, 2010, pp. 4–5). The use of the pill has enabled a man to enjoy sex, free of the risk of pregnancy, and to leave the responsibility of contraception to his partner. However, while some men liked the freedom of not being liable to impregnate their partner, some found the power and autonomy the pill gave to their partner an affront to their masculine ego (May, 2010, pp. 8–10). For the man, loss of responsibility for contraception has been accompanied by loss of control of contraception. This loss of control has become even more apparent, in recent years, as contraceptive services have become more likely to be provided by female practitioners. Also, along with control over her fertility, the pill gave a woman control over her career and lifestyle, which her partner may have found threatening.

Consequently, the pill has had an impact on the marriage relationship, and roles in marriage. One popular argument often put forward is that oral contraception has fuelled the sexual revolution which has taken place since the 1960s, and has undermined marriage as an institution (Jutte, 2008, p. 111; Hartmann, 1995, p. 189). However, this is controversial; historians have maintained that sexual behaviour remained conservative during the 1960s, that pre-marital sex was largely with intended spouses and that sexual excesses came to prominence in later decades (Cook, 2004, p. 271).

The consensus view is that the "sexual revolution" would have taken place anyway, and that the pill was a trigger or catalyst (Jutte, 2008, p. 111). Furthermore, there is little evidence from the history of the development of the pill that it was intended to bring about a sexual revolution. First, the pill's protagonists did not intend to downplay the role of marriage and promote extramarital sexual activity. For example, John Rock was an influential advocate of the pill, yet he was a devout Catholic and a social conservative, who disapproved of sex outside marriage, and certainly did not envisage the use of the pill to facilitate multiple sexual relationships outside marriage (May, 2010, p. 122). Second, when the pill was first marketed, its use was restricted to married women only (May, 2010, p. 59). Third, in the mid-60s, marriage was still seen as the normal environment for sex; May cites a survey done at the University of Kansas in 1964, where the vast majority of women surveyed stated that they believed pre-marital sex was wrong (May, 2010, p. 80).

Another important question considered by social commentators concerning the pill is whether the availability of the pill has led to a greater level of sexual activity with multiple partners in society. The effect of the oral contraceptive pill on sexual behaviour has been debated ever since it was first introduced. Interestingly, however, there is very little information about this in the medical literature. A study was conducted by Linken and Wiener in 1970 looking at sexual behaviour in 44 males and 89 females (1970). This study found that the contraceptive pill was a predominant form of contraception in women who were classed as "promiscuous" (in this study, by the now conservative definition: more than one partner in a six-month period). However, the fact that the pill was the most commonly used form of contraceptive for all sexually active subjects in the study does not suggest a causal link between pill use and sexual activity with multiple partners, but rather that the pill is a form of contraception used by women who have sex with multiple partners. This is consistent with Helen Brooke's observation that sexual activity with multiple partners is a symptom of some other underlying issue (Cook, 2004, p. 289). While the contraceptive pill is often associated culturally with sexual activity with multiple partners (Caal et al., 2013), and opponents of deregulation of the pill are often concerned about this (Wynn and Trussell, 2006), there is no clear evidence that the use of the contraceptive pill has increased levels of sexual activity with multiple partners, above those that naturally occur. Indeed, the uncertain relationship between the advent of the contraceptive pill and the beginning of the so-called sexual revolution (May, 2010, p. 59), and the fact that sexual behaviours did not change radically in the years after the introduction of the pill (Cook, 2004, p. 271), suggest that the oral contraceptive pill in itself has not had a negative impact on human virtue, at least in terms of sexual behaviour.

Rather than facilitating sexual activity with multiple partners, oral contraception enables planned parenthood, which has the potential to promote marital stability through the health and well-being of both partners (Thatcher, 2011, pp. 218–219). Furthermore, the availability of contraception may contribute to positive moral choices within marriage (Thatcher, 2011, pp. 218–219). May contends that the pill has enabled couples to have good conversations about sex, arguing that the pill has liberated married sex, and contributed to a greater openness about matters relating to sex (May, 2010, p. 159).

Along with Prozac and SSRI antidepressants, which will be discussed in the next chapter, the contraceptive pill is arguably the pharmaceutical product that has had the most impact on popular culture. Notwithstanding the debate about whether the pill caused the sexual revolution, the pill has become a powerful *symbol* of the sexual revolution and was associated with utopian dreams – or dystopian fears – that sex was being liberated from marriage (May, 2010, p. 72). Back in the 1960s, many women were enamoured of the idea of the pill – the legend of the pill – even if they did not actually take it (Cook, 2004, p. 282). The idea of the pill was as potent as the reality. Yet, despite the pill's promise of uninhibited sex, interestingly, the theme of sexual liberation as a result of the pill was not greatly developed in the films and popular culture of the time (May, 2010, pp. 85–87). However, Cook has argued that the pill "precipitated a transformation in sexual mores" and that, by reducing the real, social and economic impact of pregnancy, the pill transformed attitudes to sexuality (Cook, 2004, p. 7). Similarly, May has described the pill as not simply a method of contraception, but "a flash point for major social transformation" (May, 2010, p. 168). Unsurprisingly, then, because of its implications for marriage and the family, use of the contraceptive pill has become a matter of ethical controversy for the churches. The next section will discuss the Roman Catholic church's response to the development of hormonal contraception in the twentieth century.

3.3 Contraception and the Church

Because of the importance of procreation for marriage and family life, and the perceived moral implications of interfering with procreation, Christian churches have historically been opposed to contraception. Childress reports that, prior to the twentieth century, Christian churches prohibited contraception on natural law grounds because procreation is an important end of marriage, and of sexual intercourse in marriage, and that contraception prevents marriage being directed towards that natural end (Childress, 2001, pp. 288–289). Previously, I have discussed natural law, and the problems associated with it, and this section will describe how a natural law-based approach was used in the prohibition of the pill by the Roman Catholic Church.

The Roman Catholic Church has trenchantly opposed the use of oral contraception throughout its history on natural law grounds, arguing that it prevents the outworking of the moral goods of marriage in procreation (Thatcher, 2011, p. 217). Other Roman Catholic concerns with contraception are that it dehumanises women, and reduces them to mere instruments of men's desire, and also that it introduces "moral deficits" and "sinful mentalities" because it encourages selfish behaviour. The Catholic Church described "the contraceptive mentality", as one of four "sinful mentalities", along with the hedonistic mentality, the consumer mentality and the anti-life mentality (Thatcher, 2011, p. 224). The 1995 papal encyclical *Evangelium Vitae* took an even stronger approach, describing contraception as a "culture of death" (Pope John Paul II, 1995). Contraception is also prohibited because it is a sin against life; Roman Catholic theologians would argue that, because life begins with the fertilised egg, then some forms of contraception – those which prevent implantation of the fertilised ovum – are a form of homicide (Genovesi, 1996).

The Roman Catholic opposition to hormonal contraception developed during the twentieth century (Thatcher, 2011, pp. 217–224). Following the publication of Marie Stopes' book *Contraception* in 1923, there was an increasing public interest in contraception in Britain, and so the Church of England's position on contraception was considered by the 1930 Lambeth Conference of Bishops. This Conference approved the use of contraception in certain circumstances. The guiding principles were that contraception should only be used within marriage and that contraception should not be used for reasons of "selfishness, luxury or convenience", but only when parents have a moral obligation to avoid parenthood. The conference asserted that abstinence was morally superior to contracepted sex, and that there should be a morally sound reason why abstinence is impossible.

The Roman Catholic Church responded rapidly with *Casti Connubii* ("On Chaste Marriage") which asserted robustly that all contraception was a vice opposed to Christian marriage, and that the only possible option for Catholic couples wishing to avoid parenthood was abstinence. However, in due course, the safe period (rhythm method) of contraception was permitted by Catholics, as it was not considered to be acting against nature. Nevertheless, the Roman Catholic church considered any human intervention that affects fertility as a manipulation of the natural world.

It was into this religious landscape that the oral contraceptive pill was introduced in the 1960s. As stated previously, John Rock, the Catholic gynaecologist involved with the clinical development of the pill, saw the pill as a "natural" form of contraceptive, that Catholics could use with a good conscience. Consequently, during the 60s, many Catholics hoped for a change of heart from their church concerning contraception. However, their hopes were dashed with the publication of the papal encyclical, *Humanae Vitae* in 1968, which upheld the Catholic church's position on contraception (Pope Paul VI, 1968). *Humanae Vitae* specified that marital sex had two meanings: a) the reproductive, or procreative, meaning, and b) the personal, or unitive, meaning, and that there was an inseparable connection between them established by God – which humans could not interfere with using contraceptive technologies (Thatcher, 2011, pp. 221–223). Indeed, the argument of the encyclical was that, since procreation was the natural purpose of intercourse, then anything that obstructs that purpose is intrinsically evil.

Yet, despite this strong prohibition, statistics on contraception published in the 1970s suggested that a significant proportion of Catholics ignored the church's official teaching, and practised contraception anyway (Langford, 1976). May has argued that many Catholics in the US ignored the church's position on contraception in favour of simple economics and convenience (May, 2010, p. 122).

There are various problems with the prohibition of contraception on natural law grounds, as expressed by *Humanae Vitae*. Stephen Pope notes that *Humanae Vitae* has been criticised as an overly physicalist application of natural law which does not account for the complexity of individual circumstances, the importance of mutuality and intimacy in marriage and the difference between valuing the gift of life in principle and requiring this value to be expressed as openness to conception at each sex act (Pope, 2012).

Bernard Häring, one theologian who opposed the Catholic church on contraception, therefore did so on the grounds of totality (Thatcher, 2011, p. 218; Häring, 1976). Häring criticised the church's stance concerning the rhythm method and argued that biological functions could be subordinated to the good of the whole person and of community life, and therefore that contraception, as a biological intervention, had the potential to be ethically beneficial. Contraception, he argued, ensured marital stability and planned parenthood and so, in moral status, could be regarded as the equivalent of a blood transfusion, or the use of insulin in diabetes.

A key consequence of the physicalist interpretation of natural law in *Humanae Vitae* is that it leads to an atomistic view of the sexual act, without acknowledging the broader, relational context of sex in marriage as a whole. The reason for this atomistic approach on the part of the Roman Catholic Church is because, according to natural law, the good ends of sex and marriage are procreation and childbirth, and each sex act always has the potential for conception.

However, Thatcher notes – correctly, in my view – that marriage is better seen as a totality which should be open to new life, and that sexual morality should be about the flourishing of the whole person, not just the status of sex acts (Thatcher, 2011, p. 223). He also notes that this was the stance taken by Anglican bishops by the 1958 Lambeth Conference when they affirmed that humans were not bound by natural law, because of their supra-natural self-transcendence, and that contraception was morally acceptable in certain circumstances. Anglican theologian Oliver O'Donovan summarised this issue well, stating that, "To break marriage down into a series of disconnected sexual acts is to falsify its true nature" (1984, p. 77). In terms of human flourishing, O'Donovan's argument is a valid one.

Indeed, it is ironic that Catholic natural law objections to contraception insist that contraception is unnatural because of its suppression of procreation, and yet treat a marriage as a series of sex acts which do not represent the true nature of marriage, as an ongoing and integral relationship between a man and woman, thereby treating marriage in an evidently "unnatural" manner.

Thatcher also notes the wider ethical implications of the Roman Catholic Church's prohibition of contraception. There is no consideration that contraception might be used for a virtuous end; for example, a couple may postpone having children so they can pay off their student debts (Thatcher, 2011, p. 226). Furthermore, he claims that Catholic arguments about moral deficits seem harsh and judgemental, and lead people to question the relevance of the church in modern society (Thatcher, 2011, p. 212). Thatcher has argued – reasonably – that the Roman Catholic Church has lost the respect of its members, because of its intransigent position on contraception and, for this reason, its theological insights, which are often of considerable depth, are overlooked.

The approach taken by *Humanae Vitae* of separating the procreative and the unitive function of marital sex is problematic scientifically, as well as ethically. A basic understanding of the human reproductive system shows that the procreative and unitive functions of marital sex can be separated in some "natural" circumstances – for example, during the menopause, because of infertility or simply during the infertile times of the menstrual cycle – not just by artificial means, which undermines this argument as a prohibition of hormonal contraception (Genovesi, 1996, pp. 205–210).

Stephen Pope has argued that the Roman Catholic canonists have continued to invoke natural law, and to formulate their moral theology despite the significance of scientific developments of the nineteenth and twentieth centuries (Pope, 2014, pp. 13–19). Pope contends – correctly, in my view, given the current cultural context – that with a simplistic natural theology, as opposed to a Thomist understanding of natural law, creation tends to be seen in only impersonal terms, as a machine for processing and constructing moral precepts. This, however, is inimical to the notion that human beings are personal beings, created by a personal God, and are called to have a personal – and moral – relationship with God and with each other (Mascall, 1959, pp. 1–18). This argument is especially relevant for applying natural law to medical technologies that intervene in human reproduction. Consequently, the physicalist interpretation of natural law in *Humanae Vitae* ultimately presents a deficient view of marriage because it regards sex acts in marriage on an individual basis, yet does not place them within the broader context of the marriage relationship as a whole, or acknowledge their personal context.

On the contrary, the developers of the pill – and, indeed, other voices in society at the time – saw the potential of the pill to improve human flourishing, and provide real ethical benefits for individuals, and for society.

Indeed, there has been little evidence that the pill has actively led to unethical behaviour in human society, over and above routine ethical variants in fallen humanity, or has been the sole factor in the marginalisation of marriage as a human institution.

Ronald Bailey, a supporter of transhumanism, points out that the application of biomedical technology does not preclude virtuous moral behaviour (Bailey, 2013). A similar argument can be applied to the use of the contraceptive pill in the context of a loving, sexual relationship. Humans have not necessarily become less moral or loving because of the introduction of hormonal contraception.

3.4 The Pill and Transhumanism

In this and the following section, the contraceptive pill – its features and its impact on society – will be assessed against the criteria for evaluating a transhumanist development. Medical technologies may have benefits for humanity but may also be associated with risks and unintended consequences which can have a significant wholescale impact on society. Therefore, medical technologies should not be accepted uncritically simply because they exist and are available but should be evaluated carefully from a perspective of Christian theological ethics.

First, we will address the question of whether the contraceptive pill can be classified as a development that would have been "transhumanist" in its time – something that would have a significant impact on human flourishing and society as a whole, not just on individual human lives. Reviewing the history of the contraceptive pill earlier in this chapter, is there any evidence that those involved in the development of the contraceptive pill – Sanger, McCormick, Pincus or Rock – saw the pill in these terms?

It is well recognised that both Margaret Sanger and Katharine McCormick were motivated to support the development of the contraceptive pill because of their feminist ideology, and they believed that women should have the capacity of choice about fertility and childbirth (May, 2010, pp. 20–21). Sanger, especially, was motivated by her deeply held political beliefs concerning social justice and equality, and had a far-reaching understanding of the implications of birth control for humanity. As long previously as 1912, she said that she saw birth control as about "voluntary motherhood", not necessarily contraception, a view for which she was branded as a eugenicist (Daly, 2008, p. 12). Gregory Pincus, too, wanted to change the natural order, through the development of new scientific possibilities for animal and human life. Because his work was scientific, its implications for "nature" were more clearly in view for contemporary society, and this earned him the opprobrium of the academic community, the media and wider American society (May, 2010, p. 21). John Rock, the prominent clinical trialist in the development of the pill, was clearly motivated by his duty as a doctor to alleviate human suffering and improve the lives of his patients and saw the pill as a positive advance in that respect, and one that went beyond the remit and limits of interventional medicine at the time (May, 2010, p. 122).

These three protagonists all had different motivations for their development work on the contraceptive pill, and their stance was remarkable given government and scientific opposition to contraceptive research at the time, concerns in society about contraception as a legitimate social issue and about possible eugenic consequences – and, of course, the Roman Catholic Church's doctrinal opposition to artificial contraception.

However, the role of luck, or "serendipity", in drug discovery is well recognised (Block, 2004; Ban, 2006), and many new drugs have found their way to the market by a process of coincidences and unintended consequences.[3] Consequently, the motivations of the developers must be regarded as a subjective, secondary measure of whether a medicine was indeed a transhumanist development of its time. The general criteria for a transhumanist technology, as previously proposed, will provide a better foundation to determine whether a development may be classed as transhumanist, although they are themselves derived from the literature of transhumanism, and are very broad and all-encompassing. These general criteria for a transhumanist technology are a) that it is a technology, b) that it is applied to the human person, c) that it is applied to promote human flourishing and d) that it may be applied with autonomy.

First, a transhumanist development is a technology (More, 2013) – a material means of effecting a task or process, which will include any physical or chemical reaction or intervention (including pharmaceutical medicine) but may also include processes, policies and organisational methods (Bostrom, 2005). The contraceptive pill is a form of chemical or pharmacological intervention, and so is indeed a technology. Furthermore, while the components of the contraceptive pill are analogues of natural sex hormones, in the pill, they are synthetically produced and are introduced into the body artificially to elicit an effect. This undermines John Rock's view that the contraceptive pill was a "natural" product, whose use should be acceptable to the Roman Catholic church. Therefore, the contraceptive pill is undoubtedly a technology according to this criterion.

Second, a transhumanist development is a technology that is applied to a human person to exert its effect (World Transhumanist Association, 2013). At the core of transhumanism is the transformation of human biological life and experience, and the improvement of human society. Pregnancy is part of normal human function rather than a disease or disorder, and this has implications for the type of technological intervention that the pill is. Consequently, the pill is not therapeutic, because it is not taken primarily to restore human function in a person who is dysfunctional (although it has some therapeutic applications). Nor is the pill prophylactic in the true sense because it is not being taken to prevent an illness or an adverse event. Consequently, I would argue that the ability to control fertility and avoid pregnancy for social reasons is an enhancement of normal human function.

Furthermore, the use of the contraceptive "enhancement" has a wider impact than just on the woman taking the pill – as discussed, it affects her partner, and widespread use of the pill will have a wholescale effect on human society. The pill therefore fulfils this second criterion in that it is a technology that exerts its effects by being applied to the human person.

Third, a transhumanist development is a technology that is applied to the human person to promote human flourishing, by improving human function, or increasing longevity (World Transhumanism Association, 2013). As argued earlier in this chapter, the contraceptive pill has only a modest effect on longevity, but there are many health and social benefits of the contraceptive pill to human life. First, the pill has positive effects on human life and welfare that were envisaged by those who developed it. As with other forms of contraception, the pill allows a couple to make positive moral choices about when to have children and how many to have. Moreover, the pill enables a woman to have control over her body, which will have emotional and medical benefits for her. It will also contribute to the emotional well-being of the whole family which, in turn, will contribute to the stability of society. In this respect, the pill could be considered a "moral enhancement" in that it enables people to make good personal lifestyle choices. Second, as mentioned earlier, the pill has additional health benefits which are unrelated to its contraceptive effects, which include control of the menstrual cycle, reduced incidence of pre-menstrual tension, increased bone density (thus reducing the risk of fractures), among others. These health benefits constitute unintended consequences that were not considered when the pill was first launched but which have emerged in the decades since. Third, the pill also reduces the emotional and socioeconomic burden of unwanted pregnancy. Furthermore, as mentioned previously, the contraceptive pill was the first drug affecting the whole body ever to be given to a healthy population on a large scale. There is therefore considerable evidence that the contraceptive pill has indeed had a positive effect on human flourishing on a large scale and has realised some of the aspirations of its developers.

Fourth, with a transhumanist development, the human person should have autonomy in the use of the technology – in other words, the technology is not being applied in a coercive way (More, 2013). When it was first launched, the contraceptive pill was hailed as the ideal means to enable a woman to exercise choice about sex and pregnancy and for couples to exercise choice about family planning (McLaren, 1990, p. 2). At first sight, therefore, the pill has had a positive effect on the exercise of personal autonomy, defined as uncoerced self-determination. However, a closer examination of the social impact of the contraceptive pill indicates that the introduction of the pill has, in fact, had an ambiguous effect on personal autonomy – it has enabled some choices but has also taken some choices away.

The contraceptive pill has limited human choice and freedom in several ways. The use of the contraceptive pill by his partner has the potential to take choices about contraception away from the man in a relationship because, with the pill, the woman has control over the means of contraception, and the timing of pregnancy. Also, the excretion of synthetic steroids into the environment by users of oral contraceptives may mean that individuals other than pill users and their partners are exposed to these substances and their potentially harmful effects without their knowledge or consent.

There have also been concerns in the past that the contraceptive pill has been distributed in a coercive way in some third-world countries. In the mid-60s, the Johnson administration made population control (and contraception services) a key feature of the US government's foreign aid policy (May, 2010, p. 43). However, US-funded population control programmes in the developing world have been criticised for being examples of American imperialism, since the contraceptive pill was developed and marketed largely from the United States (May, 2010, pp. 23–25).[4] In addition, these programmes have been criticised from a feminist perspective. For example, Hartmann has argued that, in developing countries, women have often not been adequately screened for suitability to take the pill, that the side effects of the pill have been trivialised and that women have not been adequately informed of the risks of taking the pill (Hartmann, 1995, pp. 189–219). Furthermore, she has identified a patronising attitude with US-funded population control programmes, where there is an underlying assumption that only American (white, middle-class, male) gynaecologists can possibly be qualified to give contraceptive advice to women in the third world. These factors have all affected the extent that women in developing countries can exercise true informed consent when offered the contraceptive pill.

In fact, women themselves may experience a loss of autonomy or personal choice because they are taking the contraceptive pill. Women are dependent on a doctor or healthcare professional to prescribe the pill, and feminists have argued that the pill has therefore "medicalised" women and their fertility and made them the subject of health service intervention and assessment (Jutte, 2008, p. 111). This is especially ironic given the fact that, as stated earlier, pregnancy is not a disease or disorder. Furthermore, as mentioned previously, the pill has introduced into society the concept of the "coital imperative" – if a woman is on the pill, and the risk of unwanted pregnancy is removed, there is no apparent reason for her to withhold sex (Thatcher, 2011, p. 221). Consequently, in recent years, there has been considerable social pressure for young women to have penetrative sex with their partners in a way that was not expected in previous centuries (Thatcher, 2011, pp. 214–216; Cook, 2004, pp. 1–3). Because of the pill, women may be coerced into sexual relationships that they might not otherwise have, which undermines their personal autonomy.

In any case, when considering the contraceptive pill and its effects on personal autonomy in the context of the sexual relationship, the ambiguous nature of sexual desire itself must be acknowledged (Thatcher, 2011, pp. 57–69). On one hand, sexual desire is a pleasurable response to human beauty and physical attractiveness, and must be regarded as good, because of the goodness of creation (Genesis 1). On the other hand, sexual desire can lead to sinful behaviour and consequences (e.g., David's desire for Bathsheba (2 Samuel 11)). The crux of this ambiguity is that, by its very nature, sexual desire is about abandonment and loss of self-control – effectively, the surrender of personal autonomy. However, Christianity has – paradoxically – emphasised the importance of controlling this desire. One cannot give oneself up to desire and control that desire at the same time. Elsewhere, I define autonomy as non-coerced self-determination – "to be one's own person, to be directed by... desires ... that are not simply imposed externally upon one but are part of what can somehow be considered one's authentic self" (Christman, 2015). According to this definition, self-abandonment to sexual desire is not loss of autonomy if the desire is an expression of the person's authentic self. However, as Christman points out, if the desire is a product of "addiction" – for example, drug addiction – the pursuit of that desire may not be a truly autonomous activity because it is not an expression of the authentic self (Christman, 2015). This might also apply to sexual desire, for example, in extreme cases of sexual addiction. In any case, desire, as an internal factor affecting autonomy in the context of a sexual relationship, must be considered when evaluating how the use of the contraceptive pill might affect personal autonomy.

There is also the question of how autonomy might be used. The contraceptive pill has certainly enabled couples to have more choices about family planning. But, during the last fifty years, has the freedom provided by the contraceptive pill been used to enable people to make wise choices about family planning for the good of human welfare, or to pursue selfish desires and aims, at the expense of humanity as a whole? As stated earlier, there is little evidence that the pill has increased the incidence of sexual activity with multiple partners in society. Furthermore, some theological responses to contraception, such as that of Bernard Häring, have suggested that planned parenthood has positive moral value in that it can uphold good ethical decisions and moral agency in the individuals concerned (Häring, 1976).

Consequently, although use of the contraceptive pill may, at first sight, enhance personal autonomy for the user, I have shown here that use of the contraceptive pill in fact has ambiguous implications for personal autonomy. This is also the case for future transhumanist technologies, as I have discussed elsewhere.

3.5 An Ethical Re-evaluation of the Pill

The general criteria indicate that the contraceptive pill is a development that, in its time, resembled a transhumanist technology, albeit with ambiguity concerning the ability to use the technology with autonomy.

However, to make an ethical evaluation of the contraceptive pill, specific ethical criteria will need to be applied:

1 Is the project good news for the poor?
2 Is the project an attempt to be "like God" (in respect of Genesis 3v5) or does it conform to the image of God? (Genesis 1v26).
3 What attitude does the project embody towards the material world (including our own bodies)? And how does the technology affect the corporate "body" of society?
4 What attitude does the project embody towards past failures?
5 Does the technology enable unbridled autonomy in a negative manner?
6 Does the technology focus too much on the users' subjective experiences?

These criteria are a combination of Neil Messer's "diagnostic questions" of a biotechnology project (Messer, 2007, pp. 229–235), and Elaine Graham's theological critiques of transhumanism (Graham, 2006); I have discussed the use of these criteria elsewhere.

First, is the contraceptive pill good news for the poor? McLaren has argued that contraception has enabled women to be in control of their working life, as well as their sex life and their family life (McLaren, 1990, pp. 240–245). There is evidence that the contraceptive pill has had an impact on female poverty and hardship. In an analysis of US census data from 1960 to 1990, Browne and LaLumia demonstrated that access to the oral contraceptive pill from the age of 20 has reduced subsequent poverty among women due to unplanned pregnancy and childbirth, regardless of employment status (Browne and LaLumia, 2014). In theory, the pill has enabled women to make more choices about their working lives, to achieve career ambitions and gain a foothold in industries that have typically been male-dominated – all with wider societal implications, and potential benefits in terms of economic growth. There is little direct evidence to show that this is the case, but this theory is supported by a review of contraceptive use in Britain, which showed that the contraceptive pill was particularly popular with young women who had never had children (Szarewski and Guillebaud, 1991).

As noted previously, there have been some ethical concerns about the distribution of hormonal contraception in the developing world, concerning whether people in those countries have real freedom of choice when offered contraception services. There is evidence to suggest that, where contraceptive services are available in developing countries, they have significant effects on reducing health and welfare costs in those countries (Upadhyay and Robey, 1999). These benefits arise from the reduction of the population, which alleviates poverty and famine, and which also benefits the environment and enables development to proceed more efficiently in those countries. They also arise from the positive effects of the pill on the health of women, sparing them from unwanted childbirth. However, as I have discussed elsewhere, a key factor in whether biomedical technologies are good news for the poor is how accessible they are to the poor. As is the trend with many medicines, the costs of contraceptive pill formulations have decreased significantly since the launch of the first contraceptive pill in 1960. This has been partly due to the increased number of products available, due to the development of second- and third-generation pills with improved side-effect profiles, ensuring cost reduction due to competition. Consequently, at the current time, the contraceptive pill is more affordable for developing countries than it was when it was first introduced. Use of hormonal contraception worldwide, however, is still not universal. United Nations (UN) statistics show that, in 2011, throughout the world, an average of 63% of women who were married or partnered were using contraception (United Nations, 2013); however, this is a world average figure and ranges from 70% or more of women in Europe, North America, Latin America and the Caribbean, to only 31% of women in Africa, where less reliable traditional methods of contraception (rhythm method, douching and folk medicine) are still prevalent. These UN statistics also identified one in five women as having an unmet contraceptive need, with no access to contraception, especially in sub-Saharan Africa and the Pacific islands. Consequently, many commentators argue that there are unmet needs for oral contraception in the developing world and that wider distribution of the pill is needed (Bahamondes et al., 2015). In conclusion, on balance, the contraceptive pill is good news for the poor, dependent on whether the pill can, in fact, be made available to all world citizens in an equal and fair way.

Second, does the project conform to the image of God or does it attempt to be "like God"? Here, the answer is nuanced. At an individual level, the use of the contraceptive pill enables individuals to control their fertility and plan their families and, at a societal level, the pill and contraceptive services enable governments to exercise control over population growth. The contraceptive pill could therefore be regarded as an attempt to be "like God" in that people are using the pill to control and manipulate human life, and to have a power and knowledge which might be regarded as God-like, and in contravention of natural law, in terms of a creation divinely ordered under a sovereign creator. Concern over this level of control would be consistent with the Roman Catholic church's natural law objections to the contraceptive pill.

Conversely, to what extent does the pill conform to the image of God? For the purposes of answering this question, I would interpret conformation to the image of God as the extent to which the use of the pill, and its effects on individuals or society, reflects a comprehensive understanding of the *imago Dei*, accounting for the different theological approaches to the *imago Dei* that have been described. In Chapter 2, I argued that transhumanist biomedical technologies reflected a limited understanding of the *imago Dei*. The use of transhumanist technologies in humanity reflects an *imago Dei* that is excessively substantive, focusing on human attributes, at the expense of being relational or functional, and in a way that is individualistic and inward-looking, in eschatological terms. With that worldview, there is a danger that, instead of human beings worshipping God, because they are made in his image, they would instead worship the enhanced posthuman person as a god instead. There is a danger that human beings will look to technology for perfection rather than seek spiritual perfection and transformation in union with Christ, which the Christological dynamic of the *imago Dei* would point towards.

As described earlier, the contraceptive pill, as an enhancement, confers a specific attribute to humanity – the ability to postpone or delay pregnancy in a controllable manner. The pill may also confer other attributes on the user – for example, a regular menstrual cycle or increased bone density. Like proposed transhumanist technologies, the pill therefore does affect certain human attributes, and this does reflect a substantive theological view of the *imago Dei*. However, as seen earlier, use of the pill also has an impact on human relationships – in particular, on the relationship of men and women in marriage – and this has implications for the *imago Dei*. The *imago Dei* doctrine in Christian history has been criticised for being androcentric, because of the interpretation of Bible passages such as 1 Corinthians 11v7. For example, Mary Catherine Hilkert has argued that "the *imago Dei* doctrine has been the cause of oppression and discrimination against women in the past and needs rethinking" (Hilkert, 1995; Van Huyssteen, 2006). During the twentieth century, feminist theologians have strived to redress the balance, and have developed understandings of the *imago Dei* that are inclusive of women – for example, those of Hilkert, and also Mary McClintock Fulkerson (Fulkerson, 1997). The contraceptive pill has enhanced the marriage relationship by changing its dynamic and redressing the balance of power and influence in favour of women in marriage. Consequently, use of the contraceptive pill reflects a more gender-neutral *imago Dei* in the context of human relationships. This helps to address feminist concerns about the role of women in humanity and moves beyond previous views of *imago Dei* that are androcentric and have been subject to gender-related critique. Furthermore, I would suggest that, because the relational *imago Dei* in humanity is upheld by the effects of the contraceptive pill on relationships, this may also have a positive effect in emphasising the functional approach to the *imago Dei*; in other words, the pill may enable men and women to better exercise their specific vocations as men and women in God's world.

Third, what attitude does the project embody towards the material world (including our own bodies)? Although it has systemic effects, the contraceptive pill does not make wholesale material changes to the body in a negative way, or in a way that denigrates the body, in the way that some transhumanist technologies do – for example, mind-uploading or cybernetics. The pill mimics the actions of naturally occurring sex hormones, and so it is a biomedical technology that exerts positive effects through its actions on the human body, and therefore upholds the significance of the body. Nevertheless, the contraceptive pill does provide a technological means of regulating and manipulating the body. This may be used for good ethical ends – for example, to promote planned parenthood and provide family stability – but may also be used for ends that are not consistent with a Christian ethic – for example, the avoidance of parenthood for selfish reasons, or to enable sexual activity with multiple partners or adultery.

As previously mentioned, the contraceptive pill has only a modest effect on mortality so, as a biomedical technology, it is not opposed to human finitude in the way that some proposed transhumanist medical technologies are, such as cryogenic preservation or mind-uploading. However, as stated, the pill has benefits for individual quality of life – control over fertility, family planning, and other health benefits. Furthermore, the availability of contraception has enabled couples to participate more fully in activities outside of marriage and family life – careers, hobbies, sports and social life – with the potential social, cultural – and material – benefits that those activities might provide. Consequently, even though the contraceptive pill does not significantly prolong life and therefore affect human finitude, it does have the potential to enhance the material nature of human life, in the broadest sense. This may be ethically positive, if the material gains to society as the result of contraceptive use provide moral goods in society. However, in some circumstances, these material gains may detract from spiritual life, if they are employed in an individual, hedonistic or exploitative way.

The problem with transhumanist technologies is that they interfere with the integrity of the individual body and can therefore have a disruptive effect on the corporate body – the community (Graham, 2006). As argued here, the contraceptive pill does not have a negative material impact on the individual human body and, because of its positive effects on human relationships, it may have material benefits for the corporate body of humanity – human society in general. These benefits have been noted especially in developing countries, where the effects of contraception programmes in specific countries have been studied in detail (Upadhyay and Robey, 1999). However, the impact of the pill on the corporate body of society will be dependent on the ethical choices made by individuals, concerning contraception, relationships and family planning, and also on government policies on the availability of, and accessibility to, contraception. Thus, in relation to this criterion, the contraceptive pill does not resemble a transhumanist technology because there is evidence to indicate that the pill has positive effects on society – on humanity at a corporate level – as well as humanity at an individual level.

Fourth, what attitude does the project embody towards past failures? The development of the contraceptive pill has been a great success in many ways; as stated earlier, it has been hailed as the fulfilment of the search for the "ideal contraceptive", and as a triumph of control over human fertility, with far-reaching consequences for society, so it could be regarded as a hubristic technological development. The development of the contraceptive pill and its impact on human society has been described in fulsome terms by scholars and commentators. Because of its advantages over previous forms of contraception (namely, that it is a non-invasive method, which can be controlled by the woman), McLaren has described the pill as a "contraceptive revolution" (1990, p. 2). Cook has argued that the pill "precipitated a transformation in sexual mores" and that, by reducing the social and economic impact of pregnancy, the pill has transformed attitudes to sexuality (2004, p. 7). Similarly, May has described the pill as, not simply a method of contraception but "a flash point for major social transformation" (2010, p. 168). Furthermore, at the time of its introduction, the contraceptive pill was regarded not only as a convenient form of contraception, but as a solution to a range of socio-political problems. It was hailed as the solution to the problem of exponential population growth, a "clean", scientific solution to the problem of contraception and unwanted pregnancy. The pill was easy to prescribe, and it required no invasive or messy process, and therefore it sanitised contraception (McLaren, 1990, pp. 240–245; Cook, 2004, p. 278). Many doctors also saw the pill as a clinical approach to contraception, which was consistent with their professional ethics and aspirations.

In short, there is evidence to suggest that the contraceptive pill has indeed been adopted confidently by western society, as a panacea for various social problems, in a way that Cole-Turner has warned against (2001, p. 144). The contraceptive pill does appear to have been developed and distributed with confidence, even hubris, as a man-made innovation, rather than with humility, acknowledging the pill as a product of the natural world, which reflects a glory which does not belong to humanity. However, this confidence in the pill has to some extent been misplaced, with various unintended consequences over the years, such as the "pill scares" (the risk of blood clotting-related side effects with the pill) and the inability of the pill to protect against sexually transmitted diseases, which became apparent with the spread of HIV and more recently, the increased incidence of chlamydia.

Fifth, does the contraceptive pill enable individuals to exercise unbridled autonomy in a negative manner? I argued earlier that the effects of the pill on autonomy and personal choice are ambiguous. While the availability of the pill ostensibly gives women (and men) choice about family planning, its widespread use may, in practice, restrict men's choices about contraception, and be an instrument of coercion for women, because of the so-called coital imperative, and the exploitative distribution of the pill in certain societies. In this respect, the effect of the contraceptive pill on autonomy bears a striking resemblance to the likely effects of future transhumanist technologies on autonomy, as outlined in the transhumanism and enhancement literature – the technology may be adopted at the outset with autonomy, but autonomy may be restricted in some situations where the technology is used. Moreover, as mentioned previously here, autonomy is an ethically neutral phenomenon – it may be used to inflict selfish desires on other people, or it can be used to pursue good ethical ends. The contraceptive pill certainly does not confer unbridled autonomy on the individual.

Sixth, does the contraceptive pill focus too much on the users' subjective experiences? The subjectivism inherent in transhumanism may derive from the strong emphasis on autonomy (self-determination) in choosing enhancements, which has been a key feature of transhumanist thought (World Transhumanism Association, 2013). However, as I have discussed elsewhere, the irony is that, although transhumanist technologies enhance subjective experience, they are ultimately problematic because they objectify the human body, and treat it as an artefact rather than a human person (Cole-Turner, 2001, pp. 142–143, 147).

Some feminist writers have argued that the contraceptive pill can objectify the user – that is, render the woman using the pill an object of sexual desire (Jutte, 2008, p. 111). This is analogous to the way some transhumanist technologies – for example, cybernetics or gene alterations – treat the body as a product to be engineered. However, because the pill exerts its effects within and through the human body, in a way that does not negate embodiment, I would argue that, with the pill, the user does not become an artefact to be manipulated at will, as with some proposed transhumanist technologies. On the contrary, the pill provides benefits to the individual person which are experienced subjectively in sexual, marriage and family relationships.

The findings of this chapter indicate that the contraceptive pill conforms to the criteria for transhumanist developments in that it is a technology which is applied to the human person to exert its effects and is one that, largely, has a beneficial effect on human flourishing. Furthermore, the contraceptive pill has had a significant impact on human society, not just on the experience of the individual.

The application of the theological criteria to facilitate ethical analysis of the contraceptive pill as a pseudo-transhumanist biomedical technology yields interesting results. Unlike radical, "high-tech" transhumanist technologies – for example, mind-uploading or cryogenics – the contraceptive pill has the potential to be beneficial to the poor, because of its low cost, relative to high-tech medicine and its ability to help women on low incomes to plan their families and their working life. Unlike approaches to transhumanism that emphasise human attributes, and therefore a more substantive approach to the *imago Dei*, I have argued in this chapter that the effects of the contraceptive pill reflect an approach to the *imago Dei* that is more balanced and is relational and functional, as well as substantive. Unlike transhumanist technologies which are essentially anti-materialist, such as mind-uploading, the contraceptive pill exerts positive effects in and through the human body and its mechanisms and does not negate biological life. Consequently, the contraceptive pill may have benefits for the corporate body of society too.

In terms of subjectivity, the pill has the potential to objectify the user, as an object of sexual desire, and yet it enhances the user's subjective experience. Furthermore, given that it was planned, in part, as a means of controlling the population for socio-political reasons, rather than just as a means of preventing or delaying conception, I would argue that the contraceptive pill has been seen as the culmination of the search for effective contraception over the centuries, and so the pill has been regarded with extreme confidence, even hubris, as a triumph of human technological achievement, in a similar way to proposed future transhumanist technologies. This contrasts with a humility that derives from scientific engagement with the mysteries of nature, mysteries which reflect a glory that ultimately is not human glory.

Furthermore, the contraceptive pill raises significant questions for personal autonomy. A stated aim of the transhumanist movement is that individuals who are seeking biomedical enhancement can adopt a biomedical technology autonomously, as a matter of free, personal choice. Correspondingly, a key theological criticism of transhumanist technologies is that they enable unbridled autonomy in a negative manner. The evidence from the development and use of the contraceptive pill suggests that neither of these extremes is true. While individual users of the contraceptive pill can exercise autonomy in choosing it at the outset, various factors – for example, the impact on men's choices, the possibility of the "coital imperative" for women, equity in the marketing and distribution of the pill and indeed the ambiguous nature of sexual desire – can ultimately lead to negative effects of the contraceptive pill on personal autonomy.

In this chapter, I have argued that the contraceptive pill has some of the characteristics of a transhumanist technology, and that, while it has had various ethical benefits, it is subject to some of the ethical concerns that have been raised with biotechnology projects. I will explore these issues in detail elsewhere, but I contend that a natural law-based ethical approach is no longer adequate for the ethical evaluation of oral contraception. In the next chapter, I will focus on SSRI antidepressants and, in the same way, consider whether these might be regarded as a transhumanist medical technology, according to the general and specific criteria previously defined.

Notes

1 See Betsy Hartmann, *Reproductive Rights and Wrongs: The Global Politics of Population Control* (Boston: South End Press, 1995), p. 202. Because of their long-acting nature and the potential for non-consensual administration, there are additional ethical issues with these forms of hormonal contraception.

2 Yet by taking this stance, Margaret Sanger has also been criticised as a eugenicist, probably by her political opponents (Berkman, 2011). Her legacy, therefore, has been debated.

3 For example, cimetidine in the treatment of ulcers or captopril for the treatment of hypertension.

4 See May, *America and the Pill*, pp. 23–25. May states that the development of the oral contraceptive pill is essentially "an American story". However, given the involvement of Schering and Bayer (Germany) in the development of oral contraceptives, and the rapid launch of the Searle product and others in Britain in 1961, I would contest this claim, which could itself be regarded as American imperialism.

References

A Szarewski and J Guillebaud, "Contraception: Current State of the Art", *British Medical Journal*, 302 (1991), pp. 1224–1226.

A. Linken and R.S.P. Wiener, "Promiscuity and Contraception in a Sample of Patients Attending a Clinic for Venereal Diseases", *British Journal of Venereal Diseases*, 46 (1970), pp. 243–246.

Adrian Thatcher, *God, Sex and Gender: An Introduction* (Oxford: Wiley-Blackwell, 2011).

Angus McLaren, *A History of Contraception from Antiquity to the Present Day* (Oxford: Oxford University Press, 1990).

Bernard Häring, "New Dimensions of Responsible Parenthood", *Theological Studies*, 37 (1976), pp. 120–132.

Betsy Hartmann, *Reproductive Rights and Wrongs: The Global Politics of Population Control* (Boston: South End Press, 1995).

Brian Block, "Are Scientific Discoveries the Result of Good Luck? An Analysis of Some Pharmaceutical Discoveries Between 1920 and 1945", *Pharmaceutical History*, 34 (2004), pp. 59–64.

Clive Wood and Beryl Suitters, *The Fight for Acceptance: A History of Contraception* (Aylesbury: Medical and Technical Publishing. 1970).

Christopher Langford, *Birth Control Practice and Marital Fertility in Great Britain* (London: London School of Economics, 1976).

D. Caserta, E. Ralli, E. Matteucci, G. Bordi, M. Mallozzi and M. Moscarini, "Combined Oral Contraceptives: Health Benefits Beyond Contraception", *Panminerva Medicine*, 56 (2014), pp. 233–244.

Elaine Graham, "In Whose Image? Representations of Technology and the Ends of Humanity", in *Future Perfect? God, Medicine and Human Identity*, edited by Celia Deane-Drummond and Peter Manley Scott (London: T and T Clark International, 2006), pp. 58–61.

Elaine Tyler May, *America and the Pill: A History of Promise, Peril and Liberation* (New York: Basic Books, 2010).

Elizabeth Draper, *Birth Control in the Modern World* (London: Pelican, 1965).

Eric Mascall, *The Importance of Being Human: Some Aspects of the Christian Doctrine of Man* (Oxford: Oxford University Press, 1959).

Hera Cook, *The Long Sexual Revolution: English Women, Sex and Contraception, 1800–1975* (Oxford: Oxford University Press, 2004).

James Childress, "Christian Ethics, Medicine and Genetics", in *Cambridge Companion to Christian Ethics*, edited by Robin Gill (Cambridge: Cambridge University Press, 2001), pp. 288–289.

John Christman, "Autonomy in Moral and Political Philosophy", *Stanford Encyclopaedia of Philosophy* (2015), https://plato.stanford.edu/entries/autonomy-moral/ (Accessed April 2019).

J. Wentzel Van Huyssteen, *Alone in the World? Human Uniqueness in Science and Theology* (Grand Rapids: Eerdmans, 2006), pp. 139–143.

Jo Jones, William Mosher and Kimberly Daniels, "Current Contraceptive Use in the United States, 2006–2010, and Changes in Patterns of Use since 1995", *National Health Statistics Report*, 60 (2012), pp. 1–25.

Joyce Berkman, "The Question of Margaret Sanger", *History Compass*, 9 (2011), pp. 474–484.

Louise Tyrer, "Obstacles to Use of Hormonal Contraception", *American Journal of Obstetrics and Gynecology*, 170 (1994), pp. 1495–1498.

Louise Tyrer, "Introduction of the Pill and Its Impact", *Contraception*, 59 (1999), pp. 11S–16S.

L. L. Wynn and James Trussell, "Images of American Sexuality in Debates Over Non-prescription Access to Emergency Contraceptive Pills", *Obstetrics and Gynecology*, 108 (2006), pp. 1272–1276.

Luis Bahamondes, Valeria Bahamondes and Lee P. Shulman, "Non-contraceptive Benefits of Hormonal and Intrauterine Reversible Contraceptive Methods", *Human Reproduction Update*, 21 (2015), pp. 640–651.

Mary McLintock Fulkerson, "Contesting the Gendered Subject: A Feminist Account of the Imago Dei", in *Horizons in Feminist Theology: Identity, Traditions and Norms*, edited by Rebecca Chopp and Sheila Devaney (Minneapolis: Fortress, 1997), pp. 95–115.

Mary Catherine Hilkert, "Cry Beloved Image: Rethinking the Image of God", in *In the Embrace of God: Feminist Approaches to Theological Anthropology*, edited by Ann Graff (Maryknoll, NY: Orbis, 1995), pp. 190–205.

Max More, "Philosophy of Transhumanism", in *The Transhumanist Reader: Classical and Contemporary Essays on the Science, Technology and Philosophy of the Post-Human Future*, edited by Max More and Natasha Vita-More (Chichester: Wiley-Blackwell, 2013), p. 13.

Nick Bostrom, "Transhumanist Values", *Journal of Philosophical Research*, 30 (2005), pp. 3–14.

Nicolas Mendoza and Rafael Sanchez-Borrego, "Classical and Newly Recognised Non-contraceptive Benefits of Combined Hormonal Contraceptive Use in Women over 40", *Maturitas*, 78 (2014), pp. 45–50.

Neil Messer, *Selfish Genes and Christian Ethics: Theological and Ethical Reflections on Evolutionary Biology* (London: SCM, 2007).

Oliver O' Donovan, *Begotten or Made?* (Oxford: Clarendon, 1984).

Pope John Paul II, "The Gospel of Life: Evangelium Vitae", 1995, http://www.vatican.va/content/john-paul-ii/en/encyclicals/documents/hf_jp-ii_enc_25031995_evangelium-vitae.html (Accessed March 2020).

Pope Paul VI, "On the Regulation of Birth: Humanae Vitae", 1968, http://www.vatican.va/content/paul-vi/en/encyclicals/documents/hf_p-vi_enc_25071968_humanae-vitae.html (Accessed March 2020).

Ronald Bailey, "For Enhancing People", in *The Transhumanist Reader: Classical and Contemporary Essays on the Science, Technology and Philosophy of the Post-Human Future*, edited by Max More and Natasha Vita-More (Chichester: Wiley-Blackwell, 2013), pp. 331–332.

Ronald Cole-Turner, "Towards a Theology for the Age of Biotechnology", in *Beyond Cloning: Religion and the Remaking of Humanity*, edited by Ronald Cole-Turner (Harrisburg PA: Trinity Press International, 2001), p. 144.

Robert Jutte, *Contraception: A History*, translated by V. Russell (Cambridge: Polity Press, 2008).

Selma Caal, Lina Guzman, Amanda Berger, Manica Ramos and Elisabeth Golub, "Because You're on Birth Control, It Automatically Makes You Promiscuous or Something": Latina Women's Perceptions of Parental Approval to Use Reproductive Health Care", *Journal of Adolescent Health*, 53 (2013), pp. 617–622.

Stephanie Browne and Sara LaLumia, "The Effects of Contraception on Female Poverty", *Journal of Policy Analysis and Management*, 33 (2014), pp. 602–622.

Stephen Pope, "Natural Law and Christian Ethics", in *Cambridge Companion to Christian Ethics*, edited by Robin Gill (Cambridge: Cambridge University Press, 2012), pp. 67–86.

Stephen Pope, "Theological Anthropology, Science, and Human Flourishing", in *Questioning the Human: Toward a Theological Anthropology for the Twenty–First Century*, edited by Lieven Boeve, Yves De Maeseneer and Ellen Van Stichel (New York: Fordham University Press, 2014), pp. 13–19.

Sunny Daly, *Changing Images of the Birth Control Pill 1960–1973: A Social History of the Pill in America* (Saarbrucken: VDM Verlag Dr Muller, 2008).

Susan Davis, I. Dinatale, L. Rivera Wall and Sonia Davison, "Postmenopausal Hormone Therapy: From Monkey Glands to Transdermal Patches", *Journal of Endocrinology*, 185 (2005), pp. 207–222.

Thomas Ban, "The Role of Serendipity in Drug Discovery", *Dialogues in Clinical Neurosciences*, 8 (2006), pp. 335–344.

United Nations, "Department of Economic and Social Affairs, Population Division (2013) World Contraceptive Patterns 2013", 2013, at https://www.un.org/en/development/desa/population/publications/pdf/family/worldContraceptivePatternsWallChart2013.pdf (Accessed March 2020).

Ushma Upadhyay and Bryant Robey, "Why Family Planning Matters", *Population Reports. Series J, Family Planning Programs*, 49 (1999), pp. 1–31.

Vincent Genovesi, *In Pursuit of Love: Catholic Morality and Human Sexuality* (Collegeville, PA: Liturgical Press, 1996).

Walter Sneader, *Drug Discovery: A History* (Chichester: Wiley, 2005).

World Transhumanist Association, "Transhumanist Declaration", in *The Transhumanist Reader: Classical and Contemporary Essays on the Science, Technology and Philosophy of the Post-Human Future*, edited by Max More and Natasha Vita-More (Chichester: Wiley-Blackwell, 2013), pp. 54–55.

4 Better than Well

Prozac and Selective Serotonin Reuptake Inhibitor Antidepressants

4.1 Psychopharmacology in the Twentieth Century

Elsewhere, I have discussed the history of the oral contraceptive pill, and the Roman Catholic church's ethical objection to it on natural law grounds. I have evaluated the pill against objective criteria to determine whether, in its time, it constituted a transhumanist technology, and whether ethical issues associated with future transhumanist technologies have been observed with the use of the pill in human society since its development.

I have shown that the contraceptive pill resembled a transhumanist biomedical technology in general criteria, that as a pharmacologically active pharmaceutical product, it is a technology, it is applied to the human body to exert its effects and has a positive effect on human flourishing. However, as with proposed future transhumanist biomedical enhancements, the effects of the pill on personal autonomy are ambiguous – it can have negative as well as positive effects on personal autonomy. Furthermore, the pill seems in danger of objectifying the human body (in making the body an object for sexual desire), yet at the same time, the pill leads to a heightened subjectivity on the part of the user, where subjective, individual experiences of sex and relationships become more significant as societal norms. Unlike some proposed future transhumanist technologies, the contraceptive pill as a medical technology upholds human embodiment and is consistent with human bodily life and flourishing, rather than contrary to it. In general terms, the contraceptive pill may be good news for the poor, in terms of its potential effects on poverty and working patterns among women. However, there are potential ethical concerns with the pill surrounding its equitable distribution and use in different countries and cultures.

In this chapter, I perform a similar analysis with selective serotonin reuptake inhibitor (SSRI) antidepressants, another development in pharmaceutical medicine which took place during the "therapeutic revolution" years (1950–1990). SSRI antidepressants were marketed in the late 1980s – for example, fluoxetine, marketed by Lilly as Prozac. Here, the term "SSRI antidepressants" is used to signify the group taken as a whole, and the term "Prozac" (the brand name for fluoxetine) is used in general terms to refer to

DOI: 10.4324/9781003290421-5

any SSRI use in popular culture (e.g., "the Prozac phenomenon"), as it is often used in that way in the relevant literature.

In the same way as my analysis of the contraceptive pill, the first section of this chapter will describe the history of SSRI development, and how SSRIs arose from previous developments in rational psychopharmacology. The second section will discuss the impact of SSRIs on society, both their therapeutic effects on patients with clinical depression and their use as mood-altering drugs in individuals who are not depressed. The chapter will go on to discuss a Christian ethical response to the use of SSRIs, engaging with the work of Catholic scholar John-Mark Miravalle (2010), which explores the treatment of depression in relation to Aquinas' classification of human attributes, and their implications for psychology. I will present a critique of Miravalle's argument. The final part of the chapter will then assess SSRI antidepressants against objective criteria for evaluation of transhumanist technologies to determine the extent to which, in their time, they could have been regarded as a transhumanist development, and to evaluate them from a Christian ethical perspective.

The development of Prozac (fluoxetine) and other SSRI antidepressants in the late 1980s was arguably the climax of the post-war rational psychopharmacology endeavour. So, for example, Lopez-Munoz and Alamo (2009) note that there have been no therapeutic advances for depression since the 1990s, and Perez-Caballero et al. (2014), contend that the use of SSRIs has, in fact, suppressed the exploration of new models of depression, and the investigation of new drugs.

Modern antidepressant drugs were developed following a serendipitous discovery after the Second World War that led to the development of specific, targeted drug therapies for depression (Shorter, 2009, pp. 11–33). The Swiss pharmaceutical company Roche had acquired a large amount of hydrazine-containing rocket fuel from the German military in the aftermath of the Second World War and was investigating several hydrazine-based drugs for their anti-tubercular properties. However, they fortuitously discovered that one of them, iproniazid, had a positive effect on patients' moods, and therefore had potential as an antidepressant instead (López-Muñoz and Alamo, 2009; Shorter, 2009, p. 53). Iproniazid became the first of a new class of monoamine oxidase inhibitors (MAOI) for the treatment of depression. This set the scene for research in the late 1950s and early 1960s, and the development of the so-called "monoamine hypothesis" of depression (López-Muñoz and Alamo, 2009; Shorter, 2009, p. 68), which stated that the underlying cause of clinical depression is a depletion in the levels of serotonin and noradrenaline in the central nervous system (Healy, 2004, p. 9). This led to the development of drugs which prevented the re-uptake of noradrenaline and serotonin in the brain – the tricyclic anti-depressants, amitriptyline and imipramine. During the 1960s and 1970s, various tricyclic antidepressants were launched, such as trimipramine, clomipramine, nortriptyline and others. These tricyclic antidepressants were a significant breakthrough in the treatment of depression because they enabled people who had debilitating depressive illnesses to live relatively normal lives when previously they would have been unable to function normally in society. However, these tricyclic agents had pharmacological effects in all parts of the body, not just in the brain, and therefore had many physiological side effects – for example, increased heart rate, palpitations, sedation, blurred vision and dry mouth – side effects which could be marked at high doses. Such side effects therefore limited the dose that could be given and made it difficult to treat patients with severe depression with high doses. The side effects also meant that tricyclic antidepressants were toxic in overdose and, given the propensity for depressed patients to consider suicide and use their drugs as the means, this was a serious problem.

However, following new work by Carlsson and colleagues in 1969 on the effects of antihistamine structure on serotonin depletion in the brain, the focus of research moved to antidepressants that specifically affected mechanisms in the brain mediated by serotonin, rather than noradrenaline. The thinking was that these serotonin-selective agents might be as effective as antidepressants, but with a more favourable side-effect profile than the tricyclic antidepressants.

Another important feature of the treatment of depression from the 1960s onwards was the increasing classification of personality characteristics as subtypes of depressive illness. The mental illness classification, the Diagnostic and Statistical Manual of Mental Disorders (DSM), was first introduced in 1952, as a means of classifying various specific psychiatric disorders, a task made particularly urgent by the number of veterans returning from the Second World War exhibiting a variety of symptoms of mental illness. However, as more detailed knowledge of psychopharmacology became available, the DSM classification became more granular, with an increasing number of different disease categories. Schermer et al. (2009) note that no less than four hundred new disease categories have been added to the DSM since its introduction in 1952. The DSM therefore became more catch-all in its categories and what had previously been regarded as character or personality attributes were increasingly listed by the DSM as subtypes of depressive illness. So, for example, Harvard psychiatrist Joseph Glenmullen notes that "perfectionism" has come to be included under the penumbra of depression in the DSM classification (2001, p. 194). This implied that all behaviour had a biological or biochemical cause and could therefore be "treated" with antidepressants – which is the so-called "biological model" of depression treatment (Glenmullen, 2001, p. 194).

The biological model of depression has been subject to considerable criticism because it is in apparent conflict with a person-centred approach to mental healthcare. Glenmullen claims that the biological approach to psychiatry has led to an inversion of the diagnostic process (2001, pp. 193–194). Rather than medicines being developed to treat diseases and to meet the needs of the person, instead diseases were being modelled on the drugs produced by the pharmaceutical industry that could be used to treat them. This argument is valid, in my view, given the high-throughput screening approach adopted by the pharmaceutical industry in the search for new therapeutic candidates in psychopharmacology. Furthermore, Glenmullen argues that the biological approach to psychiatry leads to mechanistic, rather than holistic, treatment, and is therefore reductionist in nature (2001, p. 192). He states that the biological model of depression has been cited as "proof" that depression is genetically inherited, but he argues – persuasively – that claims about the genetic causation of depression cannot be proven, due to non-equivalence of animal models and the use of surrogate endpoints in studies. He therefore dismisses theories of genetic predisposition of depression, based on the biological model of depression, as ideologically driven "Darwinian propaganda", albeit in a somewhat polemic manner.

Irish psychiatrist David Healy is another trenchant critic of the biological model of depression; he claims that the disease modelling in this way encourages biological treatment of "diseases" that are essentially social problems, rather than pathological illnesses (2004, p. 255). Healy argues that, from an ethical perspective, this modelling paradigm represents a slippery slope to social engineering and ultimately eugenics. While this is a sweeping claim, it is not without foundation. In a similar way, Ronald Cole-Turner has identified the reductionist tendency of the biological model of depression, arguing that, with psychopharmacology, humans are reaching out for molecular solutions for what are essentially spiritual problems (2001, p. 144).

These criticisms of the biological model are valid but, in my view, the polarisation between the biological model of depression and person-centred mental healthcare is a false dichotomy. A nuanced approach, accounting for both biological and person-centred factors, is more helpful. This recognises that, on the one hand, mental disorders may be grounded in real biological – neurochemical – characteristics but, on the other, they cannot simply be reduced to neurochemistry, and that both aspects must be understood to enable high-quality and truly person-centred care.

It was in an environment of rapidly developing psychopharmacological knowledge, together with an increasing willingness to embrace a biological model of psychiatry, that the SSRI antidepressants were developed, as "rational" antidepressants. Based on the previous work on serotoninergic actions of antihistamines, Bryan Molloy, a research chemist at Lilly Research at Indianapolis, US, developed a range of phenoxy-phenylpropanolamine molecules, which were structural analogues of antihistamines. Among these was the compound, LY-110 140, which was named fluoxetine in 1975, and which would eventually be marketed as Prozac (Healy, 2004, pp. 22–24; Hillhouse and Porter, 2015). However, although fluoxetine was discovered and its pharmacology investigated in the mid-1970s, it did not emerge on the market as a new antidepressant until 1988. This was for several well-documented reasons (Shorter, 2009, p. 170; Healy, 2004, p. 32). First, as was typical with the rational drug discovery process at the time, fluoxetine was just one of many compounds being screened by Lilly for antidepressant properties and, because it appeared to have only mild effects on mood but marked alerting and stimulant properties, it was not immediately recognised as an obvious candidate for marketing as an antidepressant (Healy, 2004, p. 32). Second, because of the social and financial costs of the Vietnam War, escalating healthcare costs and a distrust of scientists that had arisen during the Nixon era, there was little federal government funding for psychopharmacology research in the United States by the end of the 1970s, despite the increasing diagnostic complexity of mental disorders, as previously noted (Healy, 2004, p. 33). The third crucial factor was that the clinical trial methodology at the time of its discovery did not adequately demonstrate fluoxetine's antidepressant activity (Shorter, 2009, p. 188). Following its initial development, fluoxetine was tested against placebo (an inactive tablet) for antidepressant activity, as was standard practice at the time, but the trials showed that fluoxetine was no more effective than placebo in six out of eight clinical studies (Shorter, 2009, p. 189). However, it was not appreciated then that there was a high placebo response rate in all clinical trials of antidepressants – in other words, a patient with depression will respond to an inactive placebo, as a purely psychological effect. Once this fact was established, new antidepressants were trialled against other antidepressants instead of just a placebo, and the clinical trial required that the active agent should be superior to the comparator was relaxed (Healy, 2004, p. 34). Trials of fluoxetine under this new methodology gave a very different picture of the drug. When compared with the established tricyclic antidepressant imipramine, fluoxetine was shown to be at least as effective as imipramine as an antidepressant, but with considerably fewer side effects because of its serotonin-specific action.

Therefore, Lilly Pharmaceuticals finally had the positive clinical evidence – and marketing messages – about fluoxetine, and it was marketed as Prozac in the United States in 1988, and then in the United Kingdom in 1989. At about that time, several similar SSRI antidepressants were launched – fluvoxamine (branded Faverin) by Solvay, sertraline (branded Zoloft (US) and Lustral (UK)) by Pfizer and paroxetine (branded Paxil (US) and Seroxat (UK)) by GlaxoSmithKline (GSK). All the medicines in this class have had a profound impact on the treatment of clinical depression. However, Prozac has been the biggest-selling drug of the class and has become the most well-known – with an impact on popular culture, as well as on medicine. This impact will be explored in the next section.

4.2 The Elvis of Pharmaceuticals – the Social and Cultural Impact of SSRIs

Peter Kramer, the psychiatrist and author of the iconic book, *Listening to Prozac*, claims that, once on the market, Prozac was popular "like no previous antidepressant" (1993, pp. 1–21). Sales of Prozac were estimated as $125 million in 1988, during the drug's first year on the market, and then $350 million in 1989 (Shorter, 2009, p. 198). Two years after its launch, there had been 650,000 prescriptions for Prozac (Kramer, 1993, pp. 1–21; Stapert, 1994). Furthermore, Stapert estimates that, by 1993, 8 million people were taking Prozac and, by 1994, 10 million people, mainly in the United States, were taking it (Stapert, 1994).

There were several factors behind the massive success of Prozac. First, as stated previously, Prozac fulfilled an unmet clinical need for an effective antidepressant, but without the side effects and toxicity of older drugs. Because of these properties, Prozac was safer if taken in overdose, compared to older agents, and this was important, given that mortality due to suicide in patients treated with antidepressants was not only a tragic loss of human life and potential, but a major public health issue for society. Prozac's low toxicity in overdose was exploited heavily in Lilly's promotional campaign for the drug (Donoghue, 2008).

Second, Lilly's marketing of Prozac in the United Kingdom was aligned to the national "Defeat Depression" campaign, which highlighted the financial and social disease burden of depression, encouraged health professionals to be on the alert for signs of untreated depression, and shamed sceptical clinicians into actively treating the disease (Donoghue, 2008). The net result was that Lilly appeared to be promoting a disease, rather than a treatment, and this was criticised by opponents of the biological model of depression, referred to earlier, who accused Lilly of "disease mongering" (Schermer, 2009, pp. 75–87). Nevertheless, this led to a greater awareness of depression, and a greater willingness to prescribe an "ideal" antidepressant.

Third, psychopharmacology commentator John Donoghue argues that Prozac was launched at just the right time (2008). In both the United States and the United Kingdom, the late 1980s were a time of economic buoyancy, he argues. Society was undergoing rapid change, there was an optimistic mood and attitudes to mental health and emotional well-being were changing. Donoghue claims that, in the late 80s, people were more willing than ever before to openly express emotional pain and distress. Furthermore, Mauro cited the constitutional right to happiness in the US Declaration of Independence and claimed that, in the US in particular, many people began to feel that this right to happiness could be definitively realised via the use of Prozac and SSRIs (Mauro, 1994). Nevertheless, Carl Elliott has wisely challenged this notion of universal happiness, arguing that "happiness" is not thwarted by clinical depression, but by what he describes as existential "alienation" from the world, due to its suffering and difficulties, and that antidepressants and psychiatry cannot in themselves provide a resolution for this alienation (Elliott, 2000).

Fourth, in his critique of SSRIs, Glenmullen has argued that Prozac, as the "optimum" antidepressant, was able to thrive in the insurance-based US healthcare system in the early 1990s (2001, p. 217). Antidepressant drugs were a relatively cheap means of treating depression in comparison with counselling/therapy, where practitioner time was costly. Furthermore, the overall improved cost-effectiveness profile was especially true with the SSRIs, with their improved safety profile compared with older tricyclic agents. Health Maintenance Organisations (HMOs), the commissioners of healthcare services in the United States, could therefore establish depression treatment protocols for provider physicians to follow, and the pharmaceutical industry could negotiate significant bulk purchase deals with the HMOs for the use of their branded antidepressants. Consequently, the use of Prozac and other SSRIs became particularly widespread in the US health system during the 1990s.

Possibly because its relative safety, combined with the increasing number of subtypes of depression in expanding disease classifications, within a few years of its launch, fluoxetine began to be prescribed to people who were not profoundly clinically depressed, people who were functionally well – but who wanted to feel "better than well" (Healy, 2004, p. 263). This practice – together with its implications for society and for medical ethics – was explored by psychiatrist, Peter Kramer, in his seminal book *Listening to Prozac*, published in 1993 (Kramer, 1993). Kramer describes a patient named Tess, a woman who had many problems – an abusive parent, an unhappy marriage and a stressful working life – and who had what he described as "soft signs" of depression, but who otherwise presented well, and may have been concealing her illness (1993, pp. 1–6). Kramer wanted to give his patient the best possible treatment, so he cautiously prescribed Prozac, which was then a relatively new agent. Within two weeks, Tess had changed profoundly; not only was she no longer depressed, but she had increased energy and enhanced personal confidence.

Kramer went on to describe how fluoxetine could improve energy and confidence in other patients, and he describes fluoxetine as "cosmetic psychopharmacology", the equivalent of cosmetic surgery on the personality (1993, p. 273). Kramer suggests that fluoxetine and SSRIs could therefore be used to "treat" personality traits that had not previously been considered illnesses – for example, shyness, timidity, fastidiousness, low self-esteem and many others (1993, pp. 18–20). While Kramer was not necessarily advocating the use of fluoxetine in all these cases, he was saying that, because of their broad-ranging actions, SSRI antidepressants – and the prospect of psychotherapeutic enhancement – could not simply be ignored by society (1993, p. 20).

Listening to Prozac became an international bestseller and was a key factor in Prozac having a wider significance in society, far beyond the treatment of depression. The social implications of Kramer's work have been discussed at length. John Donoghue described how fluoxetine did not just treat depression, but "offered opportunities for pharmacological personality reconstruction", thus medicating unhappiness (2008). In his review of the social and cultural impact of Prozac, Elliott has claimed that Prozac has become "the Elvis of pharmaceuticals", an American cultural icon, "talked about on chat shows, on the celebrity circuit and in magazines" (1996). Mauro describes the cultural phenomenon of Prozac as a lifestyle drug in America (1994). As mentioned previously, he discusses the constitutional right to happiness and argues that the authors of the US Declaration of Independence probably did not envisage laboratory-manufactured drugs as the ultimate means of happiness.

However, David Healy – unsurprisingly, given his opposition to the biological model of depression – has cautioned against the "Prozac phenomenon" and the cosmetic psychopharmacology movement, saying that the popular notion that fluoxetine is a lifestyle drug that will make a person feel "better than well" is an urban myth, with its roots in the mistaken assumption that low serotonin levels always lead to depression (2004, p. 263). Healy argues – correctly, in my view, if somewhat pedantically – that fluoxetine does not make every person who takes it consistently "better than well", and that neuroimaging and pharmacogenetics tests are needed to fully understand a person's baseline personality disposition and to tailor psychopharmacological treatment accordingly. Similarly, Stapert argues that the "better than well" effects of fluoxetine that Kramer describes are serendipitous (Stapert, 1994). However, the use of fluoxetine as a mood enhancer has become part of the wider phenomenon of neuroenhancement – the use of drugs to enhance mental performance - which is widespread in American society (Brukamp and Gross, 2012). Other examples of this might include students using modafinil to reduce fatigue, or methylphenidate to improve alertness.

Commenting on the popular perception of fluoxetine as a panacea for all known mental flaws, Mauro suggests that "perhaps the bad news for Prozac is that there is no bad news" (1994). However, in the years following its launch, several drawbacks were noted with Prozac. First, not every patient treated with fluoxetine responds immediately to treatment; clinical trials indicate that only about 30% of patients have an immediate initial response to SSRI antidepressant treatment (Halfin, 2007). Second, because of its alerting properties, fluoxetine has the potential to cause anxiety and wakefulness, which can be distressing for patients (Lucas, 1992). Third, and most seriously, from 1990 onwards, reports began to emerge of SSRI antidepressants being associated with suicidal ideation in certain types of people, which was perceived as a worsening of depressive illness in these people (Healy, 2004, p. 39).

4.3 The Drug and the Soul – Christian Engagement with the Prozac Phenomenon

While the theological and ethical response of the Roman Catholic church to oral contraception is well-documented, as I have discussed elsewhere, there has been less theological engagement with SSRI antidepressants. Furthermore, theological and ethical discussion about the use of SSRI antidepressants was not a response to the actual launch and initial use of Prozac and other SSRI antidepressants in the late 1980s. Instead, it was a response to cosmetic psychopharmacology, and the "Prozac phenomenon", which came later in the mid-1990s, popularised by Kramer and colleagues, and the subsequent use of SSRIs by people in Western society who wanted to feel "better than well".

The most significant contribution to a theological and ethical understanding of SSRI antidepressants is from the American Roman Catholic scholar, John-Mark Miravalle, in his 2010 book, *The Drug, The Soul and God: A Catholic Moral Perspective on Antidepressants* (Miravalle, 2010). In this section, I will evaluate this publication at some length.

Miravalle examines the contemporary use of antidepressants in light of Thomas Aquinas's categories of human attributes. He presents an integrity ethic to support the use of antidepressants as an adjunct treatment but not as a substitute for the use of talking therapy to understand the thought processes underlying depression. Miravalle's approach is analogous to the Roman Catholic church's natural law objections to the contraceptive pill.

Miravalle argues – contentiously, in my view – that a Thomist account of psychology is more holistic than that of modern medical psychiatry, and provides a fuller understanding of the nature of depression because it is based on the Thomist categories of human attributes (Miravalle, 2010, p. 24). According to Aquinas, Miravalle argues, depression falls into the category of sorrow (2010, p. 26).[1] Sorrow is a form of passion, which is always a response to a certain perception of reality. In terms of Thomist ontology, sorrow is a sensitive, rather than a rational, appetite; in other words, while sorrow may not always be apprehended rationally, it elicits a sensory response (Miravalle, 2010, p. 27). Moreover, Miravalle states, the cause of sorrow may be the experience of a perceived evil, but the reality is that the evil is no more than a lack of, or an inappropriate absence of, a good (Miravalle, 2010, p. 36), analogous to an Augustinian approach to sin. Consequently, Miravalle concludes, sorrow, as a passion, is not necessarily a bad thing of itself, because it cannot be identified directly with the evil that causes it (2010, p. 38). Instead, sorrow is an aversion to a form of evil, and is therefore a reasonable and appropriate human response.

Nevertheless, Miravalle argues that, according to Aquinas, passions have a moral aspect and can be controlled, either through self-restraint or by practising that which is good (2010, pp. 31–32). Consequently, passions do not lessen the freedom – and therefore moral culpability – of any action arising from them. Therefore, according to Aquinas, the person who desires moral good will neither seek to eliminate the passions, nor give them free rein, but use them to strive for the good (Miravalle, 2010, p. 33).[2] Miravalle states that, although sorrow is a form of pain, it is not a self-indulgent gloominess; instead, he argues from Thomas, appropriate sorrow is a virtue, and sorrow can be an impetus for people to better themselves (2010, p. 37).

Miravalle then examines the treatment of depression from the standpoint of integrity – the wholeness of the human person. He rightly states that it is not possible to divorce ethical norms in human life from the need to encourage human flourishing. He describes the basic moral principle of integrity – that a person should act consistently in all areas of life, and at all levels (Miravalle, 2010, p. 44). Miravalle argues, however, that not all areas of human fulfilment need to be pursued to the same extent, citing the moral good of celibacy in the priesthood, which forecloses the possibility of married life and procreation. The problem with this argument, however, is that it could, in fact, be used to support the use of contraception, as a means of preventing conception and birth of children, to achieve moral goods in other areas of life, or a greater overall moral objective in life.

Miravalle then turns his attention to the Roman Catholic teaching on oral contraception (2010, p. 50). He cites the inseparable link between the procreative and unitive functions of marriage described in *Humanae Vitae* as an example of the principle of integrity (Miravalle, 2010, p. 50).[3] He states the central tenet of the encyclical, that "marriage and conjugal love are by their nature ordained towards the begetting and education of children and that contraception rids sexuality of its procreative nature and therefore contradicts the nature of man, woman and marriage" (Miravalle, 2010, pp. 51–52).[4] Miravalle argues from this that, just as "the personal functions of sexual union and procreation are not to be disfigured or robbed of their proper ends... nor ... are the personal functions of the emotions, specifically sorrow, to be disfigured or robbed of their proper ends" (by antidepressants) (2010, p. 54).

Miravalle's overall conclusion is that the antidepressant culture of the post-Kramer era is "the product of a misunderstanding of, or a non-awareness of, the meaning and significance of suffering" (2010, p. 144). Contemporary secular society, he argues, sees pleasure as the ultimate good and sorrow as the ultimate evil, and so depression has been demonised. For this reason, he claims, the cultural response is to treat depression at all costs. Consequently, in a fast-moving society which looks for rapid results and where people do not have the patience for considered analysis and reflection, there will be a temptation to use drugs, because they are convenient, and have a rapid onset of action. However, from a Thomist perspective, sorrow is not innately an evil, and there is a need for the depressed person to regain balance by re-forming their judgements according to reality, and then re-aligning their emotions in line with those judgments (Miravalle, 2010, p. 62). Miravalle argues that antidepressants prevent this re-alignment, leading to a state of internal disharmony – a variance between cognition and emotion.

Miravalle concludes that, although the use of antidepressants is not "intrinsically evil" (2010, p. 59), in that they have an important role in the treatment of urgent symptoms of depression, they are no substitute for the use of psychotherapy to deal with the root cause of the person's sorrow and should only ever be used in conjunction with psychotherapy. He quotes the guidance of the Pontifical Council for Pastoral Assistants; "Drug therapy is helpful if it does not obfuscate or interfere with the healing of a root problem" (Miravalle, 2010, p. 75).[5] Miravalle's dispute does not seem to be with the therapeutic use of antidepressants *per se*, but the "antidepressant culture" that Kramer envisages, where the drugs are used indiscriminately to induce "better than well" personality changes. Miravalle's advocacy of antidepressants only as an adjunct to psychotherapy is supported by clinical trial results with SSRIs, which show that, while there is little difference in efficacy between antidepressants and psychotherapy in short-term use, psychotherapy has greater efficacy in long-term treatment (Glenmullen, 2001, p. 189).

However, there are some significant problems with Miravalle's approach. First, of particular note is Miravalle's absolute rejection of any biological model for depression – that is, that depression might be due in part to a chemical imbalance or a genetic predisposition, as discussed earlier in this chapter – which he expresses at various points in the book (Miravalle, 2010, pp. 12–14, 20, 45, 59, 70, 86). Miravalle has good reasons to downplay the role of a biological model of depression; it is at odds with his Thomist metaphysics because it assumes that human behaviour arises substantially from the operation of the material human body. Indeed, Miravalle is probably keen to avoid any notion of biological reductionism, as many Christian commentators would be when faced with scientific developments with significant social and ethical implications for human life. Whereas psychiatrist Glenmullen rejects the idea of genetic inheritance of depression as ideologically driven "Darwinian propaganda" on scientific grounds (2001, p. 189), Miravalle most likely rejects reductionism on religious grounds, because of his commitment to Roman Catholic natural law-based morality.

However, Miravalle's complete rejection of the biological model of depression is out of step with a scientific understanding of antidepressant action, in the light of the monoamine hypothesis and subsequent developments in psychopharmacology, as described previously here. There are indeed problems with the biological model for depression – for example, inability to measure levels of noradrenaline and serotonin *in vivo*, the use of surrogate endpoints in animal studies and the difficulties of quantifying results (Hillhouse and Porter, 2015). However, the biological model cannot simply be ignored or discounted. While response factors to antidepressants are complex and cannot be easily correlated to effects on specific biochemical systems, other evidence from psychopharmacology – for example, the role of thyroid hormone and cortisol in the regulation of depressive illness – indicates that non-neuropharmacological, biological factors are indubitably involved in the pathology of depression (Glenmullen, 2001, p. 189).

Interestingly, in his acknowledgement of the psychological effects of SSRIs, Miravalle seems to implicitly accept that the action of these antidepressants has a biological basis (Miravalle, 2010, p. 86). In doing this, Miravalle is advocating a dualism of the human person, which is consistent with Aquinas' classification, but is not aligned with more recent theological anthropologies which account for scientific understandings of humanity and advocate a non-dualistic view of the human person – for example, the non-reductive physicalism of Nancey Murphy (1998), or the dual-aspect monism of John Polkinghorne (1998, pp. 49–65).

Second, Miravalle's natural law-based arguments concerning the use of SSRI antidepressants are flawed. His stated objective is to apply the same natural law argument to SSRI antidepressants that has been used previously to oppose hormonal contraception (Miravalle, 2010, pp. 2–3, pp. 50–55). The teleology of the natural law approach seems to appeal to Miravalle (2010, pp. 24, 45). However, for Miravalle, this teleology appears to be predetermined and therefore seems to restrict both self-determination (and therefore the exercise of moral agency of the individual through personal autonomy) and also human creativity. Miravalle argues that "man does not create himself but rather finds himself and the world around him to have a definite structure, with conditions for perfection and flourishing already determined" (2010, p. 57). He claims – strikingly – that "man cannot change his structure, so cannot reinvent conditions for fulfilment and that he can but accept them". Miravalle's assertion here is in marked contrast to the transhumanist notions that morphological freedom (ability to exist in different forms) is eminently possible, that human nature is infinitely malleable, and that human beings can change themselves at will through unrestricted personal autonomy. Given the conflict I have described elsewhere between natural law and transhumanism, Miravalle's approach here is unsurprising. But Miravalle seems to contradict himself when he claims that man can make choices (2010, p. 57); for Miravalle, these choices seem to be restricted to abstract moral choices framed in the traditional natural law discourse of the Roman Catholic church.

A related problem with Miravalle's argument is his selective use of natural law. He defends the use of analgesics for the treatment of physical pain, arguing that it is important to suppress pain to enable normal bodily function (2010, pp. 78–79). He then asks (rhetorically?): why would one suppress soul pain? The answer, however, would be for the same reason as one would suppress physical pain – to enable normal functioning and provide humane treatment of a suffering person. He also defends the consumption of alcohol, stating that alcohol is consumed for many reasons, not just its mood-altering properties (Miravalle, 2010, pp. 78–79). However, many people undoubtedly consume alcohol for its mood-altering properties, and possibly not for any other reason. Miravalle's approach here is interesting in the light of Peter Kramer's claim that, with the non-therapeutic use of Prozac, the boundaries between licit and illicit drug use are blurred and that people use street drugs all the time to feel good (1993, p. 16).

Third, Miravalle readily dismisses a number of what he terms "inadequate objections" to antidepressant use (2010, p. 60). These include, for example, a) the fact that depression may be an adaptive trait and may have some positive personality benefits, for example in driven, creative and artistic people, b) the concept of pharmacological Calvinism (the idea that using drugs is a sign of weakness, and that they must be avoided in order to "toughen up" in life) and, c) that antidepressants may be a tool for cultural manipulation and oppression, a consequence envisaged by Peter Kramer (1993, pp. 269–272). These objections to antidepressant use by an individual person may be "inadequate" in Miravalle's view, from the standpoint of Catholic natural law, but they cannot be dismissed easily when considering the wider societal implications of the use of antidepressants – for example, fair distribution of antidepressants in society, or the impact of antidepressant use on cultural expectations in society. These are issues I will discuss in the next section of this chapter. Indeed, the notion of "pharmacological Calvinism" is highly relevant to Miravalle's own remarks concerning "soul pain", as opposed to physical pain, and how it should be treated.

The issue of cultural oppression through the widespread use of specific medical interventions has huge implications for social ethics. Widespread non-therapeutic use of SSRI antidepressants may mean that more individuals will have a positive outlook on life as their default mood. This will adjust the prevailing culture concerning, for example, bereavement or justice in the workplace. If people taking SSRI antidepressants as an enhancement do not grieve in the same way as in previous generations, there will be an increased expectation that people will be able to handle a loss and "move on" more easily, which would be unfair and unkind to the unenhanced person. The church would need to take this into account in its bereavement ministry. If people taking SSRI antidepressants as an enhancement are likely to be more assertive and driven in the workplace, this may lead to a changed perception of what behaviour is fair and reasonable in the workplace, which would be disadvantageous to the unenhanced person.

Here, Miravalle sets out an argument against cosmetic psychopharmacology with SSRI antidepressants firmly based on Aquinas' understanding of human nature and a Roman Catholic natural law-based approach to moral reasoning. However, if the wider clinical and social experience of SSRI antidepressant use is considered, various significant ethical flaws in the argument become clear. This suggests that a broader approach to the ethical evaluation of psychopharmacology is needed. The next section will assess the use of SSRI antidepressants according to the general and specific criteria for transhumanism, to determine the extent to which Prozac and SSRI antidepressants can be regarded as transhumanist biomedical technologies and their ethical implications.

4.4 SSRIs and Transhumanism

Development of Prozac and other SSRIs was the result of previous scientific advances. In the same way that the development of the contraceptive pill was dependent on a reasonable understanding of reproductive hormonal activity and the ability to produce sex hormones synthetically, so SSRI development was dependent on the establishment of the monoamine hypothesis of depression and an understanding of the neurotransmitter actions of serotonin.

However, the motivations of the developers were different. With the contraceptive pill, the developers arguably had a vision of the positive benefits of the pill on society, a vision that was realised with the social impact of the pill after its launch. By contrast, Prozac was developed as a potential antidepressant and there is no evidence that the implications of non-therapeutic use in society were considered at the time of its development. This was mainly because depression is a disease, whereas pregnancy is not. However, it was also because of the scientific and regulatory framework in the pharmaceutical industry at that time, which was very different to the culture of the industry when the contraceptive pill was launched. Despite Lilly's objective of developing an effective, modern antidepressant, Prozac's "better than well" effects, and their cultural impact, were essentially serendipitous (Stapert, 1994), I would argue that Peter Kramer, with his exploration of the wider use of Prozac for "cosmetic psychopharmacology", and its potential social, political and ethical implications, saw the transhumanist potential of Prozac more clearly than the industry inventors of the drug (Kramer, 1993, p. xv). Nevertheless, from a perspective of the pharmaceutical industry, the development of Prozac was, to an extent, a serendipitous process, and any intentions on the part of the pharmaceutical company will be secondary to an objective evaluation of whether Prozac resembled, in its time, a transhumanist technology.

Using the general criteria from the transhumanism literature, to what extent were SSRI antidepressants transhumanist in character? These general criteria for a transhumanist technology are 1) that it is a technology, 2) that it is applied to the human person, 3) that it is applied to promote human flourishing and 4) that it may be applied with autonomy.

First, as a chemical agent, which exerts an effect on the human body – and, in this case, on the human brain – SSRI antidepressants are indeed a technology; a material means of effecting a task or process. However, with SSRI antidepressants, especially in the light of the debate about the biological model of depression, it is fair to raise a query about what exactly that task or process is. At the basic level, the process could be defined as the relief of depression by enhancing the levels of serotonin in the brain.

Second, regardless of possible therapeutic processes, SSRI antidepressants are clearly a technology that is applied to the human person, in order to effect those processes. For example, Kahane and Savulescu describe the use of SSRI antidepressants such as citalopram for moral enhancement and claim that the ethical implications of this are no less important than the use of radical – and biologically invasive – forms of biomedical enhancement which might be available in the future (2015).

Third, are SSRI antidepressants, as a medical technology, applied to human beings to improve human function, increase longevity and promote human flourishing? SSRI antidepressants are effective in relieving clinical depression, a potentially distressing and debilitating medical condition (Donoghue, 2008). In addition, SSRI antidepressants have the potential to enhance attention, energy and alertness (Glenmullen, 2001, p. 212). Furthermore, studies suggest that SSRI antidepressants may improve quality of life, as well as symptoms of depression (Yang et al., 2017), and that relief of depression with SSRI antidepressants is associated with improved quality of life and daily physical and mental functioning (Lin et al., 2013). In addition, SSRI antidepressants have a direct effect on longevity in some specific cases, where their reduced toxicity prevents a depression-related suicide by attempted overdose. There are therefore various strands of evidence to suggest that Prozac and SSRI antidepressants have largely a positive and beneficial effect on human flourishing.

Fourth, does the human person using SSRI antidepressants have autonomy over their use? Are SSRI antidepressants used in a way that is not coercive? Given the history and experience with SSRI antidepressant use, the findings here are highly debatable. In current Western healthcare systems and culture, with their emphasis on informed consent to treatment, people considering treatment with SSRI antidepressants ostensibly have autonomy – as uncoerced self-determination – to make an individual, informed and free choice about treatment at the outset. This is also the case with the contraceptive pill, and indeed with some of the proposed future transhumanist biomedical developments, as discussed previously.

However, I would argue that there may be subsequent scenarios where personal autonomy might be eroded in people taking SSRI antidepressants. An individual may choose to use a psychoactive drug in an ostensibly autonomous, self-determined way at the outset, but that autonomy may be impaired subsequently by the effects of the drug, which may affect future decisions – either any subsequent decision to discontinue the drug, or life choices while taking the drug. For example, a person's autonomy might be impaired in cases of suicidal ideation as an adverse effect of SSRI antidepressants; these are well-documented, but thankfully rare (Healy, 2004, p. 40). In a similar way, autonomy might be affected by involuntary effects of the drug; drug-induced diminished responsibility was cited as a defence for Wesbecker, a man from Kentucky, who went on a shooting spree, while being treated with Prozac (Healy, 2004, p. 64). As well as these extreme examples, SSRI antidepressants may also be associated with withdrawal effects on routine use, where a person may experience adverse effects when discontinuing the drug (Price et al., 1996; Schatzberg et al., 1997). Whether there is a specific dependence syndrome with SSRIs, as there was with benzodiazepines, has been extensively debated (for a summary see Nutt, 2003). Nevertheless, this withdrawal effect may influence the willingness of patients to take the drug and raise concerns about its safety (Shelton, 2006).

Kramer considers the unintended consequences of Prozac on human characteristics in *Listening to Prozac* (Kramer, 1993, p. 13), which are also relevant to whether the medicine can be used with autonomy in the real world. He states that society is comfortable with the idea of someone taking a drug to make small differences to their own life, but less happy for a drug to be an agent of change at a wider societal level. He considers how society might change if more people were taking a drug which, for example, enhanced their sexual appeal, or improved their business acumen. Taking one example, Kramer surmises that, if over-seriousness and introspection could be "cured" using Prozac, then society might lose its taste for brooding, melancholic, artistic people, and this would have far-reaching implications for the arts and popular culture (1993, p. 18). In addition, Kramer considers whether more widespread use of Prozac as a "mood brightener" might lead to harsher cultural expectations concerning time to grieve after a bereavement (1993, p. 254). He also wonders how use of Prozac for personality enhancement might lead to a re-negotiation of the doctor-patient relationship (Kramer, 1993, p. 13). These observations are consistent with more recent debates about the use of SSRI antidepressants for moral enhancement. While moral enhancement with SSRI antidepressants is clearly a different proposal to the treatment of depression with SSRI antidepressants, the dividing line between therapy and enhancement is often indistinct. Furthermore, the doctrine of double effect comes into play. A medical technology may have two effects; it may act as a therapy in one scenario, but an enhancement in another (Waters, 2006). The doctrine of double effect would apply here as it would provide an ethical defence for a practitioner who gives a therapeutic intervention that is intended as a therapy, but which then acts unintentionally as an enhancement. The doctrine of double effect applies to the "better than well" personality effects of SSRI antidepressants, when they are prescribed primarily to treat depression, in the same way as the contraceptive action of the contraceptive pill when it is used therapeutically to regulate the menstrual cycle

Moreover, observations concerning autonomy in the treatment of individual depressed people with SSRIs support Sparrow's concerns about autonomy in society when SSRI antidepressants are used for enhancement (2014). SSRI antidepressants may confer personality advantages on individuals who take them, which may lead to inequity between the enhanced and the unenhanced in society, and give rise to abuse of power, injustice and oppression in society.

The method of distribution of SSRI antidepressants may also affect personal choice concerning whether to take the medicine. As discussed previously, the US healthcare system has been able to distribute SSRI antidepressants widely, so that they are an easily affordable medical intervention which is quicker and cheaper to implement that psychotherapy, and this may have exerted pressure on many stressed Americans to avail themselves of SSRI antidepressant treatment, simply because it is available. This raises ethical concerns because it could be construed as coercion of patients by health commissioners and providers. Furthermore, since the system is such that the uninsured do not have access to these treatments, the system may be regarded as unjust, in the light of the ethical principle that a government should provide an adequate level of healthcare to all its citizens.

To summarise the situation with SSRIs and autonomy, while individuals may exercise apparent autonomy when commencing SSRI antidepressant therapy, this autonomy may be impaired at subsequent points in therapy. This may be due to a direct psychopharmacological effect, such as the specific adverse effect of suicidal ideation, or the effects of SSRIs on the individual's personality, or it might be due to indirect effects, for example, changes in cultural expectations or development of oppressive social tendencies due to widespread use of SSRI antidepressants.

In conclusion, SSRI antidepressants resemble a transhumanist technology, according to these general criteria for transhumanist technologies, with the crucial feature that their impact on personal autonomy is ambiguous, a similar finding to that concerning the contraceptive pill.

4.5 An Ethical Re-evaluation of SSRI Antidepressants

But how do SSRI antidepressants measure up against the theological criteria for ethical evaluation of biomedical developments? They are as follows:

1. Is the project good news for the poor?
2. Is the project an attempt to be "like God" (in respect of Genesis 3v5) or does it conform to the image of God? (Genesis 1v26).
3. What attitude does the project embody towards the material world (including our own bodies)? And how does the technology affect the corporate "body" of society?
4. What attitude does the project embody towards past failures?
5. Does the technology enable unbridled autonomy in a negative manner?
6. Does the technology focus too much on the users' subjective experiences?

These criteria are a combination of Neil Messer's "diagnostic questions" of a biotechnology project (2007, pp. 229–235), and Elaine Graham's theological critiques of transhumanism (2006); I have discussed the use of these criteria elsewhere.

First, is Prozac good news for the poor? The economic costs of depression, as a debilitating disease, are well-recognised (Kessler, 2012). Halfin estimates that the direct cost of depression treatment (in a US context) is \$3.5 million per 1000 patients (2007). This figure is based on patients on health insurance plans, so does not account for the cost to society of untreated depression in those who do not have health insurance. Furthermore, Halfin notes that depression is often underdiagnosed, and that the actual social and economic burden of undiagnosed depression is much higher, even in the insured population.

Donoghue and Pincus note that depression is likely to be associated with considerable indirect costs, because of impaired relationships, absenteeism and reduced productivity at work, and health costs that are not related directly to the treatment of depression (2007). Furthermore, in their review of the economic burden of depression, Lane and McDonald rightly argue that any evaluation of the economic costs of depression should account for not just the acquisition costs of antidepressants, but the overall value of the treatment, in terms of long-term efficacy, improved compliance, and reduced accident potential (1994). Wilde and Benfield note that economic studies that focus primarily on the acquisition cost of ingredients are from the perspective of the cost to the payor, not the cost to the patient (1998). Consequently, while these studies provide evidence of the cost-effectiveness of SSRIs to health providers, they do not demonstrate any direct financial benefits to the individual person receiving the therapy. Consequently, although, in theory, SSRI antidepressants certainly will have a positive impact on the lives of poor and marginalised people, there is less direct evidence to show this.

In an American study of low-income and minority women, Miranda et al. found that the use of antidepressant medication, as opposed to psychotherapy or community support, was associated with better outcome gains, in terms of treatment of depression (2003). This suggests that ensuring access to, and cost-effective distribution of, SSRI antidepressants in low-income populations in the United States, or other Western countries has the potential to make a significant difference to depression treatment and associated quality of life for poor people. A study by Souetre et al. in France has examined the effects of depression on work loss (absence from work), and the impact of four antidepressant therapies (including fluoxetine (Prozac)) and placebo (1993). This study, unsurprisingly, noted a positive correlation between depression severity and the risk of work loss/absence, and found that fluoxetine treatment was associated with the best antidepressant response, and the lowest level of absence from work. However, the power of this study is diminished by having five study groups, the demographics of the participants was biased towards women and those in urban areas, and it is unclear on how these results were weighted according to work type and professional characteristics.

The costs of depression to society are well-recognised, and the costs of antidepressants for health providers have been studied extensively. Furthermore, the benefits of antidepressant use – both as therapy and enhancement – largely by middle-class professionals – have been discussed in the medical and popular literature. In theory, SSRI antidepressants will have benefits in poor and marginalised populations and there is some evidence available to demonstrate this, but this evidence is limited compared to the considerable body of evidence about economic benefits to health providers. In my view, this represents an important area of opportunity, both in terms of health provision to the poor and marginalised, especially in developing countries, and research into the benefits of that provision.

Second, is the project an attempt to be "like God" (with reference to Genesis 3v5) or does it conform to the image of God? This can be argued both ways. On one hand, SSRI use for cosmetic psychopharmacology - to remould someone's personality, as envisaged by Kramer, and change their nature – is indeed an attempt to be "like God". For John-Mark Miravalle, with his natural law objections to the sole use of SSRI antidepressants in depression, and his claim that SSRI antidepressants short-circuit the link between cognition and emotion and thus undermine the good ends of human life, indiscriminate use of SSRI antidepressants certainly appears to be an attempt to be "like God".

On the other hand, however, use of SSRI antidepressants responsibly enables humans to conform more closely to the image of God because their use aligns with a theological understanding of the *imago Dei* that is functional and relational, not just substantive. The natural law approach to therapies, which the Roman Catholic church has used as the basis of its moral theology to date, is based on the idea that human nature is fixed, unchanging and immutable (Pope, 2014), and this reflects a substantive approach to the *imago Dei* – that is, the image of God in humanity consists of innate attributes of the substance of the human person. This notion has been challenged scientifically, by both the theory of evolution and experimental behavioural studies (Pope, 2014). On the contrary, functional and relational approaches to the *imago Dei* emphasise both human function (in terms of vocation or calling in the world) and human relational capacity as aspects of the image of God, rather than just substantial nature. These approaches to understanding the *imago Dei* in humanity align with the observed benefits of SSRI therapy. SSRI therapy improves human biological and mental function (Lin, 2013), and thereby improves a person's relationships with others, and enables their meaningful and positive engagement with human society. These two factors enable a person to fulfil their vocation from a Christian perspective of human flourishing.

The distinction between biological function and vocational function (the functional approach to the *imago Dei*) should be noted. Biological function alone is an ethically neutral concept – a functioning human body can be used for good or bad ends. Nevertheless, as well as being itself a good of human wholeness and integrity, restoration of biological function is a prerequisite for a person to achieve their full potential in society, and to be able to exercise their true vocation in the world. Restoration of human function with antidepressants therefore supports human vocation and is consistent with a functional approach to the *imago Dei*.

Furthermore, as seen from the work of Peter Kramer, SSRIs have wide-ranging effects on mood and personality, and therefore have an impact on human relationships (Kramer, 1993, p. 7). Kramer's work highlighted several examples of cases where taking Prozac had an impact on individual relationships. First, in his case study of his patient, Tess, Kramer described how Tess had had a history of parental abuse, and this caused her to seek "degrading" relationships on an ongoing basis, at cost of her well-being (Kramer, 1993, p. 2). However, treatment with Prozac enabled Tess to be energised and confident, which had a positive effect on her relationships. Second, Kramer cites the example of individuals who take Prozac to improve their alertness and performance at work, which has an impact on their working relationships (1993, pp. 28, 94). Third, Kramer described the case of Mrs B, who was prescribed Prozac for compulsive behaviour (hair pulling), but who found that the drug made her more content with her personal life, and less anxious and needy about her romantic relationships (Kramer, 1993, p. 267). In her study of the use of SSRI antidepressants among university students, both therapeutically and for personality enhancement, McKinney and Greenfield cite the case of Natalie, a student who began treatment with Prozac with much reluctance, due to negative attitudes from her family, but who found that treatment with the drug was a liberating experience, which radically changed her relationship with her family (2010). Indeed, there are indications that antidepressants do not just have an impact on interhuman relationships, but on a person's relationship with God; Stapert describes the case of Marjorie, a woman taking Prozac, who discovered a "fresh sense of God" as her treatment proceeded (1994). The use of SSRI antidepressants therefore also reflects a relational approach to the *imago Dei* as well as a functional one.

To summarise, there is evidence that the use of SSRI antidepressants supports a view of human nature consistent with a comprehensive understanding of the *imago Dei*. SSRI antidepressant use supports functional and relational aspects of the image of God in humanity, and is not just concerned with substantive human attributes, which is the focus of many transhumanist technologies and proponents of transhumanism.

Third, what attitude does the project embody towards the material world, including our own bodies, and what impact does it have on the corporate body of society? Like oral contraception and some proposed future medical technologies, such as medical nanotechnology and cryogenics, but unlike some other proposed technologies, such as mind-uploading, SSRI antidepressants are affirming of the material world and bodily life, in that they exert positive effects which facilitate human flourishing in and through the material processes of the human brain and body, rather than as a therapeutic placebo or as a biotechnology that deprecates the human body. Because they are used for their effects on mood and personality, the use of SSRI antidepressants, as material technologies, could reinforce a dualistic approach to humanity, with separate rational and material (bodily) aspects of human life. However, precisely because there is some biological basis for depression, depression has somatic symptoms. The treatment of depression therefore has somatic benefits; as stated earlier, SSRI antidepressants improve attention, energy and alertness, as well as improving mood. Consequently, the positive effects of SSRI antidepressants improve mental function and uphold the integrity of the individual body. This may, in turn, have a positive impact on the corporate body of society through individual bodily function and activity, thereby improving overall human flourishing.

However, there is some evidence here that the positive effects of SSRI use for the individual do not necessarily benefit society, and that the effects of SSRI use on the corporate body of society may, in fact, be ambiguous. As argued by Kramer, SSRI antidepressant use may lead to cultural redefinition of important human experiences such as bereavement, which may change the dynamics of the doctor-patient relationship, both of which may have negative consequences for society (Kramer, 1993, pp. 13, 254). Sparrow argues that the use of SSRI antidepressants as a form of moral enhancement in society has the potential to reduce the autonomy of some people, depending on how the drugs are distributed and used in society, because the enhancers would be wielding power over the unenhanced, which may lead to injustice and oppression (Sparrow, 2014).

Fourth, what attitude does the project embody towards past failures? As described previously here, SSRI antidepressants have been hugely popular in Western society, in terms of both consumption and commercial sales. They therefore have become significant in popular culture. However, the popularity of something does not necessarily equate to pride or hubris concerning its availability and use. Bottled mineral water is popular, both in terms of consumption and commercial sales, but it can hardly be regarded as the pinnacle of human technological achievement.

Just as the oral contraceptive pill has been described as the "ideal" contraceptive, so Prozac was developed as the "ideal" antidepressant, with good efficacy in the treatment of depression, combined with a favourable side-effect profile and lack of toxicity in overdose. With reduced withdrawal potential compared to benzodiazepines, SSRI antidepressants were an advance on the "past failure" of benzodiazepines in psychopharmacology, and there is some evidence that clinicians were more wary about psychotherapeutic prescribing after the benzodiazepine scandal (King, 1992; Healy, 2004, p. 34). The development of SSRI antidepressants seems to represent the climax of rational psychopharmacology, in that there have been no therapeutic advances for depression since the 1990s (López-Muñoz and Alamo, 2009), and the use of SSRIs has suppressed the exploration of new models of depression, and the investigation of new drugs (Perez-Caballero et al., 2014). This itself might be evidence of technological hubris and triumphalism.

However, Prozac's status as a cultural phenomenon, rather than just a medicine for depression, suggests that many people saw Prozac as a panacea for society's ills and had elevated expectation of its value to society. Carl Elliott describes how Prozac became an American cultural icon and was featured prominently in the popular media – in magazines, on the celebrity circuit and on chat shows (1996). One such magazine article, by Mauro, declared that "the bad news for Prozac might be that there is no bad news", and that it really is a panacea (1994). Notwithstanding what might be regarded as cultural and media hype, not related directly to the use of the drug, there is certainly some evidence that SSRI antidepressants have been regarded by society with hubristic pride.

Fifth, does the technology enable unbridled autonomy in a negative manner? The availability of SSRI antidepressants gives people the option for treatment of depression, when in previous generations, no treatment option existed, and people ostensibly have choice about their treatment at the outset. However, as I argued at length earlier, the impact of SSRI antidepressants on autonomy are ambiguous, and the course of SSRI antidepressant treatment is by no means associated with "unbridled autonomy". In any case, autonomy is an ethically neutral phenomenon – it may be used to inflict selfish desires on others, or it can be used to pursue good ethical ends. SSRI antidepressants may be used for good ethical ends – to enhance mental function so that a person can be more effective in their job or relationships and thereby contribute positively to society – or for bad ethical ends – for hedonism and self-indulgence.

Sixth, does the technology focus too much on the users' subjective experiences? As I have discussed elsewhere, the irony is that, although transhumanist technologies have the potential to enhance the personal subjective experience of human life, because of their radical enhancement effects, they are problematic because they ultimately objectify the human body, so that the body is in danger of becoming an artefact to be engineered and manipulated at will, rather than a human person (Cole-Turner, 2001, pp. 142, 143, 147). SSRI antidepressants have a direct effect on the clinical course of depression in the patient – but also the large-scale treatment of depression in society affects the functioning of society and reduces the economic burden of depression. I would therefore argue that, while SSRIs do enhance the subjective experience of a person, due to their mental effects, when they are used in a widespread manner, their use affects society as a whole and so their use cannot be a wholly subjective experience. Indeed, the widespread use of SSRIs to manipulate the personality, as described by Kramer and others, is a way in which people are objectified by a technology.

Sartorius suggests that the incidence of depressive illness may increase in future, due to demographic changes, increased life expectancy and increasing incidences of iatrogenic depression (depression induced by medical treatment), and states that the use of new antidepressant treatments, which do not require extensive intervention by specialist mental healthcare personnel, will become an ethical imperative (2001). I tend to agree with this view, and therefore would argue that the need for a Christian ethical evaluation of antidepressants, and indeed other psychopharmacological advances, is important.

The ethical analysis of the use of SSRI antidepressants here represents a departure from a natural law-based ethical approach, which has characterised previous Christian responses to both the contraceptive pill and SSRI antidepressants. I have shown here that, like the contraceptive pill, SSRI antidepressants resemble a transhumanist technology, in that they are a technology which is applied to the human person and have largely had a beneficial effect on human flourishing.

Unlike transhumanist technologies that are highly technological in nature in comparison with conventional drug therapy – for example, mind-uploading or cryogenics – SSRI antidepressants have the potential to be beneficial to the poor, although evidence is, as yet, limited. Unlike approaches to transhumanism that emphasise human attributes, and therefore a more substantive approach to the *imago Dei*, the effects and benefits of SSRI antidepressants in clinical use reflect a comprehensive understanding of the *imago Dei*, which is functional and relational, not just substantive. Unlike some forms of transhumanist technologies, such as mind-uploading, which are anti-materialist, SSRI antidepressants, like the contraceptive pill, exert positive effects and benefits by working through the human body and its mechanisms, rather than by negating biological life. Furthermore, SSRI antidepressants may have a significant impact on human society as a whole – not just the experience of the individual. The effects of SSRI use are therefore both individual and corporate.

Given their success as a therapy, and their potential for "cosmetic" use following the "Prozac phenomenon", SSRI antidepressants have been regarded by some as the supreme achievement of rational psychopharmacology in a hubristic way, in a similar way to proposed future transhumanist technologies.

Most significantly, however, SSRI antidepressant use raises significant questions for personal autonomy, in the same way as contraceptive pill usage may do. A stated aim of the transhumanist movement is that individuals who are seeking biomedical enhancement can adopt a biomedical technology autonomously, as a matter of free, personal choice. Correspondingly, a key theological criticism of transhumanist technologies is that they enable unbridled autonomy in a negative manner. The evidence from the use of SSRI antidepressants suggests that, in a similar way to the contraceptive pill, neither of these extremes is true. While individual users of SSRI antidepressants can exercise autonomy in choosing them at the outset of use, adverse effects and unintended consequences with individual use, and changes in cultural expectations and societal norms if they are used widely in society, can lead to erosion of personal autonomy for the individual.

The next chapter will re-evaluate the Christian ethics of future transhumanist medical technologies, in the light of the findings from these two case studies of past therapeutic developments, the contraceptive pill and SSRI antidepressants, and will answer the research questions posed at the beginning of this book.

Notes

1 Miravalle, *The Drug, The Soul and God*, p. 26, citing Thomas Aquinas, "Summa Theologica Q23 Article 4", 2010, https://www.documentacatholicaomnia.eu/03d/1225-1274,_Thomas_Aquinas,_Summa_Theologica_%5B1%5D,_EN.pdf (accessed September 2020).
2 Miravalle, *The Drug, The Soul and God*, p. 33, citing Aquinas, "Summa Theologica, Q24, Article 1".
3 Miravalle, *The Drug, The Soul and God*, p. 50, citing Pope Paul VI, Pope Paul VI, "On the Regulation of Birth: Humanae Vitae", 1968, http://www.vatican.va/content/paul-vi/en/encyclicals/documents/hf_p-vi_enc_25071968_humanae-vitae.html (accessed March 2020).
4 Miravalle, *The Drug, The Soul and God*, pp. 51–52, citing Pope Paul VI, "Humanae Vitae".
5 Miravalle, *The Drug, The Soul and God*, p. 75, citing the Pontifical Council for Pastoral Assistants, "Charter for Healthcare Workers" (1995), 100.

References

Alan Schatzberg, Peter Haddad, Eric Kaplan, Michel Lejoyeux, Jerrold F. Rosenbaum, A. H. Young and John Zajecka. "Serotonin Reuptake Inhibitor Discontinuation Syndrome: A Hypothetical Definition", *Journal of Clinical Psychiatry*, 58 (Suppl 7) (1997), pp. 5–10.

Aron Halfin, "Depression: The Benefits of Early and Appropriate Treatment", *American Journal of Managed Care*, 13 (2007), pp. S92–S97.

Arvid Carlsson, Hans Corrodi, Kjell Fuxe and Tomas Hökfelt, "Effects of Some Antidepressant Drugs on the Depletion of Intraneuronal Brain Catecholamine Stores Caused by 4, a-Dimethyl-meta-tyramine", *European Journal of Pharmacology*, 5 (1969), pp. 367–373.

Brent Waters, "Saving Us from Ourselves: Christology, Anthropology and the Seduction of Posthuman Medicine", in *Future Perfect?: God, Medicine and Human Identity*, edited by Celia Deane-Drummond and Peter Manley Scott (London: T and T Clark International, 2006), pp. 183–195.

Carl Elliott, "The Elvis of Pharmaceuticals", *British Medical Journal*, 313 (1996), p. 950.

Carl Elliott, "Pursued by Happiness and Beaten Senseless: Prozac and the American Dream", *Hastings Center Report*, 30 (2000), pp. 7–12.

Ching Hua Lin, Yung-Chieh Yen, Ming-Chao Chen and Cheng-Chung Chen, "Relief of Depression and Pain Improves Daily Functioning and Quality of Life in Patients with Major Depressive Disorder", *Progress in Neuropsychopharmacology and Biological Psychiatry*, 47 (2013), pp. 93–98.

David Healy, *Let Them Eat Prozac: The Unhealthy Relationship Between the Pharmaceutical Industry and Depression* (New York/London: New York University Press, 2004).

David Nutt, "Death and Dependence: Current Controversies Over the Selective Serotonin Reuptake Inhibitors", *Journal of Psychopharmacology*, 17 (2003), pp. 355–364.

Edward Shorter, *Before Prozac: The Troubled History of Mood Disorders in Psychiatry* (Oxford: Oxford University Press, 2009).

Elaine Graham, "In Whose Image? Representations of Technology and the Ends of Humanity", in *Future Perfect? God, Medicine and Human Identity*, edited by Celia Deane-Drummond and Peter Manley Scott (London: T and T Clark International, 2006), pp. 58–61.

E. Souetre, H. Lozet, P. Martin, J. P. Lecanu, J. M. Gauthier, J. N. Beuzen and V. Ravily, "Work Loss and Depression. Impact of Fluoxetine", *Therapie*, 48 (1993), pp. 81–88.

Francisco López-Muñoz and Cecilio Alamo, "Monoaminergic Neurotransmission: The History of the Discovery of Antidepressants from 1950s Until Today", *Current Pharmaceutical Design*, 15 (2009), pp. 1563–1586.

Guy Kahane and Julian Savulescu, "Normal Human Variation: Refocussing the Enhancement Debate", *Bioethics*, 29 (2015), pp. 133–143.

James Mauro, "And Prozac for all …", *Psychology Today*, 27 (1994), pp. 44–50.

Jeanne Miranda, Joyce Y. Chung, Bonnie L. Green, Janice Krupnick, Juned Siddique, Dennis A. Revicki and Tom Belin, "Treating Depression in Predominantly Low-Income Young Minority Women: A Randomized Controlled Trial", *Journal of the American Medical Association*, 290 (2003), pp. 57–65.

John-Mark Miravalle, *The Drug, the Soul and God: A Catholic Moral Perspective on Antidepressants* (Chicago: University of Scranton Press, 2010).

John Donoghue, "Prozac: Is It Worthy of the Hype?", *Pharmaceutical Journal*, 280 (2008), pp. 57–58.

Julie Donoghue and Harold Pincus, "Reducing the Societal Burden of Depression: A Review of Economic Costs, Quality of Care and Effects of Treatment", *Pharmacoeconomics*, 25 (2007), pp. 7–24.

Joseph Glenmullen, *Prozac Backlash: Overcoming the Dangers of Prozac, Zoloft, Paxil, and Other Antidepressants with Safe, Effective Alternatives* (New York: Simon and Schuster, 2001).

John Polkinghorne, *Science and Theology: An Introduction* (London: SPCK/Fortress, 1998).

John Price, Patrick Waller, Susan Wood and Angus MacKay, "A Comparison of the Post-marketing Safety of Four Selective Serotonin Re-uptake Inhibitors Including the Investigation of Symptoms Occurring on Withdrawal", *British Journal of Clinical Pharmacology*, 42 (1996), pp. 757–763.

John Stapert, "Curing an Illness or Transforming the Self? The Power of Prozac", *Christian Century*, 111 (1994), pp. 684–687.

Kelly McKinney and Brian Greenfield, "Self-Compliance at 'Prozac Campus'", *Anthropology and Medicine*, 17 (2010), pp. 173–185.

Kirsten Brukamp and Dominik Gross, "Neuroenhancement – A Controversial Topic in Contemporary Medical Ethics", *Contemporary Issues in Bioethics*, (Rijeka: InTech, 2012), pp. 39–51.

Laura Perez-Caballero, Sonia Torres-Sanchez, Lidia Bravo, Juan Antonio Mico and Esther Berrocoso, "Fluoxetine: A Case History of its Discovery and Preclinical Development", *Expert Opinion in Drug Discovery*, 9 (2014), pp. 1–12.

Maartje Schermer, Ineke Bolt, Reinoud de Jongh and Berend Olivier, "The Future of Psychopharmacological Enhancements: Expectations and Policies", *Neuroethics*, 2 (2009), pp. 75–87.

Michael King, "Is There Still a Role for Benzodiazepines in General Practice?", *British Journal of General Practice*, 42 (1992), pp. 202–205.

Michelle Wilde and Paul Benfield, "Fluoxetine. A Pharmacoeconomic Review of Its Use in Depression", *Pharmacoeconomics*, 13 (1998), pp. 543–561.

Nancey Murphy, "Human Nature, Historical, Scientific and Religious Issues", in *Whatever happened to the Soul: Scientific and Theological Portraits of Human Nature*, edited by Warren Brown, Nancey Murphy and H. Newton Malony (Minneapolis: Fortress, 1998), pp. 1–2.

Neil Messer, *Selfish Genes and Christian Ethics: Theological and Ethical Reflections on Evolutionary Biology* (London: SCM, 2007).

Norman Sartorius, "The Economic and Social Burden of Depression", *Journal of Clinical Psychiatry*, 62 (Suppl) (2001), pp. 8–11.

Peter Kramer, *Listening to Prozac* (New York/London: Penguin, 1993).

Ronald Cole-Turner, "Towards a Theology for the Age of Biotechnology", in *Beyond Cloning: Religion and the Remaking of Humanity*, edited by Ronald Cole-Turner (Harrisburg, PA: Trinity Press International, 2001).

Ronald Kessler, "The Costs of Depression", *Psychiatric Clinics of North America*, 35 (2012), pp. 1–14.

Richard Lane and G. McDonald, "Reducing the Economic Burden of Depression", *International Clinical Psychopharmacology*, 9 (1994), pp. 229–243.

R. A. Lucas, "The Human Pharmacology of Fluoxetine", *International Journal of Obesity and Related Metabolic Disorders*, 16 (1992), pp. S49–S54.

Richard Shelton, "The Nature of the Discontinuation Syndrome Associated with Antidepressant Drugs", *Journal of Clinical Psychiatry*, 67 (Suppl 4) (2006), pp. 3–7.

Robert Sparrow, "Better Living through Chemistry? A Reply to Savulescu and Persson on Moral Enhancement", *Journal of Applied Philosophy*, 31 (2014), pp. 23–32.

Stephen Pope, "Theological Anthropology, Science, and Human Flourishing", in *Questioning the Human: Toward a Theological Anthropology for the Twenty–First Century*, edited by Lieven Boeve, Yves De Maeseneer and Ellen Van Stichel (New York: Fordham University Press, 2014), pp. 13–19.

Todd Hillhouse and Joseph Porter, "A Brief History of the Development of Antidepressant Drugs: From Monoamines to Glutamate", *Experimental Clinical Psychopharmacology*, 23 (2015), pp. 1–21.

Wei-Cheng Yang, Ching-Hua Lin, Fu-Chiang Wang and Mei-Jou Lu, "Factors Related to the Improvement in Quality of Life for Depressed Inpatients Treated with Fluoxetine", *BMC Psychiatry*, 17 (2017), p. 309.

5 Towards a New Therapeutic Ethic

Re-evaluation of Transhumanism

5.1 The Legacy of the Therapeutic Revolution

This chapter will re-evaluate ethical issues with future transhumanist technologies described, in the light of experience with two previous cases in pharmaceutical medicine, the contraceptive pill and SSRI antidepressants. I will begin by summarising the findings of the case studies concerning the extent to which these medicines could be classified as transhumanist developments in their time, according to the general criteria derived from the transhumanist literature, and the ethical acceptability of these technologies, based on the specific theological criteria derived from the work of Neil Messer and Elaine Graham (Messer, 2007, pp. 229–235; Graham, 2006).

Based on these findings, I will then address the four research questions proposed in this book, namely:

1 What are the various issues of theological ethics presented by transhumanist developments?
2 To what extent were past therapeutic developments transhumanist technologies in their time?
3 What were the ethical concerns with past therapeutic developments? Have these ethical concerns been warranted in the light of subsequent experience?
4 How do issues identified with previous therapeutic developments inform the evaluation of future biomedical technologies?

The answer to the first of these questions will involve an extended discussion of the theological and ethical issues that have been identified with transhumanist technologies, and will focus on four specific theological areas that were identified through analysis of the case studies as being significant areas for ethical reflection – autonomy, nature, *imago Dei* and embodiment. The final part of the chapter will then discuss how the ethical criteria for transhumanist developments proposed in Chapter 2 can be refined and developed in the light of the case study findings.

DOI: 10.4324/9781003290421-6

Both case studies of past pharmaceutical medicine – the contraceptive pill and SSRI antidepressants – arose from, and were enabled by, previous scientific discoveries. The contraceptive pill was developed in a planned and deliberate manner, and those involved in its development – Sanger, McCormick and Pincus – had a clear vision of the pill as a means of transforming human society. By contrast, the development and marketing of Prozac was more serendipitous (lucky) due to the different research methods used by the pharmaceutical industry in the 1970s and 1980s. Indeed, the potentially profound effects of Prozac on human society were not intended by its developers, who saw Prozac simply as a possible treatment for clinical depression, but instead resulted from the experience of psychiatrists – and patients themselves – of the use of Prozac as an "enhancement" for manipulating the personality to make healthy people feel "better than well", a phenomenon that has been described by scholars and commentators as the "Prozac phenomenon" (Healy, 2004, p. 263).

In both cases, there are features relating to the use of the drug that resemble those of a transhumanist technology, according to the general criteria for transhumanist developments. Both the contraceptive pill and SSRI antidepressants conform to three out of four of these criteria, in that each is a technology (a material means of effecting a task or process) which is applied to the human body to exert an effect and the effect is largely a beneficial one, as far as human flourishing is concerned. The fourth general criterion for a transhumanist development is that the human person has autonomy in the application of the medical technology. I have shown that, for both the contraceptive pill and for SSRI antidepressants, it is uncertain whether, as medical technologies, they can always be used by human beings in a truly autonomous way, with informed personal choice, arising from self-determination as a moral agent, without any form of coercion. This may be because of possible unintended consequences of the use of the medicines themselves, due to their effects and adverse effects, but may also be because of coercive influences and cultural expectations concerning the use of these medicines at an individual level. In addition, it may be because of issues of justice and equity in the marketing and distribution of these products at a societal level. I will explore these issues concerning autonomy, and their implications for ethical evaluation of transhumanism, in more depth in the next section.

Concerning the specific theological criteria for the ethical evaluation of a medical technology, I have made the following observations about the contraceptive pill and SSRI antidepressants:

- The contraceptive pill has the capacity to be "good news for the poor", in that there is evidence of clear benefits to poor people, because of the pill's ability to help women on low incomes to plan their families and their working life. In contrast, expensive, "high-tech" proposed transhumanist technologies, such as cryogenics and cybernetics, would probably, if available, only benefit a small percentage of wealthy people, and could be used to oppress the rest of the population. With SSRI antidepressants, there is evidence that they are a cost-effective way of treating depression from the health provider's perspective. However, there is limited evidence that they have direct benefits for the poor, although in theory they should, because of their low cost and recognised effects on cognitive function and quality of life. Nevertheless, with both medicines, benefits to the poor may be compromised by coercive and inequitable marketing and distribution arrangements for these drugs, or lack of access to the medicine, especially in third world health economies.

- Does the project enable humanity to conform to the image of God, or is it an attempt to be like God? I have shown that the effects of both the contraceptive pill and SSRI antidepressants in humans are consistent with a comprehensive approach to the *imago Dei* in humanity, which is functional, relational and possibly eschatological, not just substantive. This contrasts with some approaches to transhumanism that emphasise, or are solely concerned with, human attributes, and therefore reflect a largely substantive approach to the *imago Dei*, at the expense of the other approaches to the *imago Dei*. Indeed, rather than enabling humanity to fully conform to the image of God, such transhumanist technologies are a means of being like God, in that they emphasise the use of technology to manipulate, redesign and "re-create" the body at will. The past therapies described cannot manipulate the body as radically as some future technologies may be able to (for example, with cybernetic body components).
- Concerning the attitude of the project towards the material world, including the human body, both the contraceptive pill and SSRI antidepressants are affirming of bodily life in that they exert their positive effects in and through the biological human body, and therefore do not negate bodily and biological life. This contrasts with some proposed transhumanist technologies, such as mind uploading, which are essentially anti-materialist, and which deprecate the human body, and downgrade bodily experience. In addition, as shown earlier, the contraceptive pill has significant positive effects on society – the corporate body of humanity – as well as the health and well-being of the individual human body, because of its positive effects on the well-being of women, the role of marriage in society and the stability of family life. The effect of SSRI antidepressants on corporate society, due to their effects on the personalities and relationships of individuals, is more ambiguous; they may have both positive and negative effects on personalities and relationships, and the net overall effect on society is hard to evaluate. In any case, with both developments, there is the question of exactly how individuals might use the beneficial effects of the medicine on their material bodies, and in their material lives. Is the technology used for selfish, hedonistic ends or to enable the user to

make positive, selfless contribution to human society? With both the contraceptive pill and SSRI antidepressants, there is much evidence that, throughout its history, the use of the medicine has been largely directed towards good ends.

- What is the attitude of these projects to past failure? I have argued that introduction of the contraceptive pill has been regarded with hubris in some societies, as a triumph of human technological achievement. Nevertheless, the contraceptive pill did overcome some of the shortcomings of previous forms of contraception, and the protagonists in the development of the pill intended it to have a positive impact on previously significant issues in society, relating to family planning and human welfare, at both an individual and a social level. Furthermore, given their massive success as a therapy and their potential for "cosmetic" use, SSRI antidepressants have also been regarded by some as the supreme achievement of rational psychopharmacology in a way that again could be regarded as hubristic, in a similar way to some attitudes to proposed future transhumanist technologies. The fact remains, however, that, despite their faults, SSRI antidepressants were an improvement on previously available interventions. They were designed to overcome the problems of tricyclic antidepressants in clinical use, although they were not developed specifically to address social problems, in the way that the contraceptive pill was.
- Does the technology focus too much on the users' subjective experiences? The paradox is that, while transhumanist technologies enhance subjective experience because of the individualism and autonomy with which they may be applied, at the same time, they treat the body as an artefact to be engineered, and therefore they objectify the human body – in other words, they treat the body as an object. This problem is clearly present for both the contraceptive pill and SSRI antidepressants. This in contrast to medicines whose pharmacological effects on the human body are less intrusive to human personal and social experience – for example, antihypertensive agents. The pill gives women choice about pregnancy, family life and careers, and therefore enhances the subjective experience of the user. Yet the use of the pill enables fertility to be manipulated at will, which can be done at scale in society, and therefore it has the potential to treat the female body as an object to be engineered, rather than a personal subject. In relation to this, the pill may therefore also contribute to the phenomenon of objectification of the female body in sexual relationships, as described by some feminist commentators (Hartmann, 1995, p. 189; Jutte, 2008, p. 288). The mental effects of SSRI antidepressants can also increase the subjective experience of the user, positively or negatively. However, they too have the potential to objectify the human body, and treat it as an artefact to be engineered, when they are used to manipulate the personality, in a way that might be regarded as instrumentalist – i.e. it is a pragmatic intervention towards a

specific end, rather than something of moral value in itself. This contrasts with the moral value of personality changes which take place due to life experiences such as culture or education. I would therefore argue that, while SSRIs do provide a benefit to the individual person, which is subjectively experienced by that person, their use as "cosmetic psychopharmacology" is a means of treating the person as an artefact that can be (self) manipulated at will.

The two case studies of pharmaceutical medicine, the contraceptive pill and SSRI antidepressants, could be classed as transhumanist technologies, because of three specific features:

a their attributes as medical technologies, because their pharmacological effects are wide-ranging and they have profound systemic effects on the individual human body,
b the total impact they have had on society, rather than just on the health and well-being of the individuals who take them, and
c the understanding of their application to humanity as transformational medical technologies in both scholarly and popular discourse.

However, the above findings show that, when the specific theological criteria for transhumanist developments are applied to these two case studies to facilitate ethical analysis, a more nuanced picture of these technologies emerges. The two case studies resemble transhumanist developments in some respects, but not others. For example, the contraceptive pill and SSRI antidepressants could be regarded as examples of technological hubris – developments which are the height of rational, scientific development in their fields, which some medical practitioners and pharmaceutical industry personnel have taken for granted, rather than treated with awe and respect, and in which they have placed excessive confidence as panaceas for human suffering. This is similar to the uncritical optimism with which proposed radical transhumanist biomedical technologies are regarded by some transhumanist thinkers.

In other respects, however, there may be significant differences between these pharmaceutical medicine case studies and transhumanist technologies, depending on the type of technology. For example, both the contraceptive pill and SSRI antidepressants mediate their positive effects through the human body; they affirm bodily life and assume a view of the world where human bodily experience is good and of moral value. This, however, is in stark contrast to some proposed transhumanist technologies such as mind-uploading and cybernetics, which denigrate the human body, and consider it of lesser importance than mental life and cognitive function.

The issues concerning autonomy are particularly problematic. There are two issues regarding autonomy with biomedical technologies, both of which have been identified in the two case studies. First, there is the question of whether the technology can be adopted with true autonomy and second, there is the question of the capacity of the technology itself to enable or disable the personal autonomy of the user. It is a key tenet of the transhumanist movement that technologies may be applied to the human body with personal autonomy, a stance which follows logically from the roots of transhumanism in secular humanism. However, scholars such as Sparrow (Sparrow, 2014), and McNamee and Edwards (McNamee and Edwards, 2006), have questioned whether there can be true autonomy in a world of transhumanist technology, due to the way these technologies are then likely to be deployed in human society. With both the past case studies presented, the medical technology may be initially adopted by an individual with autonomy (uncoerced self-determination), but widespread deployment of the technology in human society may lead to coercive factors in how the technology is adopted and use of the technology itself may disable personal autonomy by introducing coercive factors. This suggests that autonomy is a key area for ethical reflection with future technologies and should be explored at some length in developing an ethical response to future transhumanist technologies.

The points of convergence between the ethical evaluation of the two case studies and real-world experience with these drugs in practice suggest that there are some aspects of current pharmaceutical medicine that are beneficial, of moral value and which raise no particular ethical concerns. For example, experience has shown that the contraceptive pill has indeed had a positive impact on human health and flourishing, especially in poor and marginalised populations. This suggests that there may be some aspects of some future technologies that will also be positive – consistent with the aims of pharmaceutical medicine to date, and with Christian medical ethics. In this chapter, I will explore these aspects in more detail.

5.2 The Ethical Issues of Transhumanism

As discussed in Chapter 2, given the broad scope of transhumanism, both scientifically and epistemologically, corresponding theological and ethical concerns about transhumanism have been equally broad. They have included social ethical concerns, such as the impact of immortality or extreme longevity on human social issues, such as work, marriage, housing, etc., potential for inequality of access to technologies, and social and cultural oppression due to inequity of access. As well as social ethical issues, theological concerns have been raised with transhumanist biomedical technologies by various world faith traditions, including Christianity.

Nevertheless, a review of the ethical issues associated with the two case studies presented in this project indicates there are four aspects of theological ethics arising from the analysis of the case studies using the theological criteria, which warrant extended discussion as key areas of the ethical evaluation of future biomedical technologies. These are:

a The extent to which the biomedical technology affects personal autonomy and with what outcomes (both for the individual moral agent and for the community).
b The extent to which a biomedical technology is "natural", and the appropriateness of its ethical evaluation using natural law theory. Note that this area of discussion does not directly arise from the application of the criteria to the cases, but it is a significant area of discussion given that natural law ethical objections have been raised in the past with both the contraceptive pill and SSRI antidepressants.
c The extent to which the biomedical technology supports or undermines human embodiment, material life and identity, and affirms the material body as a prerequisite for earthly human existence and life.
d The approaches to the *imago Dei* that the technology-enhanced human reflects. It is to be hoped that the various theological approaches to the *imago Dei* are reflected, since all are important in a Christian understanding of humanity.

These four areas were introduced in Chapter 2, and merit further exploration because, by the methodology of this study, they have been identified both as issues with past medical developments and as potential issues with proposed future transhumanist technologies. They therefore provide a link between past and future biomedical technologies, and thus a common platform for the ethical evaluation of these technologies. These issues will therefore be as relevant to future biomedical technologies as they have been to past medical developments. Furthermore, there are various ambiguities inherent in these areas, which are likely to be key areas of debate in Christian ethical responses to future adoption of biomedical technologies. I will now discuss each of these four areas in detail.

5.2.1 Autonomy

As discussed elsewhere, the use of transhumanist biomedical technologies raises significant questions concerning the exercise of personal autonomy. A stated aim of the transhumanist movement is that individuals who are seeking biomedical enhancement can choose to use the biomedical technology – or not – autonomously, as a matter of free, personal choice. The corresponding theological response to this, raised by Elaine Graham, is that transhumanist biomedical technologies therefore are problematic because they enable unbridled autonomy in a negative manner (Graham, 2006).

However, the evidence from the development and use of both the contraceptive pill and SSRI antidepressants suggests that, in fact, neither scenario is true and that the relationship between the use of a technology and the autonomy of the user is a complex one. While there may be ways in which some biomedical technologies can be applied with true autonomy – defined as uncoerced self-determination – there are also situations where biomedical technology may limit that autonomy when deployed at a societal level.

The capacity for a widely used biomedical technology to limit personal autonomy has been raised in respect of enhancement technologies by Sparrow (Sparrow, 2014), as I have discussed elsewhere, and has also been observed in the two case studies. The introduction of the contraceptive pill led to the so-called coital imperative where women felt compelled to have sex because there was no reason not to, since the risk of pregnancy was removed by use of the pill (Thatcher, 2011, p. 221). In addition, the methods of distribution of the contraceptive pill in developing countries in the past by some US family planning services have been criticised as coercive, in a way that does not respect the rights of local women (May, 2010, p. 43); Hartmann, in particular, has argued from a feminist perspective that women in developing countries have often been disempowered by such services, because of their lack of respect for local culture and the lack of information and choice provided to women (Hartmann, 1995, pp. 200–203). These factors have all contributed to the autonomy of these women being compromised. This is an external influence, arising from the activities of the family planning services, but may also be an internal coercive factor due to the assimilation of western attitudes. The impact on autonomy is even more significant with more recently introduced injectable and implantable forms of hormonal contraception – for example, Depo-Provera, Norplant and NexPlanon – as they therefore do not require the woman to participate in the process, so they have the potential to be administered with scant regard to the woman's personal autonomy, especially in cultures where subservience is valued in a woman. In relation to a woman's personal autonomy, there are therefore various aspects of the use of the contraceptive pill which might constitute the application of significant coercion.

There are also concerns about personal autonomy arising from the use of SSRI antidepressants in some situations. As discussed in Chapter 2, drug addiction and brain washing are two scenarios cited in philosophical literature as being problematic for the concept of personal autonomy (Buss, 2018). Both these issues are potentially applicable to the effects of SSRIs on personal autonomy in some situations. The withdrawal effects of SSRI antidepressants, due to biochemical dependence, may have a negative impact on the autonomy of users of these medicines, as they make it harder for a person to stop treatment when they want to, and may exert a psychological pressure on them to continue treatment or to dissuade them from discontinuing treatment. This scenario is essentially the "drug addiction" scenario – the individual finds it hard to stop using the drug, even though they might want to, because of the effects of the drug – and this compromises autonomy as an expression of self-determination, because the person cannot act in an entirely self-determined way due to the biochemical effects of the drug. Furthermore, in some people, the use of SSRI antidepressants may lead to suicidal ideation – the presence of suicidal thoughts independently of symptoms of depressive illness. In some rare cases, this phenomenon has been associated with criminal actions, and the drug has been cited as a factor in a legal defence of diminished responsibility (Healy, 2004, p. 64).[1] Therefore, although SSRI antidepressant use usually enables a user to be more rational, due to relief of clinical depression, in these cases, the person's rational functions are diminished, so this constitutes "brain washing", where the person's autonomy as a self-governing moral agent is compromised by an inability for rational thought induced by the drug.

In a future world of widespread, sophisticated medical interventions, one solution to the problem of negative effects of widespread biomedical technology use on personal autonomy might be to employ biomedical technologies specifically for "moral enhancement", to ensure people always make good moral choices (Douglas, 2008). I have discussed the issue of moral enhancement in Chapter 2, and SSRI antidepressants have been proposed for moral enhancement (Savulescu and Persson, 2012).

However, moral enhancement technology would actually be detrimental for autonomy, in my view, for three reasons. First, if a biotechnology "makes" a person make good moral decisions, this would be, in fact, a restriction of the concept of personal autonomy, defined as self-determination. If a person has real self-determination to act according to their desires and character, then they should have the freedom to make bad decisions arising from a flawed character or perverted desires, without the influence of mind-altering drugs. If they do not have that freedom then, even though the consequences of their immoral decisions might be bad, their personal autonomy is compromised. Even though, from a Christian perspective, it might seem beneficial to be biomedically enhanced to always make good decisions, a biomedically restricted autonomy is no substitute for good decisions that are freely made by a moral agent as an exercise of free will and with a clear understanding of personal responsibility.

Second, if the moral enhancement agent changes the individual's desires so that they always want to make the right choice then, although the person in theory has autonomy from a coherentist perspective – their actions will be aligned with their desires – their desires will arise from the neurochemical changes induced by the biotechnology, rather than from the psychological changes associated with character formation. Thus, if the person's will to act arises from the desires of their essential self, then the use of a moral enhancement agent might appear to enable personal autonomy, but in fact it undermines it. This is because, although the development of character comes from exposure to external influences as well as innate genetic factors, the external factors in character development are likely to comprise a range of experiences of the world over time, where the person has the opportunity to reflect upon and maybe challenge those experiences. This process of reaction and reflection, where a person discerns moral factors and implications in a situation as a prerequisite of making good decisions about that situation, is an important factor if moral agency is to be truly self-determined, or autonomous.

However, a moral enhancement agent would be a single external factor which may rapidly cause profound coercion of the person's autonomy, possibly coupled with a lack of insight on the part of the person concerning the technology's actions on the mind. For this reason, character change caused by moral enhancement is less valuable morally than character change due to natural formational experience and reflexivity, in respect of the exercise of autonomy. In short, the problem with biomedical interventions for "moral enhancement" is their potential to short-circuit the process of a person reacting to, and reflecting upon, a situation where a moral decision needs to be made. This issue has been identified in discussions about autonomy with potential future biomedical technologies (Sparrow, 2014), and I have shown here that this has been an issue with the two case studies of previous biomedical technologies described in this book.

Third, it is doubtful whether a moral enhancement agent can provide true conditions for good moral decision-making. Willows notes – correctly in my view – that, while moral enhancement agents can stimulate certain moral dispositions of character, they cannot help the person with either the habitual development of virtue or the personal application of *phronesis* (practical wisdom) (Willows, 2017). The reflections of Peter Kramer concerning the cosmetic use of Prozac bear this out; Kramer describes how Prozac use can give people specific characteristics such as confidence and assertiveness (Kramer, 1993, pp. 1–13), but there is no indication that the drug has any broader implications for an Aristotelian framework of virtue ethics. I would argue therefore that true character formation arises from moral agency which develops naturally by habitual practice, rather than due to biomedical moral enhancement technology.

The importance of reaction and reflection in the formation of autonomous moral agency has two important implications for the case studies presented in this book. First, the biological model of depression, as described in relation to SSRI antidepressants, has an underlying notion of reductionism, which suggests that depressive illness and other mental symptoms are solely the result of biochemical processes in the brain. This might suggest that the user of these drugs does not have conscious insight into their mental processes, and from a legal perspective, this lack of insight would undermine moral culpability for a criminal act while a drug is being taken. Conversely, if the individual had capacity and insight into their illness, taking the drug would not in itself diminish the person's moral responsibility for committing the crime. So, even if one did accept the biological model of depression, with its reductionist premise, the personal autonomy of the person being treated is genuine if they have insight into their mental state, and therefore the capacity to react to and reflect on their desires, and this is generally recognised by law in human society.

Second, although medical technologies, such as SSRI antidepressants and the contraceptive pill, may be imposed upon, or alternatively restricted in, certain countries or cultures in a way that might be coercive for the people affected at a societal level, this does not prevent individual people from taking personal responsibility and exercising personal autonomy – self-determination – to resist that coercion or to make good decisions about their health in other respects.

Experience with these case studies shows that the exercise of personal autonomy in respect of biomedical technologies has always been ambiguous. Limitations of personal autonomy are always possible with any medical technology, past or present, either due to unintended consequences or due to societal or commercial external coercion. However, in most circumstances of modern life, personal autonomy is genuine and valuable, and individuals can make real choices about how to apply technology in a liberal western state. Moreover, as I argued in Chapter 2, personal autonomy is a prerequisite of Christian moral responsibility.

However, if appropriate *a priori* choices are not made about the deployment and use of any technology, then there is the risk that technology will be assimilated uncritically into society and that, given the invasive, radical nature of some future technologies, the technology might manipulate humanity, rather than vice versa. In that situation, the technology may become dominant, and become an idol that is worshipped instead of God. It is important, then, that humanity should exercise discernment in evaluating technologies, controlling their deployment and use with appropriate regulation and public policy, to ensure that the autonomy of individuals using biomedical technologies is safeguarded. This is itself an important act of responsibility – and indeed autonomy – on the part of human society and is consistent with the human vocation to be a created co-creator, under God's authority (Hefner, 1993, pp. 255–277). God has acted freely in creating the world and he invites human creatures to exercise their will and share with him the responsibility of being creative in human society.

Saad's observation that autonomy in medicine to date has been excessively focused on the issue of consent and is insufficiently relational is an important one (Saad, 2018). With future, more radical biomedical technologies, the process of personal consent will play only a small part in the autonomy with which they are adopted. Most people will freely consent to use a technology if they experience personal benefits; this phenomenon has already been seen in the almost universal adoption of mobile telecommunications and would no doubt be seen again if, for example, retinal implants become a widely available and socially acceptable way to greatly increase visual acuity beyond current biological standards for eyesight. What will matter in future is that such technologies are introduced in such a way that the autonomy of the personal individual is safeguarded and respected in the context of the whole human community in which they are situated, not just through the atomistic process of individual, personal, informed consent. For this to happen, appropriate public policy will be needed to ensure equitable funding and adoption of such technologies, so that anyone in that society can choose to apply a technology to themselves as a free personal choice, without external coercion, and the technology adoption process supports relationships in society not just the rights of the individual.

Although I have highlighted some of the ways in which the contraceptive pill and SSRI antidepressants as biomedical technologies can compromise personal autonomy, it is fair to say that, reviewing the history of their use, both these biomedical technologies have also had liberating effects. The contraceptive pill has freed women – and couples – to make personal choices about having sex and planning pregnancies, and about the lifestyle issues that accompany these decisions. SSRI antidepressants have enabled people with depression to avail themselves of effective treatment without the debilitating side-effects that were a problem with previous classes of antidepressants. Both these technologies were advances in terms of the personal choices that they offered individual users, and the benefits of choice with these advances have been significant for humanity because of the large populations in which these drugs have been used. It is possible that the more widespread use of future, more radical, biomedical technologies might also have liberating effects for a significant proportion of the population, depending on how they are introduced.

Autonomy has ambiguous aspects in medicine – and always has – but the ambiguity of autonomy should not detract from the importance of individuals and communities making good moral decisions about all aspects of life, including the good application of medical technology. In terms of future transhumanist technologies, this will involve understanding how exactly a medical technology can interfere with personal autonomy and affect a person's agency to act morally in the world. This interference might be at the level of desire or will, or at the level of external coercive forces. Does the cybernetic body component have functionality which might act against the host's desires or will? Is the uploaded person's will or ability to act compromised by their disembodied nature? Does the distribution of either technology in society restrict how different individuals and groups in society exercise personal autonomy, in relation to each other? These problems will be addressed by users having a comprehensive knowledge about the technology and its consequences – and by developers being honest with users about the features of the technology, within the limits of current experience. Nevertheless, both these approaches might be limited by any unintended consequences of the technology. Furthermore, it is important that governments, health services and users consider all the implications of technology use prospectively, prior to widespread deployment of that technology. Often the adoption of technologies is driven by commercial or market factors, and governments and public bodies struggle to catch up. With something as important as personal autonomy – personally, socially and politically – it is important that a more rigorous and holistic approach is taken.

5.2.2 Nature

As discussed in Chapter 2, natural law theory proposes that what is natural in the world for a creature is directed towards what is morally good, and towards the flourishing of that creature, and that human life is naturally directed to good ends. In other words, if something is natural, or occurs naturally in the world, it must be directed towards, or be an expression of, that which is good (Pope, 2012). Thomistic natural law appears to assume that there is a teleology – a goal or end – of the universe, which some theologians claim brings it into conflict with modern, post-Darwinian biological science because this scientific approach has undermined the idea of teleology, or purpose, in the universe (Pope, 2014; Vanhoozer, 1997).

A key theme which has emerged from transhumanist scholarship is that nature is "unfinished" (Bostrom, 2005). This implies that any new biomedical technology which might enhance human attributes may have the potential to "complete" human nature. However, as discussed, this idea is problematic because it could suggest that, because of their "flaws", some people might not conform to the *imago Dei* now – which has implications for the person's current status and rights as a human being. It also implies an obligation to use technology to get all human beings to the "required" standard of function. The overall assumption is that "perfection" is something that can be determined and achieved solely by human will. However, considering the Christological dimension of the *imago Dei,* I will argue later in this chapter that all human beings fall short of perfection in Christ, as the perfect image of God (see Colossians 1v15).

I have shown in the previous section that transhumanism, with its tenet of adoption of technology with complete personal autonomy, is problematic given the ambiguities with autonomy that have been seen with previous biomedical technologies. However, transhumanism, with its underlying ethos that human life can be manipulated at will with biomedical technology, also appears to be in tension with the concept of natural law, which emphasises the concept of a fixed order of creation (Hopkins, 2013). Indeed, as previously discussed, transhumanist thinkers take the view that human nature can – and should – be manipulated by biomedical technology (for example, Bostrom, 2005). If human "nature" is indeed malleable – and medical technology to date, especially in the area of reproductive science, suggests that it is – then, in a technology-enabled world, there can no longer be an unquestionable link between the "nature" of a creature and the moral ends to which it is directed.

The two case studies of pharmaceutical medicine – the contraceptive pill and SSRI antidepressants – have the potential to manipulate aspects of human life that have previously been regarded as immutably "natural" – namely, fertility and personality respectively. Consequently, both have been criticised on natural law grounds, either by Roman Catholic theologians or by the Roman Catholic church at an institutional level. However, in the two previous chapters, I have reviewed previous experience with the contraceptive pill and SSRI antidepressants, and have described the ethical benefits of the use of these medicines in society. This analysis has highlighted the inadequacy of natural law as a sole means of ethical evaluation of these medicines. If modes of ethical evaluation other than natural law are used to evaluate the contraceptive pill and SSRI antidepressants, then it would be harder to conclude that the effects of these interventions on the human body make them "innately evil".

Furthermore, if radical biomedical technologies can alter human nature easily and extensively, as will happen in the future, then the "nature" of a person might no longer reflect good moral ends, and it would be harder to make normative claims about human nature, as Christian theology to date has largely been committed to doing (McKenny, 2018). Natural law would therefore be diminished further as a mode of ethical evaluation of biomedical technologies. The case studies presented here – the contraceptive pill and SSRI antidepressants – highlight some of the problems of the application of natural law theory to biomedical technology.

Using natural law as a means of ethical assessment of biomedical technologies is complicated by how "natural" is defined. This is seen in the two previous case studies. John Rock, the gynaecologist who did early work on the contraceptive pill, was content to regard the pill as a "natural" intervention, because it was composed of substances (oestrogen and progestogen) which resembled the reproductive hormones found naturally in the body, and which therefore mimicked their natural actions. From a scientific and medical perspective, this was a reasonable assumption. However, the church regarded the contraceptive pill as "unnatural" because it was an external agent, not originating from within the body, but which affected the normal function of the body. This was an equally reasonable assumption given the history and development of natural law theory from Aquinas onwards, but it led to a different conclusion about the acceptability of the contraceptive pill from a natural law perspective. A similar definitional issue has been at play in the development of psychopharmacology and SSRI antidepressants. During the late twentieth century, as disease knowledge of psychiatry has increased and more sophisticated treatments have become available, the DSM classification of mental health conditions has expanded, and characteristics that were previously regarded as part of normal behaviour – and therefore "natural" – have been medicalised and have been reclassified as "unnatural" disease states.

The natural law assumption is that a biological entity or process that is operating according to nature is natural and therefore directed to good ends, whereas a biological entity or process that can be manipulated at human will is "artificial". While the idea of artifice is not itself immoral in natural law, such an artifice would be immoral if it contravened natural biological processes. However, the perspective from which a situation is viewed will determine the extent to which it can be defined "natural" or "artificial". As discussed in Chapter 3, in the Roman Catholic papal encyclical, *Humanae Vitae*, the underlying assumption seems to be that a marriage consists of a series of apparently unconnected sex acts, possibly because of an overly physicalist interpretation of natural law. However, O'Donovan claims, rightly, that this assumption "falsifies" the true nature of marriage (O'Donovan, 1984, p. 77). Augustine's classic work, *On the Good of Marriage* (Augustine of Hippo, 2021 edition), which has contributed considerably to the western church's theology of marriage, places sexual intercourse within the wider context of fidelity and natural association (*societas*) between man and woman, and does not have a concept of sexual intercourse in marriage as a series of individual acts. In the light of Augustine's approach, a more "natural" understanding of marriage is as an ongoing, loving relationship in its entirety, and not merely a series of individual sexual acts.

With reference to the use of contraception, for many years, prior to the introduction of teaching on the so-called rhythm method, the official position of the Roman Catholic church was that, for married couples, abstinence was preferable to contracepted sex.[2] Yet abstinence in marriage is as "unnatural" as the use of contraception and is probably not beneficial for the marriage relationship. It is reasonable to see how, in the light of the debate following the introduction of the contraceptive pill and the publication of *Humanae Vitae,* Bernard Häring concluded that, as a determinant of morality, biological functions could be subordinated to the good of the whole person, on the principle of integrity – and the good of the whole community, on the principle of totality (Häring, 1976). On this basis, he argued that the Roman Catholic church should be open to the use of the pill on those grounds, if not on natural law grounds.

In the medical context, there are complications even in determining which biological phenomena are truly natural, always and in all circumstances. The Roman Catholic church sees the manipulation of fertility as "unnatural". However, being fertile is not always a natural state for a woman. It is perfectly natural for a woman not to be fertile at the infertile times of the menstrual cycle, or after the menopause. Defining what biological attributes and phenomena are "natural" will become increasingly problematic with the use of more radical biomedical technologies. It will be especially problematic for technologies that are a) more invasive (for example, neural threads to enable digital connectivity of the brain), b) less tangible (for example, gene therapy) or c) where there is a high degree of low-level hybridisation (for example, the use of nanotechnology for surgery and cell repair). This is because, with these technologies, it will be hard to determine what is natural or unnatural simply by observation, or even by physicochemical analysis.

From an ethical perspective, it will become more necessary than ever to regard the nature and biological function of the person as secondary and subordinate to the good of the whole person, and the welfare of the community, according to the ethical principle of totality. A biomedical technology may change human biological function, in relation to previous or "traditional" norms of biological function but could be permissible from a Christian perspective if it did not undermine the health and well-being of the whole person or compromise relationships, peace and justice in the community. Thus, for example, a new biomedical intervention that enabled human life expectancy to increase to two hundred years would have significant societal and cultural impact due to its effect on longevity, but if it did not adversely affect human well-being, or create injustices and imbalances in society (or if social policy were able to address any issues that arose) then it would not be intrinsically problematic from a perspective of Christian ethics.

As well as the problems of determining what is truly "natural" to inform the application of biomedical technologies, there is the question about whether natural law can ever be sufficient to deal with all aspects of a Christian understanding of human nature. In their discussion about contraception at the 1958 Lambeth Conference, the Anglican Bishops determined that, because of their self-transcendent nature, humans could not be wholly subject to natural law (Thatcher, 2011, p. 223). Consequently, applying only natural law principles to ethical assessment of biomedical technologies ignores a significant aspect of human experience – the way in which human beings are above nature and are seeking an understanding of the universe that is beyond their natural selves. It is this capacity that enables a human being to perceive a transcendent God, to seek and participate in the divine nature, and become more like God. As discussed in Chapter 2, the Orthodox idea of *theosis* has recently become a useful point of conversation between Christian theology and transhumanism. However, although radical biomedical technology may enable people to become more godlike, it is an artificial self-transcendence – a transcendence of their own making – rather than one achieved through relationship with the transcendent God.

A natural law approach to assessing therapies is also problematic when considering psychopharmacology and the reductionist biological model of depression. The biological model of depression in psychiatry described previously suggests that a specific medical condition is rooted in a specific biological state. However, this biological state is not typical and furthermore it is pathological, in that it causes disease and disorder. As a disorder, depression would not therefore be regarded as "natural" by natural law theorists, even though it might arise from biochemical factors, which are significant in the pathology of depression and, from a clinical perspective, cannot be completely discounted.

However, both psychiatrists – for example, Healy (Healy, 2004, pp. 255–260) – and theologians – for example, Cole-Turner (Cole-Turner, 2001, pp. 143–146) – maintain that disease states and therapeutics cannot be reduced entirely to biochemical factors. Therefore, biological factors – whether they are "natural" or not – cannot fully account for the phenomenon of depression, and its treatment. This highlights the limitations of natural law as a means of assessing the moral status of therapeutic interventions in mental health, such as SSRI antidepressants, and suggests that their use may be desirable for the alleviation of human suffering and promotion of flourishing, even though natural law moral objections might be raised about their use. This is analogous to Bernard Häring's advocacy of contraception on the principle of totality, that the biological functions of the person should be subordinated to the overall well-being of the person and the good of the whole community (Thatcher, 2011, p. 218; Häring, 1976).

An assumption often made with a reductionist approach to human biological attributes is that the person's biological attributes determine their behaviour, and this undermines the idea of morality in human behaviour (Barbour, 1998, pp. 80–81). This would suggest that a person's ability to act as a moral agent in a self-determined way is limited by their biological nature. However, I would argue that biological attributes simply represent just one level at which an individual exists as a person in the world (although, as an individual, sentient being, their biological attributes will be internally consistent with their psychological capacities). Consequently, if autonomy is the ability to act with self-determination, based on the authentic self, then the idea that a person's "authentic self" might be the sum of their biological attributes is a secondary and derivative issue in relation to the person's ability to exercise personal autonomy at a behavioural level, based on that authentic self.

Both the case studies presented – the contraceptive pill and SSRI antidepressants – have a range of biological actions which exert their positive effects on the experience of the user. Indeed, the influence of external factors that can radically undermine self-determination, such as drugs and other psychologically active biomedical technologies, has a greater impact on a person's ability to act autonomously – and therefore on their moral agency – than innate, "natural" biological attributes. Interestingly, Miravalle appeals to external factors in his argument for a natural law approach to the treatment of depression. With his Thomist argument that the sorrow of depression is a "passion", which is a reaction to an extrinsic evil, and that sorrow is meant to elicit an action from the sufferer, he argues that the "urge to better one's state of affairs ... is the *telos* of sorrow" (Miravalle, 2010, p. 40). He concludes that sorrow should be used for good in life, rather than treated with drugs. The implication is that the person with depression is somehow responsible for their disease, a view that is at odds with contemporary attitudes to mental illness, and indeed to other "natural" phenomena – such as homosexual orientation or neurodevelopmental variants like autism – for which the individual would not necessarily be regarded as morally culpable. For this reason, the natural law-based approach of Miravalle to the treatment of depression may not be appropriate in the context of either clinical therapy or pastoral ministry.

Apart from questions of definition and personal responsibility, the relationship between nature and moral value is complex when considering enhancement, as opposed to therapy. McNamee and Edwards state that one argument for use of biomedical technologies to enhance the human person to a certain standard is that, in a sense, it is fairer than accepting "natural" variations in bodily functions (McNamee and Edwards, 2006). However, this is only the case if all human beings are enhanced to the same baseline standard, which may not be easy to agree upon, or practical to implement. It is possible, though, that a definition of "natural" baseline human function could be achieved through robust public policy reflecting the consensus of society, in the same way as safeguarding personal autonomy in a technologically enhanced society. This would effectively apply a new account of normativity to human nature in a world where nature can be manipulated with technology.

In any case, even if biomedical technology is used to enhance a person so that their bodily functions and attributes are "unnatural" by previous biological and social standards, this does not necessarily prevent that person from acting in a morally virtuous way (Bailey, 2013). Conversely, a medical technology could be "natural", in that it is aligned with natural bodily processes, but the moral value of its use could still be questionable, either because it is instrumentalist – a pragmatic intervention to a specific end, rather than something of innate moral value – or because it encourages an arrogant or hubristic attitude on the part of the user towards his fellow human beings, or the world's resources. An example of this would be the use of anxiolytic agents as "chemical coshes" in agitated care home residents to sedate them for the convenience of the staff and the benefit of the service, rather than in the resident's best interest.

Although human nature cannot be entirely reduced to biological factors, it is biologically grounded, as seen in the biological model of depression. In his discussion of transhumanism and natural law, Hopkins contends that even transhumanists think that human nature is biologically grounded, or there would be no "basic" human nature to enhance (Hopkins, 2013). Nevertheless, both the case studies discussed indicate that social and cultural factors, not just biological factors, are important when considering the benefits of a medical technology for human life and flourishing. The benefits of the contraceptive pill on human flourishing are not just related to its biological effects on the individual woman's fertility, but its derivative effects on sexual relationships, family life and the role of women in society. The benefits of Prozac on human flourishing are not just related to its biological effects on an individual's mood, but its derivative effects on their motivation and relationships.

The Roman Catholic church or its moralists have argued that, with the contraceptive pill and SSRI antidepressants, the use of these technologies is immoral primarily because natural law has been contravened. However, I have demonstrated in the case studies that there are other ethical benefits associated with the use of these technologies. Use of the contraceptive pill can lead to ethical goods such as planned pregnancy, stable family life, improved health and welfare, especially for women, and more equitable sexual relationships. These benefits have been described at length in the literature since the development of the contraceptive pill (Thatcher, 2011, pp. 211–220). Similarly, use of SSRI antidepressants can lead to ethical goods such as the relief of depression, and improvement of human function and quality of life – and, significantly, the lifting of the socio-economic burden associated with depression. Again, the potential benefits of the use of antidepressants have been described extensively in the literature (Halfin, 2007). Admittedly, the ethical benefits in both cases are derived either from the anecdotal evidence of historians and commentators – for example, Elaine May with the contraceptive pill or Peter Kramer with SSRI antidepressants (May, 2010, pp. 50–80; Kramer, 1993, pp. 1–21) – or from the interpretation of economic studies in the case of SSRI antidepressants and their benefits for the poor (Donoghue and Pincus, 2007), rather than direct observation. Nevertheless, these ethical benefits have been discussed in a thorough and sustained way in the literature since these medicines were first marketed – and yet the Roman Catholic church still prohibits these medical interventions on natural law grounds, despite these benefits.

The natural law approach to ethical evaluation used with previous medical technologies, as has been the standard treatment by the Roman Catholic church, represents only one possible approach for ethical evaluation of biomedical technologies. Yet during the years of the therapeutic revolution (1950–1990), there have been few attempts by non-Roman Catholic ethicists to formulate an ethic of pharmaceutical medicine that is not based on natural law principles, and yet is explicitly Christian in character, as opposed to the prevailing secular bioethics.

There are some notable exceptions. Anglican theologian Oliver O'Donovan explored the distinction between person and artifice in the application of reproductive technologies, in his 1984 publication, *Begotten, Not Made* (O'Donovan, 1984, p. 77). In the early 1980s, the Anglican medical ethicist, Gordon Dunstan, made a theological case for downgrading the moral status of the early foetus, appealing to Aquinas's view that the foetus was not endowed with a soul until it was fully formed (Dunstan, 1984). Although Dunstan's work does not relate directly to pharmacology, and has since been contested by Jones, on both theological and scientific grounds (Jones, 2005), it was nevertheless influential in the deliberations of the Warnock Committee in 1984 (Warnock, 1984). In *Selfish Genes and Christian Ethics*, Neil Messer, a theologian of the United Reformed Church, examines six issues that arise from a Christian critique of evolutionary biology, using relevant Christian doctrines, such as creation and Christology, to develop the dialogue (Messer, 2007, pp. 1–6).[3] The overall concept that Messer explores is the possibility that human beings can redesign themselves with biomedical technology. Arising from this, Messer formulates the four diagnostic questions that could be used to assess the acceptability of a biotechnological project from a perspective of Christian ethics, and which contribute to the theological criteria used in this study.

The case studies indicate that the sole application of natural law theory in medical ethics is problematic in contemporary society, and that other factors need to be considered. The first of these is culture. Not only have cultural factors influenced the development of the contraceptive pill and SSRI antidepressants, the effects of these medicines on individual human beings, and collectively on human society, have had profound cultural implications. Cultural factors and assumptions are therefore closely linked with perceptions of the effects of a medical technology on nature and these factors will influence natural law-based ethical assessments of biomedical technologies. It may be difficult to remove cultural aspects completely from any natural law-based ethical assessment of a biomedical technology, but they must at least be accounted for.

The second of these is autonomy, as previously discussed. Both the contraceptive pill and Prozac have become widely used because individual people have been willing to adopt them with autonomy to improve their health and quality of life, irrespective of the wishes of healthcare practitioners, or the public health priorities of the state. When a medical technology is readily accessible and can be used universally, personal autonomy becomes a significant factor in whether a technology is used in a widespread manner in human society and exerts its effects on society, and considerations about the nature of a biomedical technology become of lesser significance.

The third of these is embodiment. Historically, embodiment has been regarded as a significant aspect of human life in Christian doctrine, and if human life is – and should be – biological, then there is an essential human nature, which is indeed grounded in biological features. There are some things that a human being simply cannot be, by virtue of the properties of the material from which he or she is made. There are therefore features of humanity that can serve as a baseline prior to the application of any biomedical technology. However, it is increasingly clear scientifically that this essential human nature may be biologically grounded, but it is by no means absolute. There is an extent to which the definition of human nature is arbitrary and can be manipulated by social and cultural factors.

These factors are all significant in discussions about standards for enhancement. For this reason, such standards should be owned publicly and be part of public discourse, rather than being a technical or commercial endeavour. This would be reflected in public policy; Wolbring has argued that policymakers should agree basal levels of human function, to develop an equitable framework for the regulation of enhancement technologies (Wolbring, 2010). So, while at present, public health policy decisions are concerned with preventive medicine and basic standards of human living, in future they might encompass basic standards for human function and capacities. This would then inform the activities of the health and care service, which are currently often reactive rather than proactive. Such an approach would align well with the increased significance that both human rights and distributive justice have had in medical ethics in more recent years (Jackson, 2014, p. 171). Nevertheless, such an approach may be controversial from a Christian perspective because it shifts responsibility for the definition of human nature from Christian authorities – scripture and tradition – to the secular state, where it may well be subject to political manipulation or ideological influences that are anti-religious in nature.

Nature, and what is natural, is therefore relative, and is not an absolute, measure for the evaluation of enhancement technologies. Indeed, future radical biomedical technologies – if widely distributed – may themselves change attributes that were previously regarded as natural. With this relative view of nature, other ethical benefits of a biomedical technology, regardless of its status under natural law, become more significant. As discussed in Chapter 2, both Celia Deane-Drummond and Michael Shapiro have cited the limitations and provisional character of naturalism and natural law (Deane-Drummond, 1997, pp. 100–101; Shapiro, 2013).

Natural law has had a long and venerable history in Christian moral thinking. It appeals primarily to reason, rather than to Christian revelation (or flawed interpretation of that revelation), and the universalist claim of natural law, regardless of culture and religious tradition, is therefore appealing. It also offers universal applicability and works on the basis that every rational human being has innate moral capacity (although this equally could be derived from the *imago Dei*). Consequently, natural law with its reliance on observation and reason alone aligns very well with post-Enlightenment rationalism and provides a point of contact between modern ethics and an earlier Christian tradition. This may account for its persistence in Roman Catholic moral thought into the twentieth century, and into the "therapeutic revolution" era that gave rise to the medical technologies discussed in this book. Indeed, with its alignment with rationalism and its emphasis on the virtuous life of a creature according to its nature, natural law might, at first sight, seem to be a valuable means of ethical assessment of the benefits of modern medical science.

However, because biomedical technologies can change a person's nature, determining a person's nature, and thus the good moral ends arising from that nature, is becoming an increasingly elusive goal, which is why natural law is increasingly problematic for evaluation of biomedical technologies. A review of the case studies suggests that there are two important factors in this shift in understanding of natural law. First, there is an increasing awareness of different cultural factors and assumptions that surround and affect the use of medical technologies, which detract from an understanding of the effects of these technologies on the nature of the person to whom it is applied. Second, there is the dominance of the will in modern healthcare, as elsewhere in modern society. Experience with the contraceptive pill and SSRI antidepressants has shown that citizens are willing to use medical technologies at their own convenience and for their own benefit so, in future, citizens may be willing to apply radical, highly invasive technologies, which have the potential to make profound alternations to their nature with relative speed and ease.

In addition, natural law has been closely linked with the moral theology of the Roman Catholic church, which arguably has been discredited in modern society, despite the wisdom of some of its insights, because of the church's intransigent position on contraception (Thatcher, 2011, pp. 211–212). Furthermore, the contemporary world is postmodern and has a lower view of authority than in previous centuries – especially that of the church. The contemporary world is also post-foundationalist, and the evaluation of human dilemmas is not bound up with specific *a priori* epistemic or ideological commitments in the same way that it used to be. Consequently, the sole use of a natural law ethical approach to new biomedical technologies will not meet the current needs and expectations of the world's citizens.

I would contend, therefore, that natural law may provide an initial approach to understanding the ethical implications of medical technologies, but it cannot be the basis for a full and thoroughgoing ethical evaluation of such technologies – either for therapy or for enhancement – in the context of a late modern or post-modern society. As Shapiro has suggested, a natural law discussion might provide an entry point into an ethical analysis, and would highlight assumptions about nature, identify cultural factors and enable a greater understanding of exactly how the technology interacts with the human body to exert its effect (Shapiro, 2013). But both case studies show that, because of other non-natural law based ethical factors, a fuller Christian ethical analysis of a biomedical technology requires more than just a natural law treatment.

I therefore contend that ethical evaluation of biomedical technologies should not be restricted to a natural law-based approach, such as that used with both the contraceptive pill and SSRI antidepressants in the past. Instead, a range of ethical methodologies should be used for a more comprehensive approach to the ethical evaluation of new biomedical technologies. Such an approach would need to account for ethical issues such as equity of access to, and use of, technologies and a consideration of the goods of life that medical technology should support or enable.

A comprehensive approach to biotechnological ethics would be more holistic, and therefore more in line with the current holistic approach to healthcare. Moreover, a broader approach to the ethics of biomedical therapies would, in fact, be consistent with the Roman Catholic ethical principle of integrity – that people should act consistently in all areas of human life – and that of totality – that moral decision-making should enable the flourishing of the whole community, not just the individual. This could encompass all kinds of healthcare ethical decisions, from those that are essentially clinical or scientific to those that are concerned more with culture and social convention. Such a holistic approach might be supported by many

Christian medical ethicists from Protestant traditions, but also by some Roman Catholic medical ethicists too.

Other ethical approaches which might be used include consequentialist ethics or virtue ethics, which examine respectively the consequences of use of the technology or the character of the user, rather than just the nature of the technology. Modern, secular bioethics has typically tended towards ethical decision-making based on consequentialism or situationism (Kerridge et al., 1998), with its questions of cost-utility and cost-benefit. While there are Christian critiques of consequentialism, as I have argued elsewhere, the consequences of technology implementation may not all be negative, as these past case studies demonstrate.

In particular, the role of human virtue in the ethical assessment of biomedical technologies is relatively unexplored. In his classic book *After Virtue*, Alasdair MacIntyre appeals to the renewal of the classic Aristotelian tradition of moral virtue, given the inability of modern ethical theories such as consequentialism to address the so-called existential turn, where the incommensurability of human experience seems to overshadow any attempts to make value judgements on human life using ethics (MacIntyre, 1981, pp. 256–263). Virtue has a potential important application in medical ethics – and therefore in future biomedical enhancement ethics – because it acts as a counterbalance to consequentialism and focuses instead on the qualities and attributes of the actors, rather than the materials, the situation and the social context.[4]

A virtue ethics approach emphasises the importance of virtue in the good ends of human life, as natural law does, but without the problems that arise from the use of natural law in the technological world. Indeed, there has been a growing interest in the role of virtue in contemporary medical ethics. For example, in his advocacy of virtue ethics in modern medicine, Peter Gardner asserts that the virtues of the practitioner – and their attention to the human motivations, emotional sensitivities and relationships involved in the scenario – are able to provide a fuller ethical analysis of any medical dilemma, and to lead to more creative ethical solutions than the usual appeals to either consequentialism or principlism (the idea that all scenarios in medicine can be evaluated ethically using universal principles) (Gardiner, 2003).

To conclude this section, I have argued that, despite the long-standing role of natural law in Christian ethics, a natural law-based ethical evaluation of medical technology is, on its own, deficient for the evaluation of proposed future transhumanist biomedical technologies. Natural law has not helped to present a full picture of the ethical status of past cases in pharmaceutical medicine, so is unlikely to be fit for purpose when more radical, high-tech medical technologies become available in future. A wider ethical framework is needed for the evaluation of such technologies and, in answering the proposed research questions, this book aims to lay down the foundations for such a framework.

5.2.3 Embodiment

Both the contraceptive pill and SSRI antidepressants exert their positive effects through beneficial actions on the human body, and they affirm bodily life. However, the significance of this is not wholly positive; for example, Jutte has claimed from a feminist perspective that the use of the contraceptive pill has "disembodied" women, in that it has denigrated their bodily value by rendering their bodies solely objects for male sexual desire (Jutte, 2008, p. 111), when, in fact, proper desire should be for the whole person, not just their physical body.

Indeed, it is clear from Chapter 1 that the entire project of pharmaceutical medicine to date has been linked with the necessity of human embodiment. Consequently, future transhumanist technologies which would negate the human body – for example, mind uploading – would not only be problematic in respect of Christian beliefs about the significance of the material human body, but would also be a significant departure from the trajectory of progress in medical science to date.

As discussed, both the previous cases of pharmaceutical medicine have had considerable benefits for humanity, which may be regarded as ethical goods of human life. The "un-natural" effect of these medicines on the body (as synthetic "artificial" substances that interfere with the body's "natural" functions) is a relatively small factor in the overall ethical picture of their impact on society, whether positively, in terms of benefits on human life and flourishing, or negatively, in terms of possible deficits in terms of equitable distribution and coercion in their use. Furthermore, the "un-natural" nature of these previous medicines is insignificant indeed, compared to proposed future transhumanist technologies which would be radically disembodying, such as mind uploading, which would be the ultimate in "unnatural" interventions.

I have argued elsewhere that, from a Christian ethical perspective, embodiment is an important, and probably necessary, prerequisite for human flourishing, because it is the ground for authentic human experience and identity. Consequently, technologies which completely negate bodily life are not compatible with Christian ethics on the grounds of the importance of embodiment. The more marginalised the human body is from human personhood, the less applicable the medical ethical principles and methods which have been developed to date will be to the evaluation of more radical future biomedical technologies. This is because these principles are largely predicated on the biological body as the object of medical interventions.

However, apart from potential biomedical technologies which completely disembody the human person, such as mind uploading, there are various medical technologies that are "in-between" full embodiment and complete disembodiment, such as cybernetic organs, prostheses and implanted devices. Such technologies turn a fully biological human being into a hybrid or cyborg. Elaine Graham has claimed that, in purely technological terms, hybridisation is not a new concept, and that humans have always been "mixed up" with their technologies (Graham, 2006). While Katherine Hayles rejects the idea of the disembodied mind, she highlights the fact that the hybridised person – composed of both human tissues and synthetic materials – has important ontological implications for what it means to be human (Hayles, 1999, pp. 1–5). These implications, in turn, have potential political consequences concerning personal identity and status in society.

This is not an issue with either of the case studies in this book, or even with some current inert prosthetic organs or other components, because these technologies are relatively limited, and their effects focused, but it may become an issue in future with the use of more extensive and sophisticated cybernetic technologies. This suggests that, while the effect on the body is only one aspect of the overall impact of biomedical technological intervention, the technical ability to manipulate and adapt the human body should not be deployed without corresponding evaluation of the ethical impact of such manipulation on the individual person and on the society of which the person is part. As discussed previously, this ethical evaluation should not be based solely on natural law, but should use other methodologies. And, once that evaluation has taken place, once again, the role of public policy will be important for the regulation and management of technology adoption, because this will account for the needs of all citizens and the resources available in an equitable way.

5.2.4 Imago Dei

Exactly how humans bear the image of God is an important element of a Christian understanding of what it means to be human, and for this reason, the *imago Dei* has been explored as the key to human distinctiveness, both in the light of modern evolutionary biology (Van Huyssteen, 2018) and in the light of possible future artificial intelligence (Herzfeld, 2002, pp. 25–27). As introduced in Chapter 2, there has been much debate about how the scriptural motif of the *imago Dei* should be understood, and four broad approaches have been proposed – substantive, functional, relational and eschatological (Herzfeld, 2002, pp. 25–27; Burdett, 2018). These are all interlinked theologically and are all important in providing a comprehensive, rounded account of human life in theological anthropology. A major criticism of radical transhumanist technologies, such as mind-uploading or genetic enhancement, is that, in terms of their assumptions about human life, they reflect a substantive view of the *imago Dei,* because of their emphasis on human attributes and individualism, and they downplay functional or relational understandings of human life.

However, I have shown in the case studies that both the contraceptive pill and SSRI antidepressants have ethical implications for human life that are consistent with a functional – or vocational – and a relational view of human life. The effects of these two previous medical technologies on human life are therefore more consistent with a comprehensive understanding the *imago Dei* than the likely effects on human life of proposed future technologies, which emphasise a substantive approach to the *imago Dei*, at the expense of the other approaches. Strikingly, this is despite the widescale effects the use of these medicines has had on society, effects that I have argued give them the appearance of transhumanist technologies.

For future biomedical technologies, it will be important to assess their effects on human lives – individually and corporately – to ensure they will not undermine any aspect of humanity that is important for the *imago Dei*. Future biomedical technologies may certainly enhance human attributes – for example, intellect, creativity ability or aesthetic capacity – and thus support a largely substantive view of the *imago Dei*. According to Kramer and advocates of cosmetic psychopharmacology, SSRI antidepressant use for personality enhancement already enhances – and privileges – some human attributes such as assertiveness and mental acuity. Depending on future scientific discoveries, such psychopharmacological enhancements might also eventually include more profound "spiritual" attributes such as self-transcendence and awareness of God. In either case, there will certainly be a demand in future for biomedical enhancement technologies, precisely for the attributes they confer.

But the question for future biomedical technologies will be whether application of the technology will enable a person to conform to aspects of the *imago Dei* other than the substantive. First, will the biomedical technology affect relationships in human society? Will it affect either the extent and quality of interpersonal relationships, the distribution of communities or the cohesion of society at a regional, national or international level? Some neural and psychological enhancements may have benefits for the quality of relationships, but any technology that facilitates extreme individualism and oppression in society is likely to have a negative effect on relationships.

Second, will the biomedical technology affect human function – that is, the ability of a person to fulfil the vocation to which God has called them in the world? While a functional approach to the *imago Dei* is about human vocation rather than about biological/physical functioning of the human body, nevertheless human bodily function in an embodied world is a necessary pre-requisite of vocational flourishing. Vocational flourishing may be horizontal or vertical in direction – towards the world or towards God. It may be about an individual fulfilling their unique purpose in what they do with their time and talents to serve the world, or it may be about their worship and prayer and their willingness to serve God *in* the world. In either situation, relationships are also involved with vocational function. Many enhancements of biological and mental function may assist a person in fulfilling their vocational function, but some technologies may enhance some aspects of human (biological) function at the expense of others, and these might interfere with a person's vocational function.

Another concern with transhumanism related to the *imago Dei* is that of idolatry (Van Huyssteen, 2006, pp. 139–143). The application of radical biomedical technology of human devising to a person potentially makes that person and their attributes idols – artefacts that are worshipped instead of God. This is essentially the concern expressed by O'Donovan, where an enhanced individual becomes an artefact that has been engineered, rather than a personal subject (O'Donovan, 1984, pp. 1–6, 13). There is therefore a sense in which the enhanced person is no longer made in the image of God, but in their own image, according to their own will; Noreen Herzfeld discusses this concept of *imago hominis* in her work on the implications of computer artificial intelligence for the *imago Dei* (Herzfeld, 2002, pp. 25–27).

This notion of idolatry can be identified with the application of the two technologies in the case studies. Because the contraceptive pill enables women to have control over their fertility, this in turn allows them to control other aspects of their lives – for example, their sexual life, relationships or career. These aspects of life may assume increased significance for the person and could lead to a situation where the person "worships" their lifestyle, as an idol, instead of God. Also, as discussed in Chapter 3, a feminist critique of the contraceptive pill is that it contributes to the objectification of women – it can make a woman's body (rather than her whole self) the object of a man's desire, making her an "idol" to him. Similarly, when used for cosmetic psychopharmacology, SSRI antidepressants can manipulate and control the personality, which may lead to the user becoming preoccupied with their personality traits in an inward-looking, individualistic, self-centred way. This might detract from an awareness of God and a selfless willingness to serve him in the world.

Several theologians take the view that creatureliness cannot be separated from technology (Graham, 2006). Indeed, Graham contends that human beings enact the *imago Dei* when they engage in technological innovation, and that human beings have always been hybridised – mixed in – with the technologies they use (Graham, 2006). In addition, as we have noted, Hefner proposes the notion of the human being as "created co-creator" i.e. that human beings have the agency to bring about a good future from their current nature (Hefner, 1993, p. 27). The inevitability of the interplay between human life and technology in a technological world, as suggested by these theologians, is at odds with the idea that biomedical technology is needed to complete a "deficient" *imago Dei* in humanity because of the difficulty of identifying the "deficiency" and the effects of technology when the relationship between human life and technology is so intricate.

The key issue here is the status of the unenhanced human being. If all humanity undeniably bears the image of God now – however that might be understood – then an ethically acceptable biomedical technology (past or future) should be a potential enhancement of the *imago Dei*, so that the person *more clearly* bears the *imago Dei*, rather than a remedy that is needed to complete a deficient *imago Dei*, or to rectify a flawed *imago Dei*, at the current time. For a person to bear more clearly the *imago Dei*, then substantive, functional and relational aspects of the *imago Dei* will be more clearly identifiable in that person's life. However, there will also be an eschatological element – that the person is more directed towards a future life that glorifies God, and is lived in the presence of God. This would be a true *theosis* – participation in the divine – and this would be seen in how the technology affects the person's ability to make good ethical decisions about their life, and to use their life in the service of God and the world. This move towards a future life that glorifies God is analogous to the increase in Christlikeness as the believer is transformed by the Holy Spirit and filled with the virtuous gifts of the Holy Spirit. This is quite different to the self-mediated, directionless eschatology proposed by the transhumanism movement (Waters, 2006a, pp. 123–125).

The contraceptive pill and SSRI antidepressants exert their good effects in and through the body, and I have argued already that both can have a positive effect on the functional (vocational) and relational aspects of human life. I have shown in the case studies that both these technologies have the potential to enrich relationships, individually and in society, and to help to make good decisions from a Christian perspective, which would align with a functional (vocational) approach to *the imago Dei.*

Similarly, future enhancements such as laser eye surgery or a cybernetic arm may improve function (vocation) and relationships and thus improve experience of biological life (although they may be associated with other ethical issues) but the important question from a Christian perspective will be the extent to which these enhancements support – or undermine – an eschatological trajectory, a Godward approach to life; in other words the development of the relationship with God and the Christ-like character, and the sense in which humans are proceeding to a shared destiny with God.

One of the ethical evaluation criteria here is: is the project an attempt to be like God, or does it conform to the image of God? (Messer, 2007, p. 231). When future, transhumanist biomedical technologies, such as mind-uploading, cybernetics and cryonics, are evaluated against this question then the concerns expressed by theologians seem to be warranted. Transhumanist biomedical technologies do indeed seem to be individualistic, concerned only with the attributes of the individual person. They do indeed seem to provide an alternative eschatology to that of Christian belief, one which is over-realised and does not address human moral responsibility and the reality of sin. Transhumanist technologies affect human functioning in society, and so it might be supposed that this has a bearing on the functional approach to the *imago Dei.* However, the effects of these technologies on human function serve only the individual to whom the technology has been applied, with no concept of the individual's vocation as God's agent in the created world, which is the central component of a functional account of the *imago Dei.*

When considering the contraceptive pill, the answer to the question about whether the technology is an attempt to be like God, or whether it conforms to the image of God, is rather more nuanced. In the control that it affords the user over their menstrual cycle, fertility and family planning, and thereby on their marriage, family and working life, the pill does indeed have far-reaching effects, and could be used to enable users to manipulate their fertility – and their lifestyle – and to be "like God" in terms of the control they exercise over a natural aspect of human biological life. This contradicts the notion of divine order in human life, which underpins the Roman Catholic Church's natural law objections to hormonal contraception. In this respect, the contraceptive pill resembles a proposed future transhumanist technology. However, it should be noted that, while the pill can interrupt the fertility process, it does not change or abolish the process. If the pill is discontinued, then conception and birth still take place in the same (natural) way afterwards, despite the use of the pill. On the contrary, some of the most radical transhumanist technological interventions – for example, mind uploading and cybernetic implants – appear to be, to all intents and purposes, irreversible. The effects of transhumanist technologies on human life are therefore likely to have more radical implications for the *imago Dei* in humanity than past medical developments.

Transhumanist technologies are individualistic and focused on human attributes and therefore their use would reflect a largely substantive approach to the *imago Dei*, and an alternative, privatised eschatology to that offered by the Christian hope. However, while the contraceptive pill does indeed affect certain human attributes – namely the ability to become pregnant, and positive metabolic actions – its effects have different implications for the way humans image God. The potentially beneficial effects of the contraceptive pill on marriage, family and society are consistent with a relational *imago Dei* in humanity, where the *imago Dei* is grounded in human relationality, with God and with each other. Furthermore, the *imago Dei* envisaged by the positive effects of the contraceptive pill – most notably, greater equality and mutuality in the marriage relationship – counteracts previous feminist criticisms that formulation of the *imago Dei* has, in the past, had androcentric tendencies (Fulkerson, 1997). Indeed, the impact of the contraceptive pill on human relationships at all levels downplays an *imago Dei* that is overly focused on human attributes.

The answer to the *imago Dei* question – being like God or conforming to the image of God – is similar for SSRI antidepressants, as for the contraceptive pill – and again, is distinct from future transhumanist biomedical technologies. Cosmetic psychopharmacology, as envisaged by Peter Kramer and supporters of the "Prozac phenomenon", is where the person chooses to remould their personality and change the kind of person they are at their own instigation, by technological means. This would be a more radical means of personality change than, for example, counselling or personal development, and would be applied with greater control and will power, so could be seen as an attempt to be like God. However, because the effect of SSRI antidepressants on the human person – personality alteration – is more subtle than that of the contraceptive pill on fertility, the effects of

SSRI antidepressants are harder to identify or control than the pill, and may therefore be more far-reaching than expected. Nevertheless, like the contraceptive pill, the use of SSRI antidepressants supports human flourishing in a way that is consistent with a comprehensive understanding of the *imago Dei*, rather than one which only has substantive attributes in view and in which the eschatological dimension has been undermined. This is due to the positive effects of SSRI antidepressants on human relationships, as described by Kramer (Kramer, 1993, pp. 2, 28, 94, 267), and their ability to restore biological function in those debilitated with severe depression. These, in turn, have positive effects on an individual's ability to engage with the world, and to exercise a vocation of service to God in the world, which would be the outworking of a functional approach to the *imago Dei*.

There are two caveats here. First, the clinical data concerns restoration of biological and mental function in patients with depression but does not extend to objective functional improvement in otherwise healthy individuals who might use SSRI antidepressants for personality enhancement. Nevertheless, such functional improvements can be inferred from Kramer's clinical vignettes, for example, the use of SSRI antidepressants giving patients the confidence and self-esteem to tackle negativity and problems in their personal or professional life (Kramer, 1993, pp. 2, 28, 94, 267). The positive impact of a person's life and activities on their community and professional contexts links clearly with the vocational concept at the heart of the functional approach to the *imago Dei*. Second, improvements in functional ability and relational capacity may not necessarily lead to the spiritual response that might be expected in a person who reflects different aspects of the *imago Dei*. A spiritual response might be defined as flourishing, generous and realistic relationships with oneself and with other human beings, which reflect both a rich and vital relationship with God, and a functioning that is concerned with living out a divinely given vocation for humanity of service in the world (which the interpretation of the functional *imago Dei* as a "royal representative" would entail). Whether or not an individual has true autonomy, they still have responsibility for how they live their life in relation to God and to his Kingdom, when "enhanced" with an SSRI antidepressant.

Having considered these four theological domains of autonomy, nature, embodiment and the *imago Dei* in detail, I conclude that these four areas are a rich source of reflection concerning the ethical permissibility and desirability of medical technologies, both past and future. I have shown that "nature" is part of this assessment process, but it is insufficient on its own because, in a world of biotechnological enhancements, nature is supremely malleable, its normative function cannot be assumed, and it excludes social and cultural issues with technology use. In a technological world, where nature is less significant because of its malleability, personal autonomy in decision-making about technology assumes a correspondingly greater significance, and good public policy is needed to negotiate equity issues with technology use at a societal level. Human embodiment is important because biomedical technologies that negate the body are not consistent with a Christian attitude to life, and the more marginalised the human body is from human personhood, the less applicable the medical ethical principles and methods which have been developed to date will be to the evaluation of more radical biomedical technologies in future. Finally, the *imago Dei* analysis of new biomedical technologies will assess whether the biotechnology-enhanced person will reflect a comprehensive Christian understanding of human life, and identify any eschatological issues associated with the technology. This is important given the critique that, compared with the Christian destiny envisaged by an eschatological approach to the *imago Dei*, transhumanist biomedical developments present an alternative, realised, self-centred eschatology instead.

Consideration of all four domains together provides the basis for a more detailed and nuanced ethical evaluation of previous medical technologies, developed during the "therapeutic revolution" years of the twentieth century, and will provide an adequate framework for the ethical evaluation of future, transhumanist biomedical enhancements.

5.3 Transhumanism and the Therapeutic Revolution

In Chapter 1, I stated that pharmaceutical medicine in the second half of the twentieth century made "stirring advances" (Woolf, 2001). However, some of these advances have not just improved individual lives, but have had implications for the whole of society. From the early twentieth century when Lorand first perceived the far-reaching biological effects of hormonal therapy (Davis et al., 2005), pharmaceutical medicine has entertained the possibility of radically changing the quality, conventions and experience of human life. As noted previously, David Healy has remarked on the potential of both the contraceptive pill and psychopharmacology to bring about large-scale social change; the pill changing the sexual order of society, and psychopharmacology changing the social order (Healy, 2000).

To what extent were these two past developments, in their time, transhumanist technologies? The developers of the contraceptive pill were primarily motivated by the socio-political implications of its use in society, and its potential benefits for social progress. Margaret Sanger envisaged the radical social implications of the pill, Katharine McCormick put forward the money to fund it and Gregory Pincus was courageous enough to lead the scientific development of the pill in the face of opposition from the prevailing academic culture. Indeed, these three factors – vision of a better future, significant financial outlay and willingness to extend the accepted boundaries of current practice – are the key elements in the development of proposed future transhumanist biomedical technologies (More, 2013, pp. 1–8).

In contrast, SSRI antidepressants were the product of a much more institutionalised and mature drug development process in the 1970s and

1980s. Prozac was marketed primarily as a therapeutic advance for the treatment of depression, and it was only after its launch that Peter Kramer and others saw the potential of Prozac and the SSRI antidepressants to transform society on a large scale, due to their subtle effects on personality.

However, are these past cases of pharmaceutical medicine transhumanist in character according to the objective general criteria for a technology presented in Chapter 2? I contend that they are. Both past cases are technologies, in the broadest sense – a material means to effect a process – and they exert their effects on and through the human body to achieve a largely positive effect on human flourishing.

The response to the criterion about applying the technology with complete autonomy is rather more complex. The ability to apply a biomedical technology to the human body with unbridled autonomy is a key tenet of the transhumanist movement. Consequently, whether a biomedical technology can be applied and used autonomously would be a significant factor in the classification of any biomedical technology as "transhumanist". However, I have found that the role of autonomy in the use and application of biomedical technologies – past and future – is rather more ambiguous than transhumanist scholars admit to. Elsewhere, I have defined autonomy as self-determination in personal decision-making, so that the person can act as a moral agent, with minimum interference of external factors. Furthermore, in previous chapters, I have demonstrated that all the technologies discussed in this book – medical technologies from the past, the contraceptive pill and SSRI antidepressants, and the proposed transhumanist technologies of the future – may be applied with autonomy at the outset, but that there may be loss of autonomy due to unintended consequences at a later stage of their use. These unintended consequences may be due to external factors – coercion at an individual level and social pressure and, in the case of SSRI antidepressants, possibly the effects of the drugs themselves (the dependence and withdrawal effects, or diminished responsibility due to atypical reactions).

Application of specific theological criteria to the two case studies highlights some of the ethical concerns about radical biomedical technologies. The contraceptive pill and SSRI antidepressants have benefits for the poor, although the evidence for this is sparse at present for SSRI antidepressants, and there may be issues with accessibility to the contraceptive pill in some parts of the world. However, comparing the costs of these drugs with the likely costs of radical future biomedical technologies at an early stage of commercialisation, current medicines are more universally available and more equitably distributed than some potential future technologies are likely to be. Consequently, these two past medical developments are good news for the poor, in comparison with some of the proposed future proposed transhumanist technologies.

The contraceptive pill and SSRI antidepressants both have the potential to change human life and flourishing in a way that aligns with a positive and comprehensive view of the *imago Dei*. The effects of SSRI antidepressants are not just focused on human attributes but contribute to human flourishing in a way that is also consistent with other approaches to the *imago Dei*. The contraceptive pill has the potential to affect society in a way that addresses gender imbalances, and which therefore reflects a less androcentric view of the *imago Dei*. In these respects, these drugs are not like future transhumanist technologies. However, these drugs might be said to be like future transhumanist technologies in that they can be used to enable the individual or practitioner to "be like God" and "play God" in manipulating fertility or personality at will.

Both the contraceptive pill and SSRI antidepressants exert positive effects of human flourishing and experience in and through the human body. In this respect, these drugs are decisively unlike some proposed future transhumanist technologies, such as mind uploading and cybernetics, which have a negative view of bodily human life, and which deprecate the role of the human body in human life and flourishing. Furthermore, both the contraceptive pill and SSRI antidepressants have objective benefits for human society corporately, due to changed cultural expectations, as well as benefits for the health, well-being and subjective experience of the individual. In this respect, these drugs are distinct from many of the proposed, future transhumanist technologies, which assume an individualistic, privatised approach to technology use, rather than one where medical technology is deployed according to public policy for the good of society.

There is evidence that both drugs have, during their history, been regarded by some commentators as triumphs of scientific medicine and panaceas for social problems, suggesting an overconfidence in their effectiveness and use in human society, which might be seen as technological hubris. In this respect, these drugs resemble to some extent more radical future transhumanist developments, which are often treated as radical solutions to profound human problems (McNamee and Edwards, 2006).

Finally, concerning the balance between the subjective experience of the user and the objectification of the user, both the contraceptive pill and SSRI antidepressants have the potential to enhance the subjective experience of the user, but also to objectify the user, and emphasise their status as an artefact rather than a personal subject.

To conclude this section, both these previous technologies have shown some – but not all – of the features of proposed future transhumanist technologies. As pharmaceutical medicines, these developments work in and through the human body to exert a positive effect on human life and experience, and so they work on the assumption that the human body is a prerequisite to human life and experience, unlike some proposed future technologies such as mind-uploading and cybernetic hybridisation.

However, as noted previously, transhumanism uses biomedical technology to go beyond modernity's project of transforming the world through culture and education. Consequently, as medical technologies available globally, the contraceptive pill and SSRI antidepressants do resemble future transhumanist biomedical technologies in as much as they have the potential to change society primarily by biomedical means. Medical technologies are often seen as a panacea for all sorts of social problems (McNamee and Edwards, 2006; Cole-Turner, 2001). This has been noted throughout this project with both past medical technologies and potential future transhumanist technologies. The reality, however, is that, while future biomedical technologies may well have a widespread impact on human society, and hopefully a positive one, they cannot solve all of society's problems – and the problems they will solve will be determined by safeguards around how they are developed, and policies about how they will be funded and distributed.

Many transhumanist thinkers have described proposed transhumanist technologies in general terms, and have suggested what impact they might have on future human life. However, they have not envisaged in any detail how these technologies might be developed scientifically and made available to human society. The two case studies here, the contraceptive pill and SSRI antidepressants, indicate that the radical biotechnologies of the future, with profound effects across the human population, will emerge from current medical technology research and probably be enabled by various scientific, organisational, commercial and socio-political factors.

5.4 Past Controversies and Future Hopes

As described in Chapter 1, many new medicines were developed during the therapeutic revolution years of the twentieth century. Many of these medicines – for example, antibiotics and cardiovascular medicines – have had profound effects on medical outcomes, human health and well-being, and yet Christian ethics has largely been silent about their innovation and use. The notable exceptions to this relative lack of engagement of Christian ethics with pharmaceutical medicine have been the Roman Catholic church's official opposition to the contraceptive pill on natural law grounds, and a similar response by Roman Catholic scholar, John-Mark Miravalle, to the "Prozac phenomenon" following the introduction of SSRI antidepressants (Miravalle, 2010).

The interesting aspect of this is that, logically, a natural law objection could be raised for the use of *any* non-natural, "artificial" medical intervention of human devising, be it a drug or a surgical procedure. However, the Roman Catholic Church has only developed and expressed this argument against those medicines that have significant non-medical and social implications, hence their concerns with the contraceptive pill and SSRI antidepressants. Nevertheless, despite the robust articulation of the natural law position on contraception by the Roman Catholic church in *Casti Conubii* in 1930 and again in *Humanae Vitae* in 1968, the evidence indicates that many Roman Catholic couples are ignoring the teaching of their church and using forms of hormonal contraception for purely pragmatic reasons of fertility control and family planning in a developed, modern, industrial/post-industrial society (Langford, 1976, pp. 26, 34, 51).

Both the medical technologies described in the case studies in this project – the contraceptive pill and SSRI antidepressants – have been controversial in western society at, or since, their introduction. But have the ethical concerns that were raised at the time been warranted in the light of subsequent experience?

The adoption of the contraceptive pill took place slowly, due to the relative conservatism of society in America and Britain in the early 1960s, compared to the current time. The adoption of Prozac and the SSRI antidepressants was more rapid, possibly due to the recognised therapeutic need for these drugs in the clinical treatment of depression, as alternatives to older agents, and the maturity of both the therapeutic revolution and the drug discovery process by the late 1980s.

With the introduction of the contraceptive pill in 1960, and its increasing use in the United States, opponents claimed that use of the pill would lead to eugenic population control, a breakdown of marriage as an institution and as a social good, increased sexual activity with multiple partners and the subversion of relationships (May, 2010, pp. 37, 57, 71). Similarly, concerns were expressed about SSRI antidepressants after their launch – at first, these were medical concerns about adverse effects such as alerting reactions, withdrawal effects and suicidal ideation, and then subsequently, there were philosophical and theological concerns about the wider societal implications of SSRI personality "enhancement", following the publication of Peter Kramer's *Listening to Prozac*.

Both the contraceptive pill and SSRI antidepressants had a cultural impact on society at, or after, their introduction. The contraceptive pill was associated in the popular imagination with the sexual revolution, and SSRI antidepressants with the growth of the "better than well" Prozac phenomenon. Yet, for both agents, their use has become normative, and they have been largely assimilated into twenty-first-century culture. Indeed, neither agent now is dominant in its area of pharmacology, in the way it once was. Long-acting contraceptive implants are now an important alternative to oral contraception, and cognitive behavioural therapy (CBT) is an important alternative treatment to SSRI antidepressants in many patients with depression. Many of the medical and social concerns about both the contraceptive pill and SSRI antidepressants have been found to be unwarranted, based on the experience of use that has accumulated since their launch.

First, concerning the contraceptive pill, by and large, the pill has not been used by governments to exert eugenic population control, largely because it needs to be taken voluntarily by the user.[5] This argument has, however, been levelled, and with good reason, at the way injectable forms of hormonal contraception have been distributed in developing countries, and within some sections of society in first world countries (for example, women with mental disabilities) (Hartmann, 1995, p. 202). Indeed, it has been suggested that oral contraceptive products have, in the past, been distributed in some developing countries in an imperialistic and patronising manner by agencies funded by governments of affluent western countries, in a manner that could be considered coercive (Hartmann, 1995, p. 189). Consequently, although the concerns about the use of the contraceptive pill for eugenics and population control have not been warranted during the history of its use, concerns of this nature should not be ignored with future technologies, given the importance of autonomy in the use of biomedical technologies, as argued earlier in this chapter.

Second, contrary to the fears of some commentators who were opposed to the contraceptive pill at its launch, marriage remains an important social feature in western society, and there is no direct evidence that hormonal contraception alone has had an appreciable impact on population trends in marriage. Following the introduction of the pill in Britain in 1961, the number of people getting married each year in Britain continued to rise until 1970 (Tranter, 1996, pp. 93–95). Although there was a decline in the number of marriages taking place in Britain between 1972 and 2009, population research has suggested that this was due to people delaying marriage and, while the number of couples cohabiting increased during this time, in many cases this was a precursor to marriage (McLaren, 2013). Moreover, between 2009 and 2012, the number of marriages in Britain actually increased, most likely due to factors unrelated to contraception, such as changes in immigration controls and delayed marriages following the 2007/2008 financial downturn (Tranter, 1996, pp. 93–95).

Third, despite the obvious expectation of an increase in commitment-free sex following introduction of the contraceptive pill, there is scant evidence that the availability of hormonal contraception alone has led to an increase in sexual activity with multiple partners in society (Black and Sykes, 1971). Indeed, in her commentary on the history of contraception, Cook argues that sex is legitimised by love, and quotes Helen Brook, founder of the Brook Advisory Service, who said that "if you are promiscuous, there is a reason for it. Promiscuity is a symptom of something else" (Cook, 2004, p. 278). Furthermore, the social history of contraception in the middle decades of the twentieth century indicates that, despite popular perception, there is no clear link between the development of the pill and the beginning of the so-called sexual revolution, even though the pill has had an impact on popular culture. Yet the ability to control conception and to limit family size have the potential to reinforce moral agency and responsibility on the part of would-be parents. Moreover, planned parenthood, the potential outcome of effective contraception, is an ethical good, as it has the potential to promote marital stability through the health and well-being of both partners (Häring, 1976).

Similarly, with the Prozac phenomenon, following the publication of Peter Kramer's *Listening to Prozac*, detractors envisaged the use of Prozac and other SSRI antidepressants for dystopian mind control, in a way which might have far-reaching implications for both human society and for medical ethics (Elliott, 2000). Yet these concerns have proved unfounded too. Despite protocol-based use of SSRI antidepressants in large populations by US health maintenance organisations (HMOs), for reasons of financial cost-effectiveness, there is no evidence that there have ever been any organised programmes of social control using these drugs. Furthermore, fears concerning the adverse social effects of these drugs are not matters of immediate concern for individuals being treated with SSRI antidepressants, whose priority is an effective clinical treatment for depressive illness. And, indeed, as argued in Chapter 4, many people receive treatment with SSRI antidepressants and enjoy significant benefits of that treatment, in terms of alleviation of depression and improved welfare as a result.

With their concerns about the use of both the contraceptive pill and SSRI antidepressants, the Roman Catholic church has applied natural law objections only to those medical interventions that have a social implication, or where conflicts with the church's doctrine are anticipated. I would argue that the Roman Catholic church's ethical treatment of therapeutics has therefore been selective, and that it has not applied the same natural law theory to all "unnatural" biomedical developments, as logic would dictate. Yet, in both these past cases where natural law objections have been applied, social concerns relating to the therapies have largely not been warranted, but also the positive ethical benefits of these therapies have often not been acknowledged.

As already argued at length, natural law is deficient on its own as a tool for ethical evaluation of biomedical technologies. It is not surprising therefore that modern secular bioethics has drawn heavily on consequential ethical thought, in dealing with therapy assessment and health resource allocation and distribution (Bryant et al., 2005, p. 23). Yet this approach too is potentially problematic from a Christian perspective, due to perceptions of human good, difficulties with calculating the quantum of good in different situations and the possibility of conflict of consequentialism with Christian duty (Messer, 2006, p. 80). As discussed earlier in this chapter, an approach to biomedical decision-making based on virtue – the virtue of the actors (technology users and healthcare practitioners), rather than the nature of the technologies or the consequences of their use – has considerable potential for future ethical evaluation of biomedical technologies because it aligns with the New Testament concept of the fruits of the Spirit (Galatians 5).

As previously cited, Ronald Bailey has argued that the application of biomedical technology does not preclude virtue on the part of the human actors in the scenario (Bailey, 2013). Similarly, I would argue that the virtues of marital love and commitment are not necessarily diminished by the routine use of the contraceptive pill and that use of the pill does not have a bearing on the moral quality of a marriage or parental relationship. By contrast, the methodology of the Roman Catholic Church's natural law argument against the contraceptive pill, as expressed in *Humanae Vitae*, does seem to devalue the quality of a marriage, as noted by Oliver O'Donovan in his criticism of the atomistic approach of the Roman Catholic stance on contraception, with its focus on individual sex acts (O'Donovan, 1984, p. 77). Similarly, the use of SSRI antidepressants *per se* to alter mood or personality attributes does not necessarily preclude virtuous actions on the part of the user. Nevertheless, it is possible for both these – and other biomedical technologies – to be deployed, applied and used in a non-virtuous way.

5.5 Re-evaluating Transhumanism

This section examines the implications of the ethical issues with previous medical developments for the ethical evaluation of future biomedical technologies. Kahane and Savulescu are right to make the connection between the use of currently available medicines – for example, the SSRI antidepressant, citalopram – and potentially more radical, future transhumanist technologies (Kahane and Savulescu, 2015). They make the point that current medicines are already used for "enhancement", and that the ethical issues are similar to those that will be seen when future biomedical technologies are widely used for enhancement. Therefore, they contend that the subtle enhancements that are already available (for example, the use of citalopram to attempt moral enhancement) are as significant ethically as more radical enhancements which may become available in the future. This is reasonable, as the use of current medical technologies provides ethical models for the use of future medical technologies, even though their effects might be modest compared with more radical future transhumanist enhancement technologies. However, Kahane and Savulescu make the incorrect assumption, in my view, that because an ethical issue has already been identified and discounted with current pharmaceutical medicine, it is therefore of no significance and may be discounted in any future evaluation of biomedical technologies. Ethical issues are fundamentally concerned with what is a good way of living human life, rather than just the effects of the novel application of technology. There is therefore no reason to suppose that the same ethical issues will not arise in human society at any point in history, irrespective of what technologies are being deployed. Furthermore, possible new ethical issues, arising from unintended consequences of new biomedical technologies, cannot be discounted. This section will look at how the ethical issues from the past case studies might influence and inform the ethical evaluation of future biomedical technologies.

I contend that some of the good ethical ends offered by transhumanist technologies – longevity, better biological function and improved quality of life – have, at least in part, already been achieved by pharmaceutical medicine, during the therapeutic revolution years of the twentieth century. This would include, for example, the impact of specific cardiovascular medicines, cancer chemotherapies and biological agents for autoimmune disorders. However, many previous developments in pharmaceutical medicine have not directly addressed the enhancement of human capacities. This is partly because they have been developed by the pharmaceutical industry in the context of medicine and therapy. Nevertheless, as seen here, some medicines have been far-reaching in their influence, and have transformed society, as well as individual lives. Perhaps because of the contribution of the modern research-based pharmaceutical industry to human health and well-being, the overall benefits of pharmaceutical medicine are rarely questioned in mainstream western society, despite periodic criticism of the selective, capital-driven efforts of the industry by health professionals and the press.

On the contrary, however, in popular culture, future transhumanist technologies are frequently regarded with suspicion, and those who advocate them are accused of "playing God". There may be several reasons for this. First, proposed future transhumanist technologies are often enhancements, rather than therapies – their primary purpose is to enhance human function, rather than as therapies for disease. The development and introduction of such technologies is therefore not associated with medicine or healing, or discussed in the context of healthcare, in the way that medical technology has been to date, but instead is seen as an attempt at "deification" or becoming more like God. This is significant because, as discussed, the use of therapy to alleviate suffering has a perceived moral and emotional imperative, and there is arguably a duty on the part of the state's healthcare system to provide such therapies. However, the use of enhancements in a healthy person is not associated with the same moral imperative, or perceived obligation of state provision. Consequently, the use of medical technologies for enhancement is not only ethically distinct from their use for therapy, but their use "feels" different culturally, and therefore is treated differently in popular discourse.

Second, because they are "enhancements", transhumanist technologies may appear to be "unnatural" in the context of current culture and the current evolutionary stage of humanity. Given that natural law arguments have been prominent in the past in Christian ethical assessments of reproductive technologies, this has heightened cultural suspicion about radical biomedical technologies. However, as previously stated, as the use of radical and invasive biomedical technology increases in society, the ethical significance of whether a technology is "natural" or not will correspondingly diminish.

This is particularly relevant in the field of cybernetics. At present, various artificial prostheses – artificial hip or knee joints, cardiac pacemakers or vascular stents – are routinely implanted into the human body for medical purposes, and they present no major ethical concerns for users on the grounds of how "natural" they are. Widespread use of more extensive cybernetics – for example, robotic organs or limbs – and indeed the development of the cyborg (composite human body and machine) – are extensions of these current medical interventions and may well be adopted in a gradual manner. When such biomedical technology interventions are more commonplace, other ethical issues will come to the fore, and whether the technology is "natural" will become of lesser relevance.

Nevertheless, the importance of social context in medical science should not be at the expense of realism in the task and objectives of science. Critical realism is an established epistemological point of contact between science and religion in general (Southgate, 2011, pp. 15–19; McGrath, 2004, pp. 139–153), and the concept of critical realism is important to understand the truth claims of science. Critical realism recognises that science is useful because it describes a real world, rather than an ideal one (i.e. it is not entirely a social or ideological construct) but that social and cultural factors do have a bearing on scientific discoveries and the activities of the scientific community (McGrath, 2004, pp. 139–152). I have shown that this is the case for both the contraceptive pill and SSRI antidepressants, by demonstrating how the scientific discovery and the cultural reception of these products both arose from the historical context of their development. This is in contrast to Donna Haraway's contention that natural science is purely a social construct, with the ideological agenda of imposing the views of a male scientific patriarchy onto wider liberal society (Haraway, 1991, p. 8).

However, the fact that pharmaceutical medicine has had objective and measurable benefits for human society, as shown in the two case studies, demonstrates that biomedical science cannot be simply dismissed as a social construct, and that this critical realism is important for countering any science-religion dualism which might still arise in popular culture. Just as science is primarily about developing and testing theories about the real, natural world, rather than developing and reinforcing a social construct, so medicine is primarily concerned with the alleviation of real disease and humanitarian need and the promotion of genuine human wholeness. Science is not simply a tool for reinforcing certain ideologies in human life such as a liberal modern view of autonomy and human will.

Scientific reality is more likely to be confounded by social constructionism when considering the social impact of technologies than when considering the effects on the individual human person. That is why the ethical evaluation, as well as the medical evaluation, of future transhumanist biomedical technologies should be evidence-based, according to objective verifiable criteria, using similar methodologies to those that pharmacology has developed over the last 50 years.

Third, there are transhumanist technologies that are currently technically feasible – such as cryogenic preservation of the body and cybernetic enhancements – but are still very much in their infancy and at a prototype stage. These technologies are therefore expensive, and consequently are the preserve of the wealthiest people in society, and not in widespread use. For this reason, the use of these technologies can be perceived as exclusive and discriminatory. However, similar arguments could be made for any medical technology at an early stage of its development in western health economies, where availability of the technology is necessarily restricted and regulated. New medicines are rightly subject to rigorous regulatory controls in developed countries, and all new medicines will undergo clinical trials, and be subject to scientific – and sometimes media – scrutiny. Some of these issues relating to the introduction of a new medical technology are illustrated in Chapter 3 in the development of the contraceptive pill and opposition to its use at the outset.

Nevertheless, this cultural suspicion means that transhumanist technologies are not generally regarded as therapies – agents of healing. Consequently, as part of an ethical evaluation of these transhumanist technologies, it may be helpful to exercise a countercultural approach and consider them as therapies, rather than only as enhancements. As discussed in Chapter 2, the boundary between a therapy and an enhancement is indistinct, and similar ethical arguments concerning virtue could be applied to enhancements, as well as therapies. I have shown that the contraceptive pill is an enhancement in terms of its effects on fertility, and largely fits the general criteria for a transhumanist technology. Yet, the contraceptive pill may also be used therapeutically, as a treatment for menstrual disorders, often at the same time as it is being used for its (enhancing) contraceptive properties. SSRI antidepressants were developed as a treatment for clinical depression, but subsequently were used by some people as a cosmetic psychopharmacology enhancement to make them feel "better than well".

Brent Waters has argued that medical care is not simply concerned with avoiding (inevitable) mortality, but about exercising human virtues such as compassion and kindness in the relief of human suffering (Waters, 2006b). In fact, the same arguments could be made of transhumanist enhancements. These, too, should be about exercising human virtues in the alleviation of human suffering, rather than simply avoiding finitude.

It is often supposed that immortality is the "final solution" to all the problems of human life. However, I discussed several issues which might be problematic in the event of increased longevity in human society, conferred by widespread use of transhumanist technologies – for example, the impact on marriage, future working patterns and effects on the economy. These could all lead to new hitherto unencountered ethical dilemmas, such as various economic and environmental issues arising from a considerable extended human lifespan. Simply overcoming human finitude with transhumanist technologies – even if it was possible – would not obviate every ethical dilemma that human beings face; rather it would prolong them and introduce new issues. Two factors central to the ethical acceptability of new transhumanist technologies will be a virtuous motivation on the part of the innovators and a willingness on the part of society and the medical profession to continually monitor the societal benefits and risks of the technology for human flourishing and well-being. A crude Promethean desire for immortality and super-human attributes will be no substitute for considered, ongoing ethical discourse in society about the role and desirability of such technologies.

With therapeutic developments to date that have had a potential social impact – the pill and Prozac – the Roman Catholic church has based its ethical objections on natural law theory. I have shown however that, following real-world experience with these medicines, ethical factors other than natural law come into play – for example, the benefits of virtuous use of the medicine, and the problems of just distribution of the medicine.

For this reason, the use of the natural law approach alone, or even predominantly, in the assessment of therapeutics is a naïve way of assessing therapeutics, and a more varied ethical methodology is needed for the assessment of therapeutics now and in the future. Such an approach would account for factors such as the motivations of the user, the consequences of use of the technology and the fair use of technology in society. Using specific theological criteria, I have shown here that a future ethical assessment of medical technologies from a Christian perspective would need to examine the impact of the technology on autonomy, embodiment and on the *imago Dei*, as well as on nature. This kind of varied ethical approach is urgently needed prior to the widespread availability of radical transhumanist technologies in the future.

Just as natural law alone is an inadequate ethical approach to the evaluation of potentially radical transhumanist biomedical technologies, extreme conservatism concerning the adoption of biomedical technology (what Carl Elliott terms bio-conservatism, or "pharmacological Calvinism" (Elliott, 2000)) is an inadequate cultural response to these technologies. This is for three reasons. First, regardless of their enhancement potential, some transhumanist technologies also have considerable therapeutic potential for humanity, arguably far greater and more widespread potential than therapeutic developments to date. These might include, for example, the development of sophisticated cybernetic internal organs for transplant purposes, or the use of nanoparticles in the bloodstream to deal with the biochemical effects of blood disorders.

With all healthcare technologies, from the hygiene provisions of the nineteenth century – which might not be considered "medical interventions" by today's standards – to the specific pharmaceutical developments of the twentieth century, the relief of human suffering and improvement of human welfare has been a key objective, and a major motivation for research and progress. There is no reason why the same cultural approach cannot be adopted with future transhumanist technology developments in the twenty-first century. However, governments and research agencies would need to be proactive and intentional in identifying the policies to enable this. At various points in this chapter, relating to various ethical issues, I have highlighted the importance of public policy to ensure equitable adoption and distribution of biomedical technologies and to define acceptable minimum levels for human function, which enhancement technologies could support.

Second, because of the Christian emphasis on the goodness of creation – and the provisional goodness of natural science as a means of exploring creation – Christian critics of transhumanism can be reassured that, for all the potential benefits of biomedical technologies on human flourishing, the eschatology of transhumanism cannot ultimately deal with the problem of sin and the real need for human moral responsibility. As argued earlier, the effects of transhumanist biomedical technologies on autonomy are debatable. Consequently, biomedical technologies cannot circumvent the ethical issues associated with good human life, which are only rendered more complicated by immortality or extreme longevity, due to the extended period over which the person – in whatever morphological form – must exercise moral agency. While transhumanist enhancements may bring benefits in terms of human function and longevity, they cannot be a panacea for all human ills, and many of the prevailing moral aspects of human life – for example, the development of moral agency, responsibility for sin, living well in community and making good moral decisions in the face of new challenges – are unlikely to be affected by adoption of more radical biomedical technologies. Consequently, I would argue that the fears of strict bio-conservatives are unwarranted and should be considered in the context of the hope of the potential benefits of biomedical enhancement technologies on health and well-being.

Third, strict bio-conservatism does not do justice to Philip Hefner's notion of the "created co-creator" – the idea that human beings are created by God, and yet they also exercise a creative role with him, in science and culture (Hefner, 1993, p. 27). Concerning the capacity of humanity to co-create the world using technology, Hefner's qualification is important. Hefner states that the human destiny embraced must be "wholesome to the nature that birthed it". In other words, the future creation – or re-creation – of humanity, by either cultural or scientific means, should be good, in a way that is consistent with the original creation. So, while "human nature", in a strictly biological sense, is debatable, this consistency between origin and maturity should also be concerned with the virtues that humans have always aspired to, which have long been regarded as goods of human society, and which are still desirable in a future society where there are transformative medical technologies. Such virtues would include compassion and kindness in the alleviation of suffering (Waters, 2006b), self-restraint, generosity and neighbourly love.

The cultural implications of Hefner's theology of co-creation present an ethical dimension, and this provides a context for the church to ask important questions. For example, how can the fruits of the Spirit (Galatians 5v22–26) in human actions and personalities be experienced in a context where humans can be radically re-created by biomedical technology? How can wholeness, relationality and hope be expressed in a technological context? Strict bio-conservatism not only shuts out the potential for exploration of the therapeutic benefits of transhumanist biomedical technologies, but prevents any discourse on the potential benefits of such technologies on human flourishing, from a Christian perspective.

I contend that this space in public discourse for ethical evaluation of biomedical technologies is important and moreover is compatible with a Christian view of the world. The exact nature of the human being has, in fact, always been open to debate, both in theology, with the different approaches to the *imago Dei*, and in science, with the impact of new animal behavioural studies on understandings of the distinctiveness of humanity (Van Huyssteen, 2006, pp. 139–143). While the popular perception is that adoption of transhumanist biomedical technologies will result primarily in hitherto unexpected ethical issues, in fact many recognised ethical questions in society at present – for example, the issue of how husband and wife relate in marriage – will still be present in a technological age, and these questions will not necessarily be affected by invasive biomedical technology, as I have argued. For example, the effect of the contraceptive pill on conception does not obviate the need for ethical reflection concerning how a man and woman should relate to each other in marriage.

As mentioned, some critics of potential transhumanist technologies will point to the possible unintended consequences of radical biomedical technology. However, the history of pharmaceutical medicine – for example, the serendipity of drug discovery and idiosyncratic drug safety issues (for example, the thalidomide disaster) – shows that there have always been unintended consequences with medical developments. The possibility of unintended consequences has never been an absolute reason not to proceed with a biomedical development scientifically, nor should it be an absolute reason not to proceed ethically.

It is these unintended consequences that limit the usefulness of a consequentialist ethical approach in medical ethics, as much as natural law ethical approaches may be limited in a world where nature is technologically malleable. It is understandable that the emphasis of the Hippocratic Oath, developed at a time when there was no modern, scientific understanding of medicine, was on the actions and motivations of the practitioner, because this was the one aspect of medicine that practitioners could control.

The unpredictability of the human biological response applies equally to medical developments to date, and to proposed future transhumanist biomedical technologies. In both cases, although unintended consequences of these biotechnological interventions are unavoidable, they call for humility and a respect for the mysteries of the natural world, as expressed by the fourth specific criterion about attitude to past failures. This humility and respect should be exercised by the healthcare practitioner and, in a world of person-centred care and consumerist use of health technologies, ultimately by the person who is applying the technology to their own body.

The mechanisation of medicine with technology, and the evaluative process that surrounds it, has rendered the healthcare practitioner a functionary rather than a healer, and medicine as a form of engineering rather than an art. I would argue then that, given the limitations of natural law and consequentialism in bioethics, a virtue-based approach in future medicine might be particularly valuable because it will refocus ethical discussions on future biomedical technologies on the character and skills of the practitioner, rather than the capability of the technology.

I have shown that four specific ethical domains – autonomy, nature, embodiment and the *imago Dei* – provide a framework for a fruitful discussion of the ethical issues surrounding the contraceptive pill and SSRI antidepressants, two medicines which, in their time, had characteristics of transhumanist technologies. I would therefore recommend that any future transhumanist technologies are evaluated according to these four ethical domains. These four areas constitute common ground between Christian ethical assessment of past therapies and the process of ethical evaluation of future transhumanist technologies. Indeed, a proactive approach would be to consider these ethical domains during the process of developing and implementing any new biomedical technology which might have a far-reaching effect on human life, flourishing and experience.

5.6 Refining the Ethical Criteria for New Biomedical Technologies

In this final section, I explore how the specific theological criteria used for ethical assessment of biomedical technologies might be modified in the light of this discussion of past cases of pharmaceutical medicine to make them more incisive for evaluating future biomedical technology.

There are various possible refinements to these criteria. Whether the transhumanist technology is good news for the poor will depend on how scalable the technology is, and therefore how quickly it can be made universally available at an affordable cost for as many people as possible. A related issue is that there should be no barriers to equitable access to the technology in different countries and cultures for any reasons other than cost. A further factor concerning whether an enhancement technology is good news for the poor is the extent to which governments might subsidise it in the interests of equity of access. The question therefore might be rephrased: is the technology good news for the poor, the marginalised and for equitable distribution of regional, national or international public funding?

In terms of the second question about the *imago Dei*, it is to be hoped that applications of future transhumanist technology would enable people to fully conform to the image of God, rather than being an attempt to be "like God". It would not be permissible from a Christian perspective for a technology to actively enable a person to remodel their body and mind according to their will or whim, in their own image (*imago hominis*).

Furthermore, the enhanced person should reflect all dimensions of the *imago Dei*. A more specific question would therefore be: what kind of *imago Dei* does the technology reflect? Is it concerned entirely with human attributes – attributes of substance – or does it also reflect and uphold the relational element of what it means to be human, and the vocational aspect of humanity carrying out God's purposes in the world? Furthermore, does the technology enable the eschatological development of the person towards a destiny of Christlikeness, or does it merely aim to abolish human finitude, with no reference to its effects on a person's spiritual and moral development?

Concerning the third question, about the attitude of the technology towards the material world – including the human body – it is vital that the technology is characterised by a positive and affirming approach to the material world and to the human body for it to be acceptable from a Christian perspective. This approach will honour the remarkable significance of somatic life in Christian theology and the importance of the resurrection body in the eschatological destiny of the believer. Appropriate embodiment will ensure that the technologically transformed person can continue to participate in the sacramental – material – aspects of Christian faith. In addition to ensuring appropriate embodiment, the technology should ensure that the identity of the transformed human person is preserved, since identity is closely aligned with bodily form, both theologically and psychologically. A key question to ask of a biomedical technology is not just how will it change a person's body, but how will it change their identity? Furthermore, the right approach to the value of the individual body in relation to the material world will, in turn, ensure that the corporate body of humanity – human society – is able to flourish and is not compromised.

What about the technology's attitude to past failures? There is some evidence of scientific hubris with both case studies, and indeed with other past therapeutic developments. Christians would want the attitude of a new technology to be one of humility, and a willingness to learn from past failures. As well as the question about the project's attitude to past failures, an additional question that could be asked is: what does humility look like with this project and these people in this therapeutic scenario?

The effect of a biomedical technology on autonomy is a key line of enquiry in the ethical evaluation of technology. It is often supposed that transhumanist medical technologies enable unbridled autonomy on the part of the user. On the contrary, I have shown here that, with past medical technologies, although they may be implemented ostensibly with autonomy, autonomy may be eroded by unintended consequences in the light of ongoing experience of the technology, or by the way the technology is implemented across society. In any case, autonomy itself, while genuine in many medical situations, may be an ambiguous concept. Concerning the impact of a technology on autonomy therefore, rather than wondering what liberties the technology might *permit*, it would be advisable also to consider what aspects of human life it might *restrict*. This will enable ethicists – and indeed all stakeholders – to determine the full effects that adoption of a biomedical technology might have in a social context, and pre-empt any issues relating to oppression and coercion relating to its widespread use.

Finally, although transhumanist technologies are often thought to elevate individual subjective experiences, it is worth considering the extent to which they objectify the user of the technology – that is to say, treat the user as an artefact to be engineered, manipulated, desired or idolised. In general terms, I would suggest that the greater the imbalance between the subjective experience of the human person using the technology, and the objectification of their material body, the less likely the technology is to be acceptable to Christian ethicists, in line with Elaine Graham's reservations about this issue. Human subjectivity is important for human dignity, and this principle underpins modern clinical trial protocols. Consequently, a biomedical technology that emphasises a privatised, experiential approach to life yet objectifies the human body as an artefact to be engineered by the technology undermines that dignity. Human distinctiveness is eroded, and the human person is reduced to the status of a machine or a laboratory animal.

The final chapter of this book will now draw some outline conclusions from this discussion about a possible future ethical approach to transhumanist enhancements and present a worked example of a possible future ethical approach. It will also discuss the implications of this ethical approach for the history of medical ethics, and implications for the church and for society.

Notes

1 Wesbecker, a man from Kentucky, went on a shooting spree and killed several people while being treated with Prozac. His lawyers cited his treatment with Prozac in a "diminished responsibility" defence.

2 The Roman Catholic church may have wanted to ensure that its teaching remained faithful to Augustine's binary analysis of "marriage" versus "continence" (Augustine, *On the Good of Marriage*, 8), and were forced to place the use of contraception on the side of "continence" due to its implications for natural law.

3 See also review by Southgate (Christopher Southgate, "Book Review: Neil Messer, Selfish Genes and Christian Ethics: Theological and Ethical Reflections on Evolutionary Biology", *Studies in Christian Ethics*, 21 (2008), pp. 142–143).

4 For discussion and worked example, see Neil Messer, *SCM Study Guide: Christian Ethics* (London: SCM, 2006), pp. 121–140.

5 With the notable exception of the China "one child" policy. This was largely enforced by incentivising use of contraception although, in the 1980s, more draconian measures, such as forced sterilization and abortion, were implemented.

References

Augustine of Hippo, On the Good of Marriage, (2021). http://www.newadvent.org/fathers/1309.htm (accessed October 2022).

Aron Halfin, "Depression: The Benefits of Early and Appropriate Treatment", *American Journal of Managed Care*, 13 (2007), pp. S92–S97.

Alister McGrath, *The Science of God: An Introduction to Scientific Theology* (London: T and T Clark, 2004).

Alasdair MacIntyre, *After Virtue* (London: Duckworth, 1981).

Adrian Thatcher, *God, Sex and Gender: An Introduction* (Oxford: Wiley-Blackwell, 2011).

Adam Willows, "Supplementing Virtue: The Case for a Limited Theological Transhumanism", *Theology and Science*, 15 (2017), pp. 177–187.

Bernard Häring, "New Dimensions of Responsible Parenthood", *Theological Studies*, 37 (1976), pp. 120–132.

Betsy Hartmann, *Reproductive Rights and Wrongs: The Global Politics of Population Control* (Boston: South End Press, 1995).

Brent Waters, *From Human to Posthuman: Christian Theology and Technology in a Postmodern World* (Farnham: Ashgate, 2006a), pp. 123–125.

Brent Waters, "Saving Us from Ourselves: Christology, Anthropology and the Seduction of Posthuman Medicine", in *Future Perfect? God, Medicine and Human Identity*, edited by Celia Deane-Drummond and Peter Manley Scott (London: T and T Clark International, 2006b) pp. 194–195.

Celia Deane-Drummond, "Future Perfect? God, the Transhuman Future and the Quest for Immortality", in *Future Perfect? God, Medicine and Human Identity*, edited by Celia Deane-Drummond and Peter Manley Scott (London: T and T Clark International, 2006), pp. 168–182.

Celia Deane-Drummond, *Theology and Biotechnology: Implications for a New Science* (London: Geoffrey Chapman, 1997).

Carl Elliott, "Pursued by Happiness and Beaten Senseless: Prozac and the American Dream", *Hastings Center Reports*, 30 (2000), pp. 7–12.

Christopher Langford, *Birth Control Practice and Marital Fertility in Great Britain* (London: London School of Economics, 1976).

Christopher Southgate, "Book Review: Neil Messer, Selfish Genes and Christian Ethics: Theological and Ethical Reflections on Evolutionary Biology", *Studies in Christian Ethics*, 21 (2008), pp. 142–143.

Christopher Southgate, *God, Humanity and The Cosmos*, 3rd Edition (London: T and T Clark, 2011).

Donna Haraway, *Simians, Cyborgs and Women: The Reinvention of Nature* (New York: Routledge, 1991).

David Healy, *Let Them Eat Prozac: The Unhealthy Relationship Between the Pharmaceutical Industry and Depression* (New York/London: New York University Press, 2004).

David Healy, "Psychopharmacology and the Government of the Self", *Colloquium at the Centre for Addiction and Mental Health, Nature Medicine*, 2000.

David Jones, "Dunstan, the Embryo and Christian Tradition", *Journal of Medical Ethics*, 31 (2005), pp. 710–714.

Elaine Tyler May, *America and the Pill: A History of Promise, Peril and Liberation* (New York: Basic Books, 2010).

Elaine Graham, "In Whose Image? Representations of Technology and the Ends of Humanity", in *Future Perfect? God, Medicine and Human Identity*, edited by

Celia Deane-Drummond and Peter Manley Scott (London: T and T Clark International, 2006), pp. 58–61.
Elizabeth McLaren, "Marriages in England and Wales (Provisional), 2012", 2013, https://webarchive.nationalarchives.gov.uk/20160107154955/http://www.ons.gov.uk/ons/dcp171778_366530.pdf (accessed August 2015).
Gordon Dunstan, "The Moral Status of the Human Embryo: A Tradition Recalled", *Journal of Medical Ethics*, 10 (1984), pp. 38–44.
Guy Kahane and Julian Savulescu, "Normal Human Variation: Refocussing the Enhancement Debate", *Bioethics*, 29 (2015), pp. 133–143.
Gerald McKenny, *Biotechnology, Human Nature and Christian Ethics* (Cambridge: Cambridge University Press, 2018), pp. 1–24.
Gregor Wolbring, "Nanotechnology and the Transhumanization of Health, Medicine, and Rehabilitation", *Controversies in Science and Technology*, 3 (2010), pp. 290–303.
Hera Cook, *The Long Sexual Revolution: English Women, Sex and Contraception, 1800–1975* (Oxford: Oxford University Press, 2004).
Ian G. Barbour, *Religion and Science: Historic and Contemporary Issues* (London: SCM, 1998).
Ian Kerridge, Michael Lowe and David Henry, "Ethics and Evidence-Based Medicine", *British Medical Journal*, 316 (1998), pp. 1151–1153.
John Bryant, Linda Baggott la Velle and John Searle, *Introduction to Bioethics* (Chichester: Wiley, 2005).
Julie Donoghue and Harold Pincus, "Reducing the Societal Burden of Depression: A Review of Economic Costs, Quality of Care and Effects of Treatment", *Pharmacoeconomics*, 25 (2007), pp. 7–24.
Joseph Glenmullen, *Prozac Backlash: Overcoming the Dangers of Prozac, Zoloft, Paxil, and Other Antidepressants with Safe, Effective Alternatives* (New York: Simon and Schuster, 2001).
Julian Savulescu and Ingmar Persson, "Moral Enhancement, Freedom and the God Machine", *The Monist*, 95 (2012), pp. 399–421.
J. Wentzel Van Huyssteen, *Alone in the World? Human Uniqueness in Science and Theology* (Grand Rapids: Eerdmans, 2006), pp. 139–143.
J. Wentzel Van Huyssteen, "Questions, Challenges and Concerns for the Image of God", in *Finding Ourselves After Darwin*, edited by Stanley Rosenberg (Grand Rapids: Baker, 2018), pp. 92–106.
John-Mark Miravalle, *The Drug, The Soul and God: A Catholic Moral Perspective on Antidepressants* (Chicago: University of Scranton Press, 2010).
Kevin Vanhoozer, "Human Being: Individual and Social", in *Cambridge Companion to Christian Doctrine*, edited by Colin Gunton (Cambridge: Cambridge University Press, 1997), pp. 158–188.
Michael Shapiro, "Performance Enhancement and Legal Theory", in *The Transhumanist Reader: Classical and Contemporary Essays on the Science, Technology and Philosophy of the Post-Human Future*, edited by Max More and Natasha Vita-More (Chichester: Wiley-Blackwell, 2013), pp. 281–290.
Michael Burdett, "The Image of God and Evolution", in *Finding Ourselves After Darwin*, edited by Stanley Rosenberg (Grand Rapids: Baker, 2018), pp. 27–31.
Mary McClintock Fulkerson, "Contesting the Gendered Subject: A Feminist Account of the Imago Dei", in *Horizons in Feminist Theology: Identity,*

Traditions and Norms, edited by Rebecca Chopp and Sheila Davaney (Minneapolis: Fortress, 1997), pp. 99–115.

Mark Jackson, *The History of Medicine: A Beginner's Guide* (London: Oneworld, 2014).

M.J. McNamee and S.D. Edwards, "Transhumanism, Medical Technology and Slippery Slopes", *Journal of Medical Ethics*, 32 (2006), pp. 513–518.

Max More, "The Philosophy of Transhumanism", in *The Transhumanist Reader: Classical and Contemporary Essays on the Science, Technology and Philosophy of the Post-Human Future*, edited by Max More and Natasha Vita-More (Chichester: Wiley Blackwell, 2013), pp. 1–17.

Mary Warnock (Chair), "Report of the Committee of Inquiry into Human Fertilisation and Embryology", 1984, https://www.hfea.gov.uk/media/2608/warnock-report-of-the-committee-of-inquiry-into-human-fertilisation-and-embryology-1984.pdf (accessed September 2019).

Nick Bostrom, "Transhumanist Values", *Journal of Philosophical Research*, 30 (2005), pp. 3–14.

N. Katherine Hayles, *How We Became Post-Human? Virtual Bodies in Cybernetics, Literature and Informatics* (Chicago and London: University of Chicago Press, 1999).

Noreen Herzfeld, *In Our Image: Artificial Intelligence and the Human Spirit* (Minneapolis: Fortress, 2002).

Neil Messer, *SCM Study Guide: Christian Ethics* (London: SCM, 2006).

Neil Messer, *Selfish Genes and Christian Ethics: Theological and Ethical Reflections on Evolutionary Biology* (London: SCM, 2007).

Neil Tranter, *British Population in the 20th Century* (Basingstoke: MacMillan, 1996).

Oliver O' Donovan, *Begotten or Made?* (Oxford: Clarendon, 1984).

Peter Gardiner, "A Virtue Ethics Approach to Moral Dilemmas in Medicine", *Journal of Medical Ethics*, 29 (2003), pp. 297–302.

Philip Hefner, *The Human Factor: Evolution, Culture, and Religion* (Minneapolis: Fortress, 1993).

Patrick Hopkins, "Is Enhancement Worthy of Being a Right?", in *The Transhumanist Reader: Classical and Contemporary Essays on the Science, Technology and Philosophy of the Post-Human Future*, edited by Max More and Natasha Vita-More (Chichester: Wiley-Blackwell, 2013), pp. 345–354.

Peter Kramer, *Listening to Prozac* (New York/London: Penguin, 1993).

Ronald Bailey, "For Enhancing People", in *The Transhumanist Reader: Classical and Contemporary Essays on the Science, Technology and Philosophy of the Post-Human Future*, edited by Max More and Natasha Vita-More (Chichester: Wiley-Blackwell, 2013), pp. 327–344.

Ronald Cole-Turner, "Towards a Theology for the Age of Biotechnology" in *Beyond Cloning: Religion and the Remaking of Humanity*, edited by Ronald Cole-Turner (Harrisburg PA: Trinity Press International, 2001), pp. 143–146.

Robert Jutte, *Contraception: A History*, translated by V. Russell (Cambridge: Polity Press, 2008).

Robert Sparrow, "Better Living through Chemistry? A Reply to Savulescu and Persson on Moral Enhancement", *Journal of Applied Philosophy*, 31 (2014), pp. 23–32.

Steven Woolf, "Evidence-Based Medicine: A Historical and International Overview", *Proceedings of the Royal College of Physicians of Edinburgh*, 31 (2001), pp. 39–41.
Stephen Black and Mary Sykes, "Promiscuity and Oral Contraception: The Relationship Examined", *Social Science and Medicine*, 5 (1971), pp. 637–643.
Sarah Buss, "Personal Autonomy" Stanford Encyclopaedia of Philosophy, 2018, https://plato.stanford.edu/entries/personal-autonomy/ (accessed: April 2018).
S.R. Davis, I. Dinatale, L. Rivera Wall and S. Davison, "Postmenopausal Hormone Therapy: From Monkey Glands to Transdermal Patches", *Journal of Endocrinology*, 185 (2005), pp. 207–222.
Stephen Pope, "Natural Law and Christian Ethics", in *Cambridge Companion to Christian Ethics*, edited by Robin Gill (Cambridge: Cambridge University Press, 2012).
Stephen Pope, "Theological Anthropology: Science and Human Flourishing", in *Questioning the Human: Towards a Theological Anthropology for the 21st Century*, edited by Lieven Boeve, Yves De Maeseneer and Ellen Van Stichel (New York: Fordham University Press, 2014).
Thomas Douglas, "Moral Enhancement", *Journal of Applied Philosophy*, 25 (2008), pp. 228–245.
Toni Saad, "The History of Autonomy in Medicine from Antiquity to Principlism", *Medicine, Health Care and Philosophy*, 21 (2018), pp. 125–137.

6 Braver New World

Reimagining Transhumanism

6.1 Agents of Change – Therapy, Then and Now

This project has examined how a Christian ethical evaluation of future transhumanist biomedical technologies can be informed by reflection on the ethical issues that arose from developments in pharmaceutical medicine that took place during the therapeutic revolution years of the twentieth century (1950–1990), and which are still in routine use at the current time.

Specifically, this project has set out to answer the following research questions:

1. What are the various issues of theological ethics presented by transhumanist developments?
2. To what extent were past medical technologies transhumanist in their time?
3. What were the ethical concerns with past medical technologies? Have these ethical concerns been warranted in the light of subsequent experience?
4. How do issues identified with previous medical technologies inform the evaluation of future biomedical technologies?

These questions were explored by the comparative evaluation of two cases of past pharmaceutical medicine – the contraceptive pill and SSRI antidepressants – and of some proposed future transhumanist technologies according to objective criteria. These comprised a general set of criteria to define what might constitute a transhumanist biomedical technology, derived from the transhumanist literature, and specific theological considerations for the ethical evaluation of a biomedical technology, derived from the work of Neil Messer and Elaine Graham (Messer, 2007, pp. 229–235; Graham, 2006). The purpose of using these criteria was to determine whether the past medical developments have transhumanist features and to evaluate the ethical implications of these developments.

Using the general criteria for what might constitute a transhumanist technology, I have argued that the oral contraceptive pill and SSRI

DOI: 10.4324/9781003290421-7

antidepressants were transhumanist developments in their time according to some of the criteria, but less so according to others. The transhumanist character of these two medical technologies is borne out by their scientific history, and is illustrated by three characteristics:

a their attributes as medical technologies, because their pharmacological effects are wide-ranging and have profound systemic effects on the individual human body,
b the total impact they have had on society, rather than just on the health and well-being of the individuals who take them, and
c the understanding of their application to humanity as transformational medical technologies in both scholarly and popular discourse.

These two medicines were transhumanist in that they have had transformational effects on individual human flourishing and human society in terms of their effects on human relationships, welfare and quality of life. They were also transhumanist in the sense that they are a means of manipulating the human body with technology, and have been adopted, to some extent, with the hubris of technological achievement and human progress. However, these medicines were not transhumanist because they fell short of the radical nature of some of the proposed future transhumanist technologies, such as mind uploading and radical cybernetics, which negate the significance of bodily life, and which marginalise human bodily experience. On the contrary, both these previous cases are medicines which work in and through the human body and uphold human bodily life in their actions and effects.

Crucially, these two cases were ambiguous concerning whether they could be adopted without compromising individual autonomy. A key tenet of the transhumanist movement is that biomedical technology can be applied to the human person with the user having complete autonomy to manipulate his/her person at will, a tenet that has arisen from the roots of transhumanism in secular modernity. However, with both case studies, while the medical intervention can be applied with autonomy at the outset, there are potential unintended consequences with the use of these agents, as there are with many situations in contemporary medicine, and these have the potential to undermine the user's personal autonomy.

On application to the two case studies, the specific theological criteria for ethical evaluation of a transhumanist technology identified four major theological domains that constitute ethical issues with both present and future biomedical technologies and represent areas of contrast and debate that would enable the evaluation of future transhumanist biomedical technologies in the context of medicine to date.

These four areas are a) autonomy, b) nature, c) embodiment and d) the *imago Dei*. These four areas are key points of contact between past and present medical interventions and future transhumanist biomedical technologies, and are therefore important areas in the ethical exploration of future transhumanist biomedical technologies, to determine whether a biotechnology is permissible or desirable from a Christian perspective for use in human society.

I described the ethical concerns that have arisen with these two past cases, at the time of their introduction and since – which are largely natural law-based objections from a perspective of Roman Catholic moral theology. I argued that, during the time these medicines have been on the market, these ethical concerns have largely not been vindicated, but that both medical technologies have had positive ethical benefits for human society and flourishing and that there has been Christian ethical support for the use of these technologies from the principles of integrity and totality – the good of the whole person and of human society.

I have argued that despite its significant role in the history of Christian ethics, natural law alone is no longer a sufficient method of ethical evaluation of biomedical technologies, because medical technologies are now able to manipulate the human body in a way that undermines traditional notions of natural and unnatural. In a scientific and healthcare context where nature is less absolute and more open to manipulation, the question of whether a technology can be used with autonomy, and the effects of the technology on autonomy, will have a much greater influence on the ethical implications of the technology than any arguments derived solely from the effects of the technology on human nature.

Furthermore, with increasing use of cybernetic components, especially those that are less inert than the prostheses and implants used in medicine to date, the concept of embodiment will have increasing significance in medical ethics. The more marginalised the human person is from a physical body, the less applicable the medical ethical principles and methods which have been developed to date will be to the evaluation of more radical future biomedical technologies.

Consequently, ethical approaches other than that of natural law will need to be actively applied to the assessment of new biomedical technologies. At one level, there will be an ongoing need for a consequentialist approach, which underpins medical technology assessments at present, to deal with questions of cost-effectiveness and utility. However, virtue ethics will have an increasingly important role in future because, in a world of mechanised medicine, a virtue-based approach rightly refocuses medical ethics on the motivations, actions – and character – of the practitioner.

Furthermore, the theological criteria I have used can be refined in the light of experience with past cases, based on reflection on these cases according to the four domains of autonomy, nature, embodiment and the *imago Dei*. As a result of this, I proposed various possible refinements to the criteria.

First, whether the transhumanist technology is good news for the poor will depend on how scalable the technology is and therefore how quickly it can be made universally available at an affordable cost for as many people as possible. The question therefore might be rephrased: is the technology good news for the poor, the marginalised and for public funding?

Second, concerning the *imago Dei*, it is to be hoped that applications of future transhumanist technology would enable people to fully conform to the image of God, rather than being an attempt at deification, so a person can be "like God". The enhanced person should reflect all dimensions of the *imago Dei* – the relational and functional (vocational), as well as substantive – so a better specific question would be: what kind of *imago Dei* does the technology reflect? It will be important to consider exactly what aspects of the *imago Dei* are affected when the technology is applied, and that the eschatological dimension – the ability to grow towards a Christ-like destiny – is not compromised.

Third, concerning the attitude of the technology towards the material world – including the human body – it is vital that the technology is characterised by a positive and affirming approach to the material world and to the human body, for it to be acceptable from a Christian perspective, as this will honour the remarkable significance of somatic life, and the goodness of material creation in Christian theology. Embodiment is important to identity, and so a key question to ask of a biomedical technology is not just how will it change a person's body, but how will it change their identity? Furthermore, the right approach to the value of the individual body in relation to the material world may, in turn, help to ensure that the corporate body of humanity – human society – is able to flourish and is not compromised.

Fourth, in respect of the attitude of the technology to past failures, while there have been elements of hubris with some past medical developments, Christians would want the attitude of a new technology and its developers to be one of humility, and a willingness to learn from past failures. As well as the question about the project's attitude to past failures, an additional question that could be asked is: what does humility look like with this project and these people in this biomedical scenario?

Fifth, concerning the impact of a technology on autonomy therefore, rather than wondering what liberties the technology might *permit*, it would be advisable also to consider what aspects of human life it might *restrict*. Finally, the extent to which a technology objectifies the body, in relation to the subjectivity it affords, should be carefully considered.

6.2 Conclusions – Medicine, Ethics and Society

I now advance the following general conclusions based on the results and discussion in this study:

1 For transhumanists and pharmaceutical scientists alike, a key motivation for the development of any medical technology is to alleviate human suffering and enhance human flourishing specifically by means

of material intervention with the human body. The two past cases of pharmaceutical medicine discussed here, which demonstrate some of the characteristics of transhumanist developments, show that these two significant advances during the therapeutic revolution years of the twentieth century (1950–1990) have indeed had demonstrable benefits for human health and well-being. I would argue, therefore, that if there have been such benefits with pharmaceutical medicine to date, then even greater benefits may be possible in future, with more radical, invasive, biomedical technologies. This suggests that, while some Christians may be suspicious of medical technology, either for cultural or theological reasons, a position of extreme bio-conservatism is probably not tenable for Christians, simply because of the humanitarian implications of the possible benefits of future biomedical technologies, which would be consistent with a Christian understanding of human flourishing. Indeed, an argument for strict bio-conservativism is ultimately not consistent with Christian compassion and commitment to healing, or the church's advocacy and practice of healing ministry. Moreover, extreme bio-conservatism towards medical technologies on the part of Christian theologians or the church would not be credible to the scientific community and might inhibit dialogue between science and religion on other issues. Furthermore, regardless of Christian apologetics to the scientific community, this stance would also be counterproductive to the church's mission in the world in other respects, given the universal human appeal of compassion and humanitarianism in many societies.

2 An ethical issue which may engender caution with the exploration of radical – and expensive – transhumanist biomedical technologies in future is the extent to which they should be developed, given the current pressing medical needs in some countries of the world yet which are unmet by medical technologies that are already available, but just not accessible in those countries. Should governments and big corporations be investing considerable resources in radical biomedical technologies when diseases such as HIV and tuberculosis are still endemic in sub-Saharan Africa, due to a lack of access to medicines and services? Resources – budget and people – are not in unlimited supply – and I would venture that governments should address issues of availability and equity of access with currently available medical technologies first. Nevertheless, governments do need to have systematic and coherent policies on the funding of future biomedical technologies, for two good ethical reasons. First, such policies will serve to regulate individual and corporate innovators in an appropriately permissive way, so that innovation is not stifled, and that research and development of biomedical technologies can proceed but is directed towards humanitarian ends which support the common good. Second, such policies will manage the technology markets to ensure equity of access and that

future biomedical technologies are indeed "good news for the poor" in that they are accessible and affordable for all sections of society. This is central to an ethic of human flourishing within the Judaeo-Christian tradition; if *shalom* is defined as "universal flourishing, wholeness, and delight ... under the arch of God's love" (O'Brien and Harris, 2012) – then it should encompass just and equitable access to medical technologies across the whole of human society, as this would support the Kingdom aspiration of "good news for the poor". Some transhumanists have been less interested in the socio-cultural implications of transhumanism than others (see, for example, Moravec, 1988, p. 5), but medicine has always been a social and humanitarian venture. It will be important that robust public policy on the deployment and use of future radical medical technologies enables a comprehensive ethical analysis of those technologies that is in keeping with the aims and objectives of medicine to date.

3 As illustrated by the scientific history of the development of the contraceptive pill and SSRI antidepressants, scientific endeavour in pharmacology, as in any area of science, is not a purely abstract activity, but always takes place in a social and political context. Given the contingencies of human society, this situation is unlikely to change in future. I concluded above that extreme bio-conservatism is ultimately incompatible with a Christian ethic of healing and medical care. However, on the other hand, awareness of the social and political context of biomedical research is a powerful corrective to Christians who, perhaps because of scientific ignorance, regard science with uncritical awe and have unrealistic expectations of the possibilities of science, and who therefore may believe that religion cannot in any way influence scientific and technological "progress". The ongoing inability to completely eradicate the endemic diseases in Africa is not simply a scientific problem, it is also a cultural, financial and political problem. That is indicative of why all these factors must be accounted for when developing a comprehensive medical ethical framework for the transhumanist age. Nevertheless, the importance of social context in medical science should not be at the expense of realism in the task and objectives of science. The realistic nature of a scientific advance is possibly easier to overlook when considering the social impact of technologies than when considering the effects on the individual human person because the social context in which the technology is being used will act as a lens through which it is interpreted. The potential for social constructs is why evaluations of future transhumanist biomedical technologies – both medical and ethical – should be evidence-based, according to objective verifiable criteria, using similar methodologies to those that pharmacology has developed over the last fifty years during the therapeutic revolution years. Going forward, this evidence-based approach will help to ensure that ethical responses to new biomedical

technologies from the church, or indeed other agencies, avoid either an uncritical acceptance of technology, on the one hand, or a knee-jerk rejection of technology, on anti-scientific or cultural grounds, on the other. This study has used objective criteria to examine, and find points of ethical contact between, past and potential future biomedical technologies, to derive an evidence-based ethical approach to evaluating future biomedical technologies.

4 A survey of the scientific history and development of the two case studies presented here, and their evaluation using the general criteria for transhumanist developments, suggests that these medicines were, in many ways, transhumanist developments, by the standards of their time, even though they were not the radically invasive technologies envisaged in the future by transhumanist scholars such as mind-uploading and cybernetics. The case studies show that social and cultural concerns about what were at the time new medical technologies – for example, about how society would be affected, how relationships would be changed and how the technology might be misused – stimulated significant intellectual discourse. Similar cultural and social concerns exist now with proposed future radical transhumanist technologies. However, regardless of current popular fears and cultural concerns with future transhumanist technologies, these technologies may, in due course, yield medical and social benefits, in the same way that past medicines have. I would suggest then that a Christian ethical evaluation of a new technology should incorporate lessons learnt from past cases of medical technologies where initial fears were not vindicated, as I have done in this project. Lessons learnt from the past may help to identify and rule out any concerns that are largely social and cultural and which are not ultimately prohibitive from a Christian perspective.

5 I have noted that some scholars have attempted to reconcile transhumanism with religious belief, exploring the themes of perfectibility, immortality and Christian social concern (Campbell and Walker, 2005; Garner, 2005). Helpful as these attempts at dialogue might appear, they are superficial, in that they gloss over significant underlying differences between religious belief and transhumanist thought, especially concerning embodied life, soteriology and eschatology. The objective theological criteria used here help to analyse and identify the actual points of divergence between Christian belief and the claims of transhumanism.

6 While I have argued here that it is imperative for Christian churches to engage with technology, in terms of enquiring about it, understanding and evaluating it, churches are under no obligation to advocate the implementation of a technology if there are significant ethical concerns, either from a perspective of social justice or the distinctiveness of human life. The principle that there is no stigma in doing nothing is

well-established in medical ethics (Nutton, 1995, p. 29). Notwithstanding point (4) (above), if a medical intervention – whether past or future – is perceived to carry significant risks, then it is reasonable – and indeed ethically defensible – to employ the axiom "First do no harm" and be cautious until the risks of the technology are better understood. In the context of Christian ethics, "harm" might consist of something that hinders the fulfilment of the Kingdom of God, or which compromises loving relationships, not just something that disrupts the functioning of the biological body. Public policy on the regulation and deployment of such technologies should take all risks into account – including risks to the goods of human life, as well as medical and scientific risks, and should, where necessary, reflect the important medical ethical principle of "first do no harm".

7 Christian ethicists and churches need to have a comprehensive Christian medical ethic to apply to biomedical interventions as the transhumanist era dawns. I have argued that an approach based largely on natural law alone – as has characterised religious responses to the contraceptive pill and SSRI antidepressants – is inadequate. This is because radical biomedical technologies render the traditional demarcation between natural and unnatural indistinct. Furthermore, there are ethical benefits of these therapies that cannot be assessed by an appeal to nature alone, for example, positive impacts on human function and quality of life, and on wider society. Yet, ironically, these are the benefits that John-Mark Miravalle seems to discount as positive ethical features in his ethical analysis of SSRI antidepressants, because of his insistence on a natural law approach, aligned with the stance of the Roman Catholic church regarding the contraceptive pill (Miravalle, 2010, pp. 2–3, 50–55). A natural law approach to medical ethics only perpetuates the notion of a dualism between science and religion, and this is problematic for any dialogue between the church and the scientific community. Likewise, a consequentialist ethical approach, which has characterised much bioethical deliberation in the late modern era, and is the approach used by Julian Savulescu in his advocacy of radical biomedical technologies (Savulescu, 2009), is also flawed as a sole means of ethical evaluation of biomedical technology because it fails to account for unintended consequences of medical interventions arising from unexpected biological actions. Virtue ethics, which consider the motivations of the technology user or practitioner, are potentially valuable in modern technological medicine because they help to identify the reasons for using new biomedical technology, regardless of the nature of the technology. Furthermore, a virtue ethics approach has the potential to provide continuity between the future medical ethical issues which might be encountered with transhumanist technologies, and the ancient Hippocratic medical ethical tradition. I conclude that virtue ethics may have an increasingly important role in medical ethics in future.

8 Application of the theological criteria to the two case studies and to some future transhumanist developments has identified four ethical domains that are important points of contact between past and potential future medical technologies – autonomy, nature, embodiment and the *imago Dei*. Christian ethical evaluation of future medical technologies should therefore account for the effects of the technology on autonomy, the impact of the technology on the person's embodied state and the assumptions the technology makes about the *imago Dei*, as well as natural law. Although natural law will continue to have some value in medical ethics, as a means of framing discussions, it will no longer be a sufficient sole means of evaluating future biomedical technologies because of their potentially radical and highly invasive effects. The other areas mentioned here will have increasing ethical significance in future.

9 I argued earlier that a purely natural law-based ethic for assessment of transhumanist biomedical technologies was also inadequate because it is individualistic and atomistic and does not account for the social ethical aspects of these technologies, such as concerns over the social impact of immortality and the equitable distribution of such technologies. I would also argue that advocates of transhumanism are naïve to think that biomedical technology is able to solve social and spiritual problems, as well as medical ones, and that medical science will somehow bypass moral agency and eliminate these social ethical issues in a human population going forwards. The reality is that, even if biomedical technologies with positive benefits are universally deployed and are acceptable ethically in terms of human equity, dignity and community, human beings will still need to negotiate the day-to-day ethical dilemmas of human life regardless of technology use.

My purpose in writing this book has been to forge a connection between the ethical evaluation of medical interventions to date and proposed future transhumanist biomedical technologies, and to locate the transhumanism movement within the wider history of medicine. It therefore shows that careful analysis of previous medical developments in the modern era to date can influence our ethical understanding of potential transhumanist proposals.

By reviewing significant past medical innovations according to objective criteria for transhumanist developments and examining theological objections to transhumanism, I have shown specifically that four domains of ethical evaluation – a) autonomy, b) nature, c) embodiment and d) the *imago Dei* – provide points of contact between past and proposed future medical biomedical technologies. These are therefore important themes for ethical analysis of proposed future transhumanist technologies, to assess their acceptability from a perspective of Christian ethics. They also relate to theological concerns of other world religions.

Future work in this area would involve the application of this "four domains" ethical methodology to specific proposed future biomedical technologies. This might include current proposed transhumanist developments, such as mind uploading or gene therapy, but also future technologies that have not yet been considered. I provide a preliminary worked example of this below.

6.3 A Four Domains Ethical Method to Evaluate Biomedical Technology

As discussed here, some pharmaceutical technologies to date – for example, the contraceptive pill and SSRI antidepressants – have had significant effects on human society, as well as individual health and wellness. In the future, similar biotechnologies may be introduced, but with more radical effects. For example, in future, it may be possible to have a "magic implant" fitted which releases a combination of metabolically active nanoparticles and gene therapy components (viral victor and nucleotide substances) which would have the effect of radically extending the human lifespan to, say, 200 years, improving physical functioning during that lifespan and effectively eradicating dementia and cognitive decline. Once such an implant has been developed commercially, it could be inexpensive enough to distribute to all adults in the population, and could be fitted as a simple, minor surgical procedure at a local doctor's surgery or clinic.

Such an intervention would clearly have enormous health and well-being benefits for the individual. It would also have a profound impact on society and would present the ethical issues related to extended longevity described previously. These might concern the economic pressures of an enlarged population, availability of jobs, attitudes to work, the ability of society to change and innovate and increased pressure on marriage as a permanent, lifelong relationship and the development of alternative lifestyles as a result.

A "magic implant" would indeed have ethical implications for society, to which governments, policymakers and corporations would need to respond. However, how does this technology look when analysed according to the domains of autonomy, nature, embodiment and the *imago Dei*? In terms of autonomy, it is unlikely that such an implant acting at the biochemical level would exert effects on freedom of decision-making, unlike some psychoactive drugs. The implant could be fitted at will – but could it be removed at will, with no adverse effects other than the loss of its longevity benefits, if the user no longer wished to use it? As far as nature is concerned, the insertion of such a "magic implant" with radical whole-body systemic effects constitutes an intervention that would interfere with a person's natural attributes and function, in the same way as hormonal contraception does, if viewed from a natural law ethical perspective. However, such an intervention appears to be more aligned with the natural ends of human bodily life than, say, mind uploading or radical cybernetic remodelling, and there would be significant potential ethical benefits of the implant if it were used well by the user, as I have shown is the case with oral contraception and use of SSRI antidepressants for neuroenhancement. Therefore, the "unnatural" nature of the implant does not necessarily render the intervention unethical from a broad Christian ethical perspective. Then there is the question of embodiment. While the "magic implant" would be an invasive intervention, it would still exert positive effects in and through the human body and would enhance bodily life, rather than undermine it, as opposed to mind-uploading and radical cybernetic remodelling, which negate the body, and marginalise its significance. Indeed, drug-eluting stents and implants are already in use primarily to increase life expectancy – for example, the use of anticoagulant-eluting stents to improve life expectancy in coronary disease or stroke. These are essentially enhancements, albeit more minor than the "magic implant" proposed here, in terms of quantitative effects on longevity. Consequently, in terms of embodiment, such a "magic implant" is, in fact, similar to some of the implants used at the current time in terms of ethical status, even if its clinical utility is greater.

What are the implications of such a "magic implant" in terms of the *imago Dei*? The answer here is more complex. A "magic implant" would offer considerably extended longevity, yet with the possibility of eventual death and finitude. Such longevity has the potential to transform family and societal relationships, in the same way that hormonal contraception has done, and lead to positive opportunities for individuals to do good and improve society. This would be positive in terms of a relational approach to the *imago Dei* and would also possibly benefit a functional approach to the *imago Dei* – extended longevity would probably benefit someone's ability to serve God in the world and exercise their God-given vocation. The potentially interesting effect of such a technology is on the eschatological approach to the *imago Dei*. The question is whether the technology would enable the person to achieve their eventual destiny of Christlikeness and being with Christ after life in this world. The longevity provided by the technology might indeed help the user to grow towards Christlikeness but, if longevity became extended indefinitely, then when would the person achieve their eventual destiny of being with Christ beyond this world? The problem of delayed or alternative eschatology is a key theological critique of transhumanism.

This would be a particularly significant issue if it were possible, for example, to extend life even further by replacing the "magic implant" contents every 100 years, thus enabling the person to be effectively immortal. This would not only render obsolete many aspects of medical care in the face of human suffering, but would undermine an individual's finitude and hinder their ultimate fulfilment of a destiny with Christ beyond this world. However, it would be a man-made immortality. A situation might arise where there were insufficient implant replacements for all citizens, either due to lack of availability or funds. How then would it be decided who lives and who dies? Of course, similar ethical decisions about resource allocation are currently made about expensive treatments for rare diseases on a consequentialist basis. However, current resource allocation decisions are concerned with providing a therapy for a disease, which may only have a marginal impact on a person, whereas this future situation is about withholding a life-giving enhancement, which is much more problematic.

If, on the other hand, the "magic implant" gave a single finite increase in longevity, then the key question for potential users of such an implant would be: when and how might death come? Of course, some "magic implant" users might be killed in a road traffic accident at the untimely age of 120. There is then the question of whether there might be any adverse – or indeed potentially fatal – unintended consequences of long-term use of the implant. Unintended consequences have been a common issue in ethics of medical treatment to date, and there is no reason why this might not still be the case in future.

The analysis of the "magic implant" technology according to this autonomy, nature, embodiment and *imago Dei* framework indicates that, while a single-use medical technology which increases longevity may be culturally alien to current society and will introduce some ethical issues, it is not necessarily a technology that is unacceptable from a perspective of Christian ethics and a Christian view of human life. The key caveat is that the technology does not affect human finitude; the problem with medical technologies that confer "immortality" is that, firstly, they delay the person's realisation of their ultimate destiny in Christ and secondly, they bring with them the ethical problems of an "immortality" that is dependent on human initiative.

6.4 Transhumanism in Historical Perspective – The New Therapeutic Revolution

Earlier in this book, I described how medical ethics have developed through three phases to date – first the Hippocratic phase, characterised by an emphasis on the duties and behaviours of the practitioner; then the Renaissance phase, when ethical thinking about medicine began to focus on the techniques of medical intervention, and the consequences for the patient; and then thirdly, the Late Modern phase, which encapsulates modern bioethics, where medical ethics are not just concerned with the actions of the practitioner or the consequences of the treatment, but also about the equality of healthcare resource distribution and the impact of medicine on human rights.

From this project, I conclude that a fourth phase of medical ethics is needed to evaluate the future biomedical technology developments proposed by transhumanists. This will need to comprise a comprehensive ethical system, which will not rely on a single ethical methodology, such as natural law or consequentialism, but will allow a range of forms of ethical analysis. The transhumanist philosopher, F.M. Esfandiary claimed that transhumanism "deplores standard paradigms" (Bostrom, 2005, p. 11); it is perhaps right then that a form of ethical analysis equal to the challenges of radical transhumanist biomedical technology should also not be constrained by analysis according to any one standard ethical paradigm. The analysis of biomedical technologies described here, according to objective criteria, showing the fourfold importance of autonomy, nature, embodiment and the *imago Dei*, offers a comprehensive approach to ethical evaluation of biomedical technologies. It is an approach that is broad enough to evaluate a variety of potential future technologies, but incisive enough to identify the significant issues and gain a clear understanding of the acceptability of a technology from a Christian perspective.

This comprehensive approach does medical ethics the service of reconnecting modern bioethics with both the ancient medical ethical tradition, with its emphasis on the virtue of the practitioner, and the history of the Christian healing tradition with its emphasis on compassion in medical care. This comprehensive ethical understanding of medicine to date, which can then be applied to the future transhumanist biomedical technologies of tomorrow, would not only be a positive development for current bioethics in medical and healthcare practice, but would also refocus discourse in this area on the broader goods of human life in a postmodern world, and would set the scene for a Christian understanding of human life in its current and future postmodern technological context. It would also enable greater dialogue between scientific and religious concerns, in respect of future radical biomedical technologies.

To achieve this would constitute the full flowering of the medical science endeavour, which has so far encompassed the so-called therapeutic revolution – the growth of modern pharmaceutical medicine since the beginning of the twentieth century – and possibly even the development of empirical, iatrochemical medicine since the seventeenth century. This ethical framework would give Christians and churches the confidence to reject the cultural stereotypes of biomedical enhancement, characterised by science fiction motifs and "brave new world" ideology, and to embrace those forms of biomedical technology which have the potential to alleviate human suffering and improve human well-being, but which do not undermine the dignity and distinctiveness of human life from a Christian perspective. Radical biomedical enhancement technologies are neither an absolute evil to be rejected at all costs, nor are they a panacea for every medical and social disease. The reality is that they are somewhere in between; many technologies will have significant benefits to human health and well-being, but need not fatally compromise the autonomy, the nature, the embodied status or the *imago Dei* of the human person. Some proposed future transhumanist technologies will be found to be acceptable ethically, even if they are unfamiliar culturally. If this is the case, then these transhumanist technologies may be as beneficial for the alleviation of human suffering as some previous therapeutic technologies from the "therapeutic revolution" years of the twentieth century. With this kind of ethical approach to the evaluation of transhumanist technologies, both the church and society will be truly prepared for the enhancement revolution, which will bring more profound change to human society and will be more far-reaching than the therapeutic revolution.

References

Elaine Graham, "In Whose Image? Representations of Technology and the Ends of Humanity", in *Future Perfect? God, Medicine and Human Identity*, edited by Celia Deane-Drummond and Peter Manley Scott (London: T and T Clark International, 2006), pp. 56–69.

Graham O'Brien and Timothy Harris, "What on Earth Is God Doing? Relating Theology and Science through Biblical Theology", *Perspectives on Science and Christian Faith*, 64 (2012), pp. 147–156.

Hans Moravec, *Mind Children: The Future of Robot and Human Intelligence* (Cambridge, Mass: Harvard University Press, 1988).

Heidi Campbell and Mark Walker, "Religion and Transhumanism: Introducing a Conversation", *Journal of Evolution and Technology*, 14 (2005), pp. i–xv.

John-Mark Miravalle, *The Drug, The Soul and God: A Catholic Moral Perspective on Antidepressants* (Chicago: University of Scranton Press, 2010).

Julian Savulescu, "The Human Prejudice and the Moral Status of Enhanced Beings: What Do We Owe the Gods?", in *Human Enhancement*, edited by Julian Savulescu and Nicholas Bostrom (Oxford: Oxford University Press, 2009), pp. 211–250.

Neil Messer, *Selfish Genes and Christian Ethics: Theological and Ethical Reflections on Evolutionary Biology* (London: SCM, 2007).

Nick Bostrom, "A History of Transhumanist Thought", *Journal of Evolution and Technology*, 14 (2005), pp. 1–25.

Stephen Garner, "Transhumanism and Christian Social Concern", *Journal of Evolution and Technology*, 14 (2005), pp. 29–43.

Vivian Nutton, "Medicine in the Greek World: 800–50BC", in *The Western Medical Tradition 800BC–1800AD*, edited by Lawrence Conrad, Michael Neve, Vivian Nutton, Roy Porter and Andrew Wear (Cambridge: Cambridge University Press, 1995), pp. 11–38.

Glossary

This section provides a glossary of key technical terms used in the discourse of transhumanism, science and religion. I hope that this will be a helpful reference for both students who are at an early stage of their studies and for more experienced readers for whom this is not their specialist area.

Autonomy the ability of a person to govern themselves and act in a self-determined way, unhindered by internal or external coercive factors.

Bio-conservativism a cautious or wary approach to widespread use of biotechnology, as opposed to a liberal or permissive approach (as might be seen in advocates of transhumanism).

Consequentialism the ethical approach that considers the consequences of an action to determine whether it is a good or beneficial action. The most well-known form of consequentialism is utilitarianism (see below).

Created co-creator the theological idea that humanity can share with God in the creative process. Therefore, when humanity devises and uses biotechnology which has an impact on the material world, humans are contributing with God to the creative process. The term was most notably formulated by American theologian, Philip Hefner.

Enhancement a biotechnology that does not just provide a therapy (treatment of a disease or deficiency) but extends normal human capacities – for example, significantly extends life expectancy.

Extropy the idea proposed by transhumanists which describes the drive to move human life beyond its current limitations and parameters.

Exocentricity (translated from Weltoffenheit in German) a term used to describe the natural dynamic movement of human nature to its destiny of life with God – an openness to the world, to each other and to our self-consciousness.

Hippocratic Oath the ancient oath where a medical practitioner will promise how he or she will or will not act. A longstanding component of medical ethics, which stresses the virtues of the medical practitioner.

Iatrochemical medicine the form of medical practice that developed in the seventeenth century which focused on the evidence-based use of chemical or physical treatments, rather than relying on the theories of medicine from the Hippocratic era. The approach on which modern pharmaceutical medicine is based.

Imago Dei Latin for "image of God". There are four main theological approaches – a) substantive, where the image of God is because of human attributes, b) functional, where the image of God is because of humanity's God-given function or vocation in the world, c) relational, where the image of God is grounded in humanity's capacity to relate to God and each other and d) eschatological, where the image of God is seen in the eschatological destiny of humanity, which emphasises Christ as the perfect image of God, and growth in Christ-likeness.

Morphological Freedom a term used by transhumanists to denote that a transhuman person is not tied to a particular bodily form, meaning that they may not take on a recognisable humanoid body shape.

Natural Law the ethical idea that the good of every organism or creature is to attain fully its natural activity, and that the functioning of every creature is directed towards good ends by virtue of their nature. Since the contraceptive pill frustrates the natural process of fertility, the Roman Catholic church has opposed hormonal contraception on natural law grounds.

Objectification where a person is treated as an object to be manipulated and engineered, rather than as a personal subject.

Pattern Identity the idea that identity can be fully described and disclosed by the informational content of a person's mind, an idea used by some scholars to safeguard the identity of the person whose mind has been uploaded.

Singularity the point in history at which, due to environmental conditions or scientific discoveries, humanity can no longer continue in its current form of existence.

Subjectivity relating to the experiences of the person, as a personal subject.

Therapy a biotechnology that treats a disease or corrects a defect, but does not extend normal human function.

Thomist relating to the thinking of Thomas Aquinas, and his approach to natural law.

Utilitarianism the form of consequentialist ethics developed by John Stuart Mill and Jeremy Bentham, which states that the right act is the one that produces the greatest good for the greatest number of people.

Virtue Ethics the ethical theory where the good of a person is derived from their personal characteristics and qualities. The virtues were described by classical thinkers such as Plato and Aristotle.

Annotated Bibliography

This section provides an annotated select bibliography of the key references in the study of transhumanism and medical ethics, designed to provide a guide to students about the content and claims of the important references.

Adrian Thatcher, *God, Sex and Gender: An Introduction* (Oxford: Wiley-Blackwell, 2011). *This reference provides a concise introduction to the response of the churches to the increasingly widespread use of contraception in the twentieth century.*

Brent Waters, *This Mortal Flesh: Incarnation and Bioethics* (Grand Rapids: Brazos, 2009). *Here, Waters provides a detailed critique of transhumanist attitudes to the body, on the basis of the doctrine of the incarnation.*

Brent Waters, "Saving Us from Ourselves: Christology, Anthropology and the Seduction of Posthuman Medicine", in *Future Perfect?: God, Medicine and Human Identity*, edited by Celia Deane-Drummond and Peter Manley Scott (London: T and T Clark International, 2006), pp. 183–195. *Here, Waters critiques the transhumanism vision, in relation to medicine, and he describes the proper aims and values of medicine.*

Brent Waters, *From Human to Posthuman: Christian Theology & Technology in a Postmodern World* (Aldershot: Ashgate, 2006). *Waters provides a sustained criticism of transhumanism from a perspective of Christian theology and, in particular, the "secular eschatology" of transhumanism.*

Celia Deane-Drummond, "Future Perfect? God, the Transhuman Future and the Quest for Immortality", in *Future Perfect? God, Medicine and Human Identity*, edited by Celia Deane-Drummond and Peter Manley Scott (London: T and T Clark International, 2006), pp. 168–182. *Deane-Drummond presents a theological critique of transhumanism in a medical context.*

Carl Elliott, "Prozac: The Elvis of Pharmaceuticals", *British Medical Journal*, 313 (1996), p. 950. *Elliot, a "bio-conservative" commentator, describes and critiques the cultural impact of Prozac and SSRIs on twentieth-century society.*

Carl Elliott, "Pursued by Happiness and Beaten Senseless: Prozac and the American Dream", *Hastings Center Report*, 30 (2000), pp. 7–12. *Elliot explores the philosophical problem with drug-induced "happiness."*

Christopher Southgate, "Stewardship and its Competitors: A Spectrum of Relationships Between Humans and the Non-Human Creation", in *Environmental Stewardship: Critical Perspectives – Past and Present*, edited by R.J. Berry (London: T and T Clark, 2006), pp. 185–195. *Southgate presents the various theological options to describe and characterise the relationship between humans and non-human creation.*

Donna Haraway, *Simians, Cyborgs and Women: The Reinvention of Nature* (New York: Routledge, 1991). *Haraway discusses how the idea of the cyborg – the human-machine hybrid – can undermine the dualisms in human life, and subvert the assumptions and processes of the natural sciences.*

Elaine Graham, "In Whose Image? Representations of Technology and the Ends of Humanity", in *Future Perfect? God, Medicine and Human Identity*, edited by Celia Deane-Drummond and Peter Manley Scott (London: T and T Clark International, 2006), pp. 56–69. *A key reference, in which Graham cites three theological concerns with transhumanism – 1) that technology enables radical human autonomy, 2) that it may disrupt the body of society, as well as the individual body, and 3) that it promotes subjectivism in human experience, while at the same time objectifying the human body.*

Elaine Tyler May, *America & The Pill: A History of Promise, Peril & Liberation* (New York: Basic Books, 2010). *A detailed philosophical, social and cultural history of the contraceptive pill, written from an American perspective.*

Francis Fukuyama, *Our Posthuman Future: Consequences of the Biotechnology Revolution* (New York: Farrar, Strauss and Giroux, 2002). *A classic and popular critique, describing the implications of transhumanism for equality and human dignity.*

Guy Kahane and Julian Savulescu, "Normal Human Variation: Refocussing the Enhancement Debate", *Bioethics*, 29 (2015), pp. 133–143. *These authors argue for a permissive approach to enhancement, making the important point that biomedical "enhancements" are already in use – for example, modafinil to aid concentration - but may not be regarded as such.*

Graham O'Brien and Timothy Harris, "What on Earth Is God Doing? Relating Theology and Science through Biblical Theology", *Perspectives on Science and Christian Faith*, 64 (2012), pp.147–156. *These authors provide a definition and discussion of the Biblical concept of shalom in a scientific world.*

Gregory Stock and Daniel Callahan, "Debates: Point-Counterpoint: Would Doubling the Human Life Span Be a Net Positive?", *Journals of Gerontology Series A: Biological Sciences and Medical Sciences*, 59 (2004), pp. B554–B559. *This reference provides a discussion of the social ethical issues associated with biomedical immortality.*

Heidi Campbell and Mark Walker, "Religion and Transhumanism: Introducing a Conversation", *Journal of Evolution & Technology*, 14 (2005), pp. i–xv. *They argue that, because both transhumanism and religious belief are concerned with human perfectibility, dialogue between transhumanism and religions is reasonable and may be fruitful in understanding both transhumanism and religion.*

Hans Moravec, *Mind Children: The Future of Robot and Human Intelligence* (Cambridge: Harvard University Press, 1988). *Moravec presents a vision for universal "mind uploading" in future, so human life is conducted in the virtual world, and emphasises the importance of morphological freedom, that humans will live life in future in whatever form they choose. He appeals to the idea of "pattern identity" to resolve the problem of disembodiment for identity.*

Julian Savulescu, "The Human Prejudice and the Moral Status of Enhanced Beings: What do we owe the gods?", in *Human Enhancement*, edited by Julian Savulescu and Nicholas Bostrom (Oxford: Oxford University Press, 2009), pp. 211–250.

In arguing for transhumanist enhancements on a consequentialist basis, Savulescu makes a secular argument against the privileging of humanity in terms of status in the world in relation to the non-human creation.

Julian Savulescu and Ingmar Persson, "Moral enhancement, freedom and the God machine", *The Monist*, 95 (2012), pp. 399–421. *These authors propose the concept of a "God-machine" as a safeguard against domination of society by a certain group in a technologically enhanced society.*

John Stapert, "Curing an Illness or Transforming the Self? The Power of Prozac", *Christian Century*, 111.21 (1994), pp. 684–687. *Stapert outlines some of the Christian concerns with Prozac and SSRI antidepressants.*

Jeanine Thweatt Bates, *Cyborg Selves: A Theological Anthropology of the Post Human* (Burlington: Ashgate, 2012). *This author provides a theological "post-anthropology" of the cyborg, and argues for the inclusion of the cyborg in humanity, with reference to creation, the imago Dei and Christology.*

John-Mark Miravalle, *The Drug, The Soul and God: A Catholic Moral Perspective on Antidepressants* (Chicago: University of Scranton Press, 2010). *Miravalle presents a case for use of SSRI antidepressants as adjunct therapy, based on Thomist psychology, and a natural law-based critique of the Prozac phenomenon.*

Leon Kass, "L'Chaim and its limits: why not immortality?", *First Things*, (2001), pp. 17–24. *Kass, another leading "bio-conservative", describes the social problems that biomedical immortality might lead to.*

Michael Shapiro, "Performance Enhancement and Legal Theory", in *The Transhumanist Reader: Classical and Contemporary Essays on the Science, Technology and Philosophy of the Post-Human Future*, edited by Max More and Natasha Vita-More (Chichester: Wiley-Blackwell, 2013), pp. 281–290. *Shapiro discusses the relationship between enhancement and therapy, and the problems of definition and use of enhancements.*

M.J. McNamee and S.D. Edwards, "Transhumanism, medical technology and slippery slopes", *Journal of Medical Ethics*, 32 (2006), pp. 513–518. *A concise article, describing the benefits and risks of transhumanism from a medical ethical perspective.*

Max More, "The Philosophy of Transhumanism", in *The Transhumanist Reader: Classical and Contemporary Essays on the Science, Technology and Philosophy of the Post-Human Future*, edited by Max More and Natasha Vita-More (Chichester: Wiley-Blackwell, 2013), pp. 1–17. *More provides an overview of the philosophy and key features of the transhumanism movement. An ideal initial text for students of transhumanism.*

Michael Northcott, "Concept Art, Clones and Co-Creators: The Theology of Making", *Modern Theology*, 21 (2005), pp. 219–236. *A critique of the "created co-creator" from a perspective of aesthetics in art and science.*

Matthew Zaro Fisher, "More Human than the Human? Towards a "Transhumanist" Christian Theological Anthropology", in *Religion and Transhumanism: The Unknown Future of Human Enhancement*, edited by Calvin Mercer and Tracy Trothen (Santa Barbara: Praeger, 2015), pp. 23–38. *Zaro Fisher argues that the uploaded mind, as a relational entity, bears the imago Dei, according to the relational approach to imago Dei.*

Nick Bostrom, "Human genetic enhancements: A transhumanist perspective", *Journal of Value Inquiry*, 37 (2004), pp. 493–506. *Bostrom advocates the use of genetic enhancements to improve human well-being and open new possibilities for humanity and deals with various objections to enhancement.*

Nick Bostrom, "Transhumanist Values", *Journal of Philosophical Research*, 30 (2005), pp. 3–14. *Bostrom explores and explains the values that transhumanists espouse, and describes how those values can be nurtured.*

Nick Bostrom, "A History of Transhumanist Thought", *Journal of Evolution & Technology*, 14 (2005), pp. 1–25. *Bostrom describes how the transhumanism movement has developed from its cultural and philosophical roots in the twentieth century and before through to twenty-first-century biopolitics.*

N. Katherine Hayles, *How We Became Post-Human: Virtual Bodies in Cybernetics, Literature and Informatics* (Chicago & London: University of Chicago Press, 1999). *A critique of disembodiment, as presented by Kurzweil, in which Hayles explores the importance of bodily life in literature and culture.*

Noreen Herzfeld, *In Our Image: Artificial Intelligence & the Human Spirit* (Minneapolis: Fortress, 2002). *A discussion of the implications of artificial intelligence (AI) for human nature, including a re-analysis of theological approaches to the imago Dei in the light of AI.*

Neil Messer, *Selfish Genes & Christian Ethics: Theological and Ethical Reflections on Evolutionary Biology* (London: SCM, 2007). *British theological ethicist, Neil Messer explores the possibility that human beings can redesign themselves with biomedical technology, and formulates "diagnostic questions" to assess the acceptability of a biotechnological project from a perspective of Christian ethics.*

Oliver O' Donovan, *Begotten or Made?* (Oxford: Clarendon, 1984). *O'Donovan engages with the ethical issues raised by reproductive technologies, such as in vitro fertilisation, identifies the problems of imposing human will on human nature, and of the body being reduced by biomedical technology to an artefact to be engineered. Here, he also criticises the Roman Catholic opposition to hormonal contraception.*

Onora O'Neill, *Autonomy and Trust in Bioethics* (Cambridge: Cambridge University Press, 2002). *An important discussion of the role of autonomy in bioethics and, in relation to this book, of the cultural and societal factors which influence how autonomy is perceived in modern medical ethics.*

Peter Kramer, *Listening to Prozac* (New York/London: Penguin, 1993). *In this seminal text, a psychiatrist discusses the potential of Prozac to treat "soft signs" of depression, and therefore to make personality adjustments, and describes the implications for society. The book which arguably started the "Prozac phenomenon."*

Ronald Bailey, "For Enhancing People", in *The Transhumanist Reader: Classical and Contemporary Essays on the Science, Technology and Philosophy of the Post-Human Future*, edited by Max More and Natasha Vita-More (Chichester: Wiley-Blackwell, 2013), pp. 327–344. *Here, Bailey argues, in relation to genetic modifications, that enhancement will contribute to human flourishing, and need not lead to inequality or preclude human virtue.*

Ronald Cole-Turner, "Towards a Theology for the Age of Biotechnology", in *Beyond Cloning: Religion & the Remaking of Humanity*, edited by Ronald Cole-Turner (Harrisburg PA: Trinity Press International, 2001), pp. 137–150. *Cole-Turner discusses the implications of biotechnology for theology, and some of the challenges that it provides theologians.*

Robert Freitas, "Welcome to the Future of Medicine", in *The Transhumanist Reader: Classical and Contemporary Essays on the Science, Technology and Philosophy of the* Post-Human *Future*, edited by Max More and Natasha Vita-More (Chichester: Wiley-Blackwell, 2013), pp. 67–72. *Freitas argues that there is a moral imperative to explore transhumanist technologies because of the negative impact of human disease on society.*

Ray Kurzweil, *The Age of Spiritual Machines: When Computers Exceed Human Intelligence* (New York: Penguin, 1999). *In this classic text, Kurzweil describes the rapidly expanding capacity of computing and capabilities of digital systems, and makes an argument for "mind-uploading", the migration of human life into a virtual world. He discusses the problems relating to disembodiment, and outlines some solutions.*

Robert Sparrow, "Better Living through Chemistry? A Reply to Savulescu & Persson on Moral Enhancement", *Journal of Applied Philosophy*, 31 (2014), pp. 23–32. *Sparrow responds to Savulescu and Persson, arguing that the concept of a "God machine" is just another means of domination, and that many people would not be free in a technologically enhanced world.*

Sarah Chan and John Harris, "In Support of Human Enhancement", *Studies in Ethics, Law, and Technology*, 1 (2008), p. 1. *These authors give a definition of an enhancement and argue that enhancement has an important role in human evolution and welfare.*

Stephen Garner, "Transhumanism and Christian Social Concern", *Journal of Evolution & Technology*, 14 (2005), pp. 29–43. *Compares transhumanism and religion from the perspective of their common concern for social welfare.*

Scott Midson, *Cyborg Theology: Humans, Technology and God* (London/New York: I.B. Tauris, 2018). *Midson develops a theological anthropology of the cyborg, and, in particular, appeals to a relational approach to the imago Dei to enable the inclusion of the cyborg in human society.*

Stephen Pope, "Natural Law and Christian Ethics", in *Cambridge Companion to Christian Ethics*, edited by Robin Gill (Cambridge: Cambridge University Press, 2012), pp. 67–86. *A concise, introductory chapter on natural law as a basis for Christian ethics, describing natural law theory from Thomas Aquinas through to the twentieth-century new natural law theorists.*

Thomas Aquinas, "Summa Theologica Q90-94", 2010, https://www.documentacatholicaomnia.eu/03d/1225-1274,_Thomas_Aquinas,_Summa_Theologiae_%5B1%5D,_EN.pdf (accessed September 2020). *The section from the Treatise on Law gives Thomas Aquinas' account of natural law (referred to in this book as Thomistic natural law).*

Thomas Douglas, "Moral Enhancement", *Journal of Applied Philosophy*, 25 (2008), pp. 228–245. *Here, the classic argument for moral enhancement – the use of biomedicine to enhance moral reasoning – is articulated.*

Ted Peters, "Techno-secularism, Religion, and the Created Co-creator", *Zygon*, 40 (2005), pp. 845–862. *Peters affirms the importance of the idea of created co-creator for humanity's application of technology to human life in a technologically enabled world.*

Wolfhart Pannenberg, *What is Man? Contemporary Anthropology in Theological Perspective*, translated by D.A. Priebe (Philadelphia: Fortress, 1970). *Pannenberg provides a classic description of the eschatological approach to the imago Dei, and used the term exocentricity (Weltoffenheit) to describe the dynamic movement of human nature to its destiny of life with God.*

World Transhumanist Association, "Transhumanist Declaration", in *The Transhumanist Reader: Classical and Contemporary Essays on the Science, Technology and Philosophy of the Post-Human Future*, edited by Max More and Natasha Vita-More (Chichester: Wiley-Blackwell, 2013), pp. 54–55. *This declaration outlines the central tenets of transhumanism, which inform the general criteria in this book, which are used to determine whether a biotechnology is transhumanist in character.*

Index

For Product Safety Concerns and Information please contact our EU
representative GPSR@taylorandfrancis.com
Taylor & Francis Verlag GmbH, Kaufingerstraße 24, 80331 München, Germany

www.ingramcontent.com/pod-product-compliance
Ingram Content Group UK Ltd.
Pitfield, Milton Keynes, MK11 3LW, UK
UKHW021308260926
475702UK00048B/862
* 9 7 8 1 0 3 2 2 4 4 0 0 6 *